Veterinary Immunology – Principles and Practice

Second Edition

Michael J. Day

BSc, BVMS(Hons), PhD, DSc, DiplECVP, FASM, FRCPath, FRCVS
Professor of Veterinary Pathology
School of Veterinary Sciences
University of Bristol
Langford, Bristol, UK

in collaboration with

Ronald D. Schultz

BS, MS, PhD, DACVM
Professor and Chair
Department of Pathobiological Sciences
School of Veterinary Medicine
University of Wisconsin-Madison
Madison, Wisconsin, USA

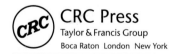

CRC Press
Taylor & Francis Group
Boca Raton London New York

CRC Press is an imprint of the
Taylor & Francis Group, an **informa** business

CRC Press
Taylor & Francis Group
6000 Broken Sound Parkway NW, Suite 300
Boca Raton, FL 33487-2742

© 2014 by Taylor & Francis Group, LLC
CRC Press is an imprint of Taylor & Francis Group, an Informa business

No claim to original U.S. Government works

Printed on acid-free paper
Version Date: 20140219

Printed and bound in India by Replika Press Pvt. Ltd.

International Standard Book Number-13: 978-1-4822-2462-7 (Paperback)

Library of Congress Cataloging-in-Publication Data

Day, Michael J., 1960- author.
  Veterinary immunology : principles and practice / authors, Michael J. Day, Ronald D. Schultz. -- Second edition.
  p. ; cm.
Includes bibliographical references and index.
ISBN 978-1-4822-2462-7 (pbk. : alk. paper)
  I. Schultz, Ronald D., author. II. Title.
  [DNLM: 1. Animal Diseases--immunology--Case Reports. 2. Immune System Diseases--veterinary--Case Reports. SF 757.2]

SF757.2
636.089'6079--dc23   2014005392

**Visit the Taylor & Francis Web site at
http://www.taylorandfrancis.com**

**and the CRC Press Web site at
http://www.crcpress.com**

Contents

Foreword

Veterinary immunology is one of the most recent, and the most important, basic and clinical sciences in veterinary medicine. Veterinary immunology became an important part of the veterinary curriculum approximately 40 years ago when most veterinary medical students were introduced to concepts of basic immunology during their first or second year of veterinary school. Clinical immunology was either a minor part of the basic immunology course or it was taught at a later time as part of the medicine courses. During the past 40 years, information regarding basic and clinical immunology in veterinary medicine has increased beyond the scope of a single course. However, this textbook, *Veterinary Immunology – Principles and Practice, Second Edition*, includes both basic and clinical concepts of veterinary immunology.

The author is a veterinary immunologist engaged in both basic and clinical research studies in immunology and immunopathology. The book provides not only the veterinary medical student, but also the graduate veterinarian, with excellent information on the basic and clinical aspects of veterinary immunology. The basic aspects of the science are made easily understandable to those with limited or no knowledge of immunology. At the same time the book provides an excellent insight into the complexity of diseases caused by or prevented via innate and/or adaptive immunity. The book is equally valuable to those with little or no understanding of clinical medicine and to those with an excellent knowledge of basic clinical medicine. This is accomplished through the author's unique presentation style in which the basic concepts of immunology are introduced and explained, often in the context of the mechanism for an immune-mediated disease or the immunological mechanism for prevention or treatment of a disease. The author has also 'sifted and winnowed' through the complexities of basic medical immunology in order to provide the reader with factual information that applies to most veterinary species. This text, unlike many introductory immunology texts available for medical students and undergraduate or graduate students in the biological sciences, does not focus on the myriad of information on the immunology of the mouse, a favourite species of many immunologists who perform *in-vivo* studies. Ironically, most immunologists are of the opinion that because the mouse's immune system is easily manipulated for *in-vivo* and *ex-vivo* immunological studies, it serves as a model for all other species. Unfortunately, this is often not true and many of the veterinary species differ significantly between each other as well as with the mouse regarding basic and clinical mechanisms of diseases caused by and/or prevented via their immune system. The species differences, when known, are defined in this text. Information on differences among species should make this text a valuable reference for all immunologists, especially those with an interest in real animal studies. Information is included on food animal species, but the focus in the clinical immunology sections is on companion animal species, especially the dog and cat. The author has published a more detailed book, *Clinical Immunology of the Dog and Cat*, which is beautifully illustrated with graphs and figures including histopathology sections of immune-mediated diseases in these species. Similarly, this text is very well illustrated, but for obvious reasons does not contain the detail found in the *Clinical Immunology of the Dog and Cat*.

I especially like this book because the veterinary immunology course taught to second-year veterinary medical students at the University of Wisconsin-Madison first presents the 'Basics of Veterinary Immunology' via eighteen didactic lectures, followed by 'Clinical Immunology' via twelve 'Clinical Correlates'. In addition, there are approximately 50 hours in the course that cover laboratory exercises such as vaccinating calves and puppies, performing clinical immunology tests for the diagnosis of diseases of companion and food animals, and other laboratory procedures (phagocytic tests, lymphocyte function tests and multiple serological tests). This book provides a very helpful way of understanding these diagnostic tests, animal immunization and immune-mediated diseases.

This second edition of *Veterinary Immunology – Principles and Practice* is a book for veterinary students worldwide. It is also an excellent review and update for veterinarians who graduated five or more years ago and want or need to know more about basic and clinical veterinary immunology.

Ronald D. Schultz

Veterinary Immunology – Principles and Practice has the simple aim of providing undergraduate veterinary students with core knowledge of veterinary immunology, while emphasizing the clinical relevance of this subject area. Veterinary students often struggle with the complexity of the immune system and find it difficult to relate immunological concepts to veterinary practice. In many universities, immunology is taught to veterinary undergraduates at a superficial level and the subject is also often delivered by basic scientists with an inappropriate focus on murine or human systems. Despite this, immunology is a key subject in the veterinary curriculum; it links together subject areas such as biochemistry, microbiology, parasitology and pathology with clinical medicine. One of the main clinical applications of immunology is the practice of vaccination, and all graduating veterinarians must have a solid understanding of the principles of vaccinology.

There are relatively few textbooks of veterinary immunology to support the delivery of undergraduate courses in this subject. I hope that *Veterinary Immunology – Principles and Practice* will fill a key niche in providing students with an affordable and practical reference that will also have relevance as they progress through a practice career. The key features of this book include:

- A sufficient level of detail of core knowledge without this being diluted by minutiae.
- Clear definition of learning objectives and bullet-point summaries of key points, with key words highlighted throughout the text in bold font and listed in a glossary.
- An affordable price for a full colour text supported by numerous diagrams and photographic images.
- An emphasis on clinical examples with a series of 15 clinical case studies that present core information related to clinically significant immune-mediated diseases. This aspect is truly unique to this text and is found in no other reference book on this subject. These case studies should very clearly indicate to the student the major clinical relevance of immunology. They provide a bridge between this book and the more practitioner-orientated *Clinical Immunology of the Dog and Cat*. Both of these texts share fundamental aspects of presentation (e.g. diagrammatic symbols), which should make it straightforward to progress from one to the other.

This book is born from the lecture course in veterinary immunology that I have delivered over the past 20 years to students at the University of Bristol. I am delighted to have had the opportunity of working with Professor Ron Schultz on this project. Ron has made insightful suggestions on the text and ensured that the content also covers the curriculum needs of students in North America. I am very grateful to Ron for sharing his vast experience in veterinary immunology and helping shape this major new resource. Both of us share a passion for this subject and the teaching of it to veterinary undergraduates. However, it is our belief that *Veterinary Immunology – Principles and Practice* will not only have relevance to the student market, but should serve as a simple reference for veterinarians already in practice.

I would like to acknowledge the support and enthusiasm for this project from Michael Manson and Commissioning Editor Jill Northcott. This is my fourth book for Manson Publishing, but the first truly undergraduate textbook. My thanks go to the production team of Kate Nardoni (project manager), Susan Tyler (illustrator) and Peter Beynon (copy editor) for their professional input into the finished product.

M. J. Day
January 2011

I was delighted with the response to publication of the first edition of *Veterinary Immunology – Principles and Practice* in 2011. The book was very well received by veterinary students and has now become the adopted text in numerous veterinary schools throughout the world. The text achieved its goal of providing a concise and affordable book supported by high-quality colour illustration. Many colleagues who teach veterinary immunology were highly complimentary about this new resource and offered constructive suggestions for changes to a second edition. Teachers of the subject were also very pleased with the opportunity, provided by the publishers, to obtain teaching sets of the images and diagrams used in the book.

Immunology is a rapidly developing subject area and in order for this textbook to remain current the text of the second edition has been widely updated with advances in knowledge since 2011. The format and style of the text remains the same, but the second edition contains around 20 new and updated figures, one new table and two new clinical case studies. New developments in fundamental and clinical veterinary immunology are reported, with expanded information on commonly used diagnostic test procedures and the inclusion of newly arising diseases such as bovine neonatal pancytopenia.

I have been delighted to have the opportunity once more of collaborating with my friend and colleague, Professor Ron Schultz, on this second edition. I would also like to acknowledge my Commissioning Editor, Jill Northcott, and the production team of CRC Press.

It is now over 15 years since I first began working with Manson Publishing on the production of my first book, *Clinical Immunology of the Dog and Cat*. This second edition of *Veterinary Immunology – Principles and Practice* would have been my sixth Manson publication, but as the final manuscript for this edition was submitted, Michael announced his retirement and the transfer of Manson Publishing to CRC Press. I would like to acknowledge my long and fruitful collaboration with Michael and wish him the very best for the future.

M. J. Day
May 2014

Abbreviations

AchR	acetylcholine receptor
AD	atopic dermatitis
ADCC	antibody-dependent cell-mediated cytotoxicity
AGD	agar gel diffusion
AIDS	acquired immune deficiency syndrome
AIHA	autoimmune haemolytic anaemia
AINP	autoimmune neutropenia
AITP	autoimmune thrombocytopenia
ALL	acute lymphoblastic leukaemia
ALP	alkaline phosphatase
ANA	antinuclear antibody
APC	antigen presenting cell
APTT	activated partial thromboplastin time
ASIT	allergen-specific immunotherapy
AST	aspartate aminotransferase
BALT	bronchial-associated lymphoid tissue
BCR	B-cell receptor
BLAD	bovine leucocyte adhesion deficiency
BLV	bovine leukaemia virus
BNP	bovine neonatal pancytopenia
BoLA	bovine leucocyte antigen
BSA	bovine serum albumin
BVDV	bovine viral diarrhoea virus
CADESI	canine atopic dermatitis extent and severity index
CALT	conjunctiva-associated lymphoid tissue
CAV	canine adenovirus
CD	cluster of differentiation
CDR	complementarity determining region
CDV	canine distemper virus
CFT	complement fixation test
C_H	constant region of the heavy chain
CH_{50}	total haemolytic complement (assay)
C_L	constant region of the light chain
CLA	cutaneous lymphocyte antigen
CLAD	canine leucocyte adhesion deficiency
CLE	cutaneous lupus erythematosus
CLIP	class II-associated invariant chain peptide
CLL	chronic lymphoid leukaemia
CMI	cell-mediated immunity
CNS	central nervous system
ConA	concanavalin A (mitogen)
COX	cyclooxygenase
cpm	counts per minute
CR	complement receptor
CRP	C-reactive protein
CTLA-4	cytotoxic T lymphocyte antigen-4
DAF	decay accelerating factor
DAMP	damage-associated molecular pattern
DAT	direct antiglobulin test
DEA1	dog erythrocyte antigen 1
DLA	dog leucocyte antigen
DNA	deoxyribonucleic acid
DOI	duration of immunity
DTH	delayed-type hypersensitivity
EAE	experimental autoimmune encephalomyelitis
EBP	eosinophilic bronchopneumopathy
ELA	equine leucocyte antigen
ELISA	enzyme-linked immunosorbent assay
ELISPOT	enzyme-linked immunospot
EPI	exocrine pancreatic insufficiency

ER	endoplasmic reticulum	Ig	immunoglobulin
ES	excretory–secretory (proteins)	*IGHA*	gene encoding the IgA heavy chain
Fab	antigen-binding fragment (of Ig)	IL	interleukin
FAD	flea allergy dermatitis	IMHA	immune-mediated haemolytic anaemia
Fc	crystallizable fragment (of Ig)		
FcR	Fc (Ig heavy chain) receptor	IMP	inosine monophosphate
FeLV	feline leukaemia virus	IMNP	immune-mediated neutropenia
FHV	feline herpesvirus	IMTP	immune-mediated thrombocytopenia
FIP	feline infectious peritonitis		
FISS	feline injection site sarcoma	iTreg	induced Treg (cell)
FITC	fluorescein isothiocyanate	IVIG	intravenous immunoglobulin (therapy)
FIV	feline immunodeficiency virus		
FLA	feline leucocyte antigen	JAK	Janus kinase
FOCMA	feline oncornavirus-associated cell membrane antigen	KCS	keratoconjunctivitis sicca
		KIR	killer cell immunoglobulin-like receptor
GALT	gastrointestinal-associated lymphoid tissue		
		KLH	keyhole limpet haemocyanin
G-CSF	granulocyte colony-stimulating factor	LAD	leucocyte adhesion deficiency
		LAK	lymphokine-activated killer (cell)
GITR	glucocorticoid-induced TNF-receptor-regulated (gene)	LFA-1	lymphocyte function-associated antigen-1
GMCSF	granulocyte–macrophage colony-stimulating factor		
		LGL	large granular lymphocyte
		LPS	lipopolysaccharide
GMP	guanosine monophosphate	M cell	microfold cell
GnRH	gonadotrophin-releasing hormone	M1/M2	subtypes of macrophages
GTP	guanosine triphosphate	MAC	membrane attack complex
GVHD	graft-versus-host disease	MAdCAM	mucosal addressin cell adhesion molecule
GWAS	genome-wide association study		
HAI	haemagglutination inhibition	MALT	mucosa-associated lymphoid tissue
HAT	hypoxanthine, aminopterin and thymidine	MAMP	microorganism-associated molecular pattern
HEV	high endothelial venule	MASP	MBL-associated serine protease
HGPRT	hypoxanthine–guanine phosphoribosyl transferase	MBL	mannan-binding lectin
		MCH	mean cell haemoglobin
HIV	human immunodeficiency virus	MCHC	mean cell haemoglobin concentration
HLA	human leucocyte antigen (human MHC)		
		MCP	membrane co-factor protein
IBD	inflammatory bowel disease	MCV	mean cell volume
IBH	insect bite hypersensitivity	MDA	maternally derived antibody
IBR	infectious bovine rhinotracheitis	MHC	major histocompatibility complex
ICAM-1	intercellular adhesion molecule-1	MMP	matrix metalloproteinase
IDST	intradermal skin test	mRNA	messenger RNA
IEL	intraepithelial lymphocyte	MS	multiple sclerosis
IEP	immonoelectrophoresis	NADPH	nicotinamide adenine dinucleotide phosphate
IFA	immunofluorescent antibody (test)		
IFN	interferon (e.g. IFN-γ)	NALT	nasal-associated lymphoid tissue

NET	neutrophil extracellular trap		**rHuIFN-α**	recombinant human IFN-α
NF-AT	nuclear factor of activated T cells		**RIG**	retinoic acid inducible gene (receptor)
NFκB	nuclear factor κB		**RNA**	ribonucleic acid
NI	neonatal isoerythrolysis		**ROS**	reactive oxygen species
NK	natural killer (cell)		**RT-PCR**	reverse transcriptase polymerase chain reaction
NKT	natural killer T (cell)			
NLR	NOD-like receptor		**SAA**	serum amyloid A
NO	nitric oxide		**SCID**	severe combined immunodeficiency/ immunodeficient
NOD1/2	nucleotide-binding oligomerization domain 1/2			
NOD	non-obese diabetic mouse		**SI**	stimulation index
NOS	nitric oxide synthase		**SLA**	swine leucocyte antigen
nTreg	natural Treg (cell)		**SLE**	systemic lupus erythematosus
NZB	New Zealand black mouse		**SLIT**	sublingual immunotherapy
OLA	ovine leucocyte antigen		**SNP**	single nucleotide polymorphism
OSP	outer surface protein		**SPC**	summary of product characteristics
OVA	ovalbumin		**SRBC**	sheep red blood cell
PALS	periarteriolar lymphoid sheath		**SRID**	single radial immunodiffusion
PAMP	pathogen-associated molecular pattern		**STAT**	signal transducers and activators of transcription
PBMC	peripheral blood mononuclear cell		**TAM**	tumour-associated macrophage
PBS	phosphate buffered saline		**TAP**	transporter protein (TAP1/TAP2)
PCR	polymerase chain reaction		**Tc**	T cytotoxic (cell)
PCV	packed cell volume		**TCR**	T-cell receptor
PEG	polyethylene glycol		**TFh**	T follicular helper (cell)
PHA	phytohaemagglutinin		**Tg**	thyroglobulin
PI	persistently infected		**TGF**	transforming growth factor
pIgR	polymeric immunoglobulin receptor		**Th**	T helper (cell)
PRR	pattern recognition receptor		**TLR**	Toll-like receptor
PT	prothrombin time		**TMS**	trimethoprim–sulphonamide
PTH	parathyroid hormone		**TNF**	tumour necrosis factor
PVDF	polyvinylidene fluoride		**TNS**	trapped neutrophil syndrome
PWM	pokeweed mitogen		**TPMT**	thiopurine methyltransferase
PWMS	post-weaning multi-systemic wasting syndrome (of pigs)		**Treg**	T regulatory (cell)
			TSH	thyroid-stimulating hormone
RAG	recombination activating gene		**UPC**	urine protein:creatinine (ratio)
RAO	recurrent airway obstruction		**VEGF**	vascular endothelial growth factor
RBCs	red blood cells		V_H	variable region of the heavy chain
RF	rheumatoid factor		V_L	variable region of the light chain
rHuGCSF	recombinant human granulocyte colony-stimulating factor		**VN**	virus neutralization
			WHO	World Health Organization
rHuGMCSF	recombinant human granulocyte–monocyte colony-stimulating factor		**X-SCID**	X-linked severe combined immunodeficiency

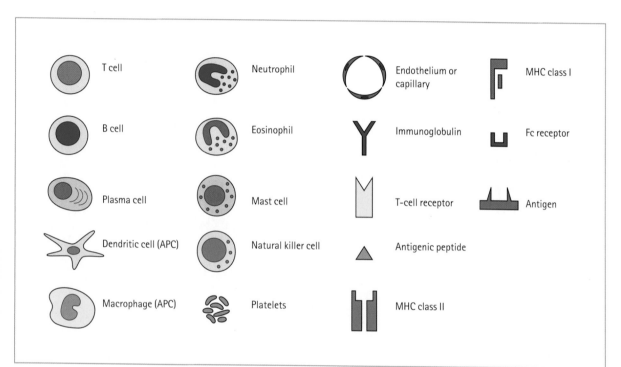

T cell

B cell

Plasma cell

Dendritic cell (APC)

Macrophage (APC)

Neutrophil

Eosinophil

Mast cell

Natural killer cell

Platelets

Endothelium or
capillary

Immunoglobulin

T-cell receptor

Antigenic peptide

MHC class II

MHC class I

Fc receptor

Antigen

CHAPTER 1

An Overview of the Immune System:
Innate and Adaptive Immunity and the Inflammatory Response

OBJECTIVES

At the end of this chapter you should be able to:
- Distinguish between innate and adaptive immunity.
- Discuss how gene duplication within the immune system provided an evolutionary advantage.
- Give examples of innate immune mechanisms of the skin and mucosal surfaces.
- Describe the main features of acute and chronic inflammation.
- List the components of the adaptive immune system.
- Understand the key role of the dendritic cell in linking innate and adaptive immunity.
- Understand why it is necessary to regulate the immune system.
- Define the concept of immunological memory.
- Briefly describe the evolution of the immune system.

INTRODUCTION

Immunology is a relatively young and rapidly developing science that has established itself as a fundamental cornerstone of human and veterinary clinical medicine. There are not many veterinary activities that do not have an immunological aspect. The husbandry of neonatal domestic livestock and the essential requirements for colostral immunity, the crucial role of vaccination in protecting the population and the individual from infectious disease, the laboratory diagnosis of a wide range of disorders, the consequences of chronic disease for immune function and the myriad of immune-mediated diseases caused by disturbance of immune homeostasis are all examples of how basic knowledge of the immune system impacts on the daily practice of veterinary medicine. The aim of this textbook is not only to provide this basic knowledge of immune function, but also to clearly relate this to clinical practice.

This chapter will briefly review the history of immunology and broadly consider the different elements of the immune system and how they interact to create a unified whole. The focus here will be on the innate immune system, with an introduction to adaptive immunity, which will be discussed in detail in subsequent chapters.

HISTORY OF IMMUNOLOGY

A perusal of the relatively short history of the discipline of immunology reveals just how integral veterinary immunology has been to the development of this science. This brief summary cannot do full justice to the progressive discoveries that have led to our current state of knowledge. Most texts record the birth of immunology, at least in the Western world, as related to the introduction of the concept of vaccination by Edward Jenner. In 1796 Jenner performed his famous experiment whereby he collected fluid from a cowpox vesicle on the hand of the dairymaid Sarah Nelmes, and inoculated this into the arm of the 8-year-old boy James Phipps. Although James developed cowpox lesions, he was protected when subsequently challenged 2 months later with virulent smallpox. It has recently been suggested that a similar experiment may have been conducted some 20 years before Jenner by the Dorset farmer Benjamin Jesty. The next major developments in immunology were attributed to Louis Pasteur, who developed vaccines to fowl cholera (1879), anthrax (1881), swine erysipelas (1892) and rabies (1885). It is noteworthy how many of the early developments in immunology related to animal diseases.

In fact, the history of immunological developments can be easily appreciated by studying a list of Nobel prizes awarded in this discipline (*Table 1.1*). These chart the progressive recognition of antibody, phagocytic cells and complement through to the current appreciation of the molecular interactions that underpin immune function. Of note is the 1996 award to Peter Doherty, a 1962 graduate of the University of Queensland School of Veterinary Science, who undertook postgraduate studies on ovine 'louping-ill' at the Moredun Research Institute in Scotland, further demonstrating the role that veterinarians have had in the development of immunology. In the current century, veterinary immunology remains a flourishing field of research with its own journals (e.g. *Veterinary Immunology and Immunopathology*), conferences and societies such as the American Association of Veterinary Immunologists (of which Dr Schultz was the first President). A major recent achievement in veterinary immunology was the declaration in 2011 that the world was free of rinderpest virus infection following successful vaccination campaigns. This is only the second occasion that a major infectious disease has been eliminated, the first being the eradication of smallpox in 1979.

TABLE 1.1. NOBEL PRIZES IN IMMUNOLOGY

1901	Von Behring	Discovery of serum antibody
1905	Koch	Immune response in tuberculosis
1908	Mechnikov and Ehrlich	Phagocytosis and antitoxins
1913	Richet	Anaphylaxis
1919	Bordet	Complement
1960	Burnet and Medawar	Immunological tolerance
1972	Edelman and Porter	Antibody structure
1977	Yalow	Development of radioimmunoassay
1980	Benacerraf, Dausset and Snell	Discovery of the major histocompatibility complex
1984	Jerne, Kohler and Milstein	Production of monoclonal antibodies
1987	Tonegawa	Mechanism of antibody diversity
1990	Murray and Thomas	Transplantation
1996	Doherty and Zinkernagel	Major histocompatibility complex restriction
2011	Steinman	Role of the dendritic cell in adaptive immunity
2011	Beutler and Hoffman	Activation of innate immunity

THE IMMUNE SYSTEM: AN OVERVIEW

As you progress through this book, it is inevitable that you will be struck by the complexity of the mammalian immune system. The principal purpose of the immune system is to provide protection from the myriad of infectious agents responsible for human and animal morbidity and mortality. The immune system is capable of responding, with varying degrees of efficacy, to all bacterial, viral, fungal, protozoal and helminth pathogens. The immune system is intrinsically involved with the inflammatory and tissue repair processes of the body; it can initiate responses to abnormal cells that arise during neoplastic transformation or that may be inappropriately transplanted into the body. Such a potent biological system requires careful management and an entire set of regulatory mechanisms to ensure that immune responses are switched off when not required, so as not to cause inadvertent damage to normal body tissue.

Occasionally, this delicate balance goes awry and the immune system makes inappropriate responses to innocuous environmental antigens, dietary antigens or components of the body, leading to the range of immune-mediated allergic and autoimmune diseases that are so important in human and companion animal medicine.

The immune system of all animal species is comprised of a standard set of building blocks that interact with each other in predictable fashion. Much more is known about experimental rodent and human immunology than that related to domestic animals, but it is possible to extrapolate many of the fundamental principles from the better explored species to our animals. That said, there are numerous intriguing species differences that have arisen during evolution and these will be discussed in the chapters that follow.

The standard building blocks of the immune system are depicted in **Figure 1.1**. Classically, the immune system is considered to be comprised of two

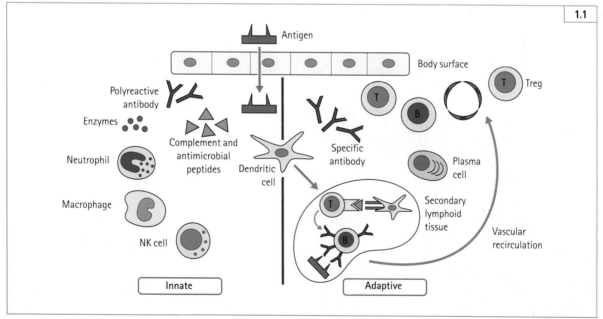

1.1

Fig. 1.1 The immune system. This diagram depicts the various components of the innate and adaptive immune systems responding to challenge by a foreign antigen. Innate immune defence is provided by epithelial barriers, resident phagocytic and specialized lymphoid cells, polyreactive antibodies and the alternative pathway of the complement system. The dendritic cell is the key link between innate and adaptive immunity and transports sampled antigen to the regional lymphoid tissue. T and B lymphocytes of the adaptive immune system are activated within lymphoid tissue and these potent and antigen-specific cells are mobilized to migrate through the vascular system to the site of antigen exposure in order to mount the effector immune response. Once antigen is eliminated, the system must be switched off by the action of specific regulatory populations of lymphocytes.

related halves: the **innate** and the **adaptive** immune responses. The innate (inborn) immune system is older in evolutionary terms than the adaptive immune system. On the evolutionary tree, even relatively primitive life forms have some form of immunity. As species evolved, the array of potential pathogens that could target those species evolved in parallel, so there was evolutionary pressure for the evolving species to develop a progressively more complex immune system in order to survive the race between host and pathogen evolution (see below). As we shall see in subsequent chapters, the increasing complexity of host immunity was largely made possible by the process of **gene duplication**, giving rise to related families of immunological molecules. Innate immunity therefore represents the earliest form of immune defence and is intrinsically interlinked with the acute and chronic **inflammatory responses**.

Innate immunity

The innate immune system is particularly active at those anatomical sites that are most likely to be the first point of contact with potential pathogens: the skin, respiratory tract, gastrointestinal tract, urogenital tract, mammary gland and ocular mucosa. The **epithelial barriers** that cover these surfaces are considered part of the innate immune system. Many of these physical barriers have a range of site-specific modifications that further contribute to their ability to exclude pathogens. For example:

- The cutaneous keratinized stratified squamous **epidermis** is a relatively inhospitable environment bathed in **sebum** and **sweat**, both of which contain numerous antimicrobial substances. Colonies of endogenous cutaneous bacteria (**microflora**) live normally on the skin and compete with any potential cutaneous microbial pathogen for space and nutrients in this environment (**Figure 1.2**).

- The **respiratory mucosa** is lined by ciliated columnar epithelial cells, the cilia of which beat in unison to transport mucus and debris upwards from the lower bronchial tree to the oropharynx, where this material can be swallowed (**Figures 1.3a, b**). This transport mechanism is often referred to as the '**mucociliary escalator**'. Glandular secretions released onto the respiratory surface contain antimicrobial substances and the population of **alveolar macrophages** patrols these spaces in the lung to remove particulate debris by phagocytosis (**Figure 1.4**).

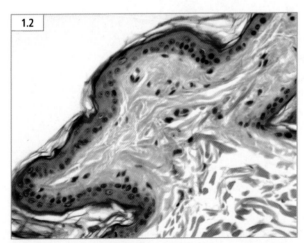

Fig. 1.2 Cutaneous innate immunity. The innate immune defences of the skin include the inhospitable nature of keratinized squamous epithelium, the secretion of antimicrobial substances in sebum and sweat, the presence of a cutaneous microflora and a range of leucocytes including the intraepithelial lymphocytes and dendritic cells (Langerhans dendritic cells) and phagocytic cells within the dermal microenvironment.

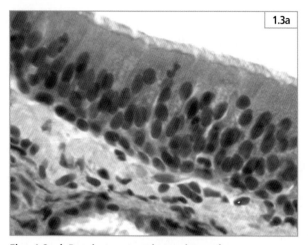

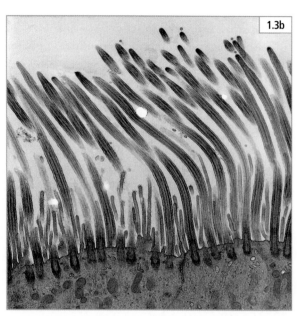

Figs. 1.3a, b Respiratory tract innate immunity.
(a) The columnar epithelial cells lining the respiratory mucosa are ciliated. The directional beating of these cilia moves particulate debris and mucus from the lower respiratory tract to the oropharynx, where it is removed by swallowing (the 'mucociliary escalator'). (b) An electronmicrograph showing the structure of the cilia. Other innate immune defences include the antimicrobial secretions of mucosal glands and the leucocytes resident in the lamina propria.

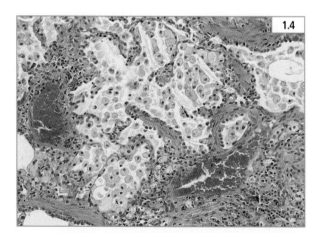

Fig. 1.4 Alveolar macrophages. A population of macrophages resides in the alveolar space and phagocytoses any particulate debris that might bypass innate defences higher up the respiratory tract. These cells develop a prominent 'foamy' cytoplasm when activated.

- The **small intestinal mucosa** has a similar epithelial barrier, with **mucus-producing goblet cells** and secreted antimicrobial substances, including the various enzymes contained within the bile (**Figure 1.5**). The **peristaltic action** of the gut wall provides continued directional movement of luminal content, which discourages local colonization by pathogens. The intestinal tract has a rich **microbial flora** that again competes with pathogens for space and nutrients in this location.

As mentioned above, these physical barriers are often bathed by secretions enriched in antimicrobial molecules that can cause direct damage to the pathogen (e.g. digestion of bacterial cell walls). These molecules include enzymes such as **lysozyme** and **phospholipase A** and small antimicrobial peptides such as the α-**defensins** and **cathelicidins** produced by Paneth cells in the crypts of the intestine and by epithelial surfaces of the skin, the oral mucosa and the respiratory and urogenital tracts. The **surfactant proteins** that coat the alveolar surfaces of the lung are also antimicrobial. Pathogens coated by these molecules (e.g. surfactant proteins A and D) are more readily removed by **alveolar macrophages** (see Chapters 3 and 5). Other secreted molecules include the **polyreactive antibodies** (see Chapter 2), which can potentially bind to a range of foreign invaders, and molecules of the **alternative pathway** of the **complement system** (see Chapter 3).

Should any potential pathogen breach this 'first line' epithelial barrier, then the innate immune system must have back-up protective mechanisms. The key to innate immunity is that these mechanisms must be readily and continually available for '**instant action**' when required. These mechanisms must be able to cope with the wide spectrum of potential pathogens that might attempt to enter the body via any of the routes described above, and so they are relatively **non-specific** in their action.

A number of leucocyte types satisfy these requirements of being continuously present, rapidly activated and non-specific in targeting pathogens. These include the phagocytic cells (**neutrophils** and **macrophages**), the **dendritic cells**, the **mast cells**, the **natural killer (NK) cells** and a specialized subpopulation of **T lymphocytes** that reside within the epithelial barriers (the **intraepithelial lymphocytes, IELs**). Together, the cells and molecules of the innate immune system can provide instant defence from infection, but this defence is relatively weak and may only be able to hold the invading pathogens at bay for short periods of time.

The collective effect of the molecules and cells of the innate immune system in responding to insult by pathogens, trauma or a local immune response is termed **inflammation**. The **inflammatory response** to such initiating stimuli is initiated by tissue resident (or sentinel) cells of the innate immune system including tissue macrophages, dendritic cells and mast cells. These cells bear surface receptors that allow them to respond to structural or secreted components of pathogens or to a range of molecules released by damaged or dying tissue cells (collectively referred to as **alarmins**). Engagement of the sentinel cell receptors leads to those cells releasing an array of soluble mediators, which are responsible for the ensuing inflammatory response. These mediators include **cytokines** and **chemokines** (see Chapter 7) and vasoactive molecules (see Chapter 3). An inflammatory response involves the accumulation of fluid, plasma proteins and blood leucocytes at the site of such insult. The aims of the inflammatory response are to neutralize the inciting cause (e.g. a pathogen), to contain pathogens and prevent their systemic spread and to promote tissue repair once the pathogen is eliminated. The inflammatory response has two distinct phases known as acute and chronic inflammation.

Acute inflammation begins within minutes of tissue insult and classically is characterized by the presence of the five **cardinal signs** of inflammation: pain, swelling, heat, redness and loss of function of the affected tissue. These changes relate to alterations in the capillary vasculature of the affected tissue. Capillary dilation (**vasodilation**) leads to increased local blood flow and reduced velocity of this flow, while increased permeability leads to the loss of fluid from blood to tissue (**oedema**) and associated loss of plasma proteins. The **endothelial cells** lining the blood vessels express surface **adhesion molecules** (see Chapter 5), which permit the adhesion of leucocytes and the migration of these cells between the stretched endothelial cells into the tissue. The first leucocytes to undergo such **extravasation** are the **neutrophils** and this migration occurs within the first few hours of the acute inflammatory response (**Figure 1.6**). In parallel with these changes, the stretching of the vessel wall exposes the collagen beneath the endothelium to the flowing blood and initiates **coagulation** involving the platelets and coagulation factors. The relevance of this mechanism is that it provides a means of preventing spread of pathogens into the bloodstream.

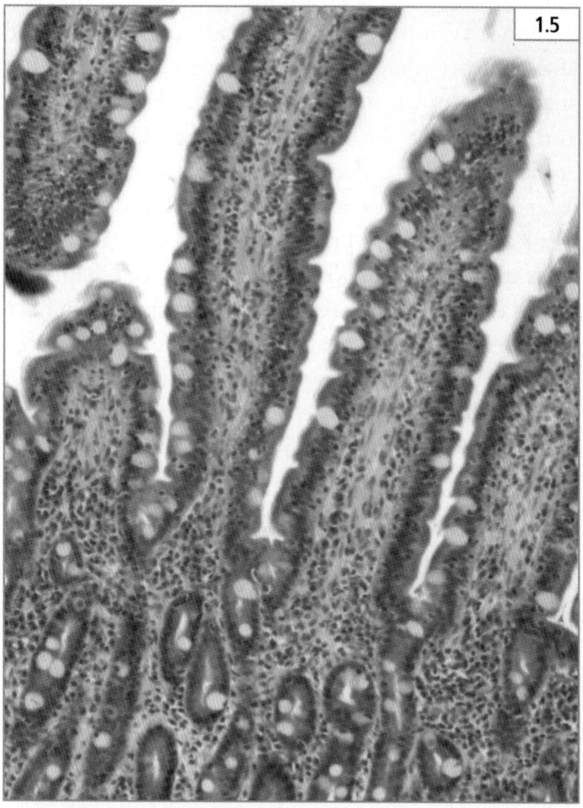

Recruited neutrophils migrate in a directed fashion towards the target pathogen in tissue via the process of **chemotaxis** (see Chapter 3). The neutrophil must then recognize and bind the target, a process that involves the engagement of surface receptors on the neutrophil by molecules expressed on the surface of the pathogen. These may be components of the cell wall of the organism or serum proteins (e.g. antibodies and complement) that have precoated the organism to increase the likelihood of recognition (**opsonization**; see Chapter 3). Following recognition the organism is engulfed by cytoplasmic extensions and drawn into the neutrophil cytoplasm in a process known as **phagocytosis**. Once in the neutrophil cytoplasm, the organism is enclosed within a vacuole (the **phagosome**). The phagocytosed organism is then destroyed via the effects of the respiratory burst or by the release of lytic enzymes and antimicrobial peptides into the vacuole.

1.5

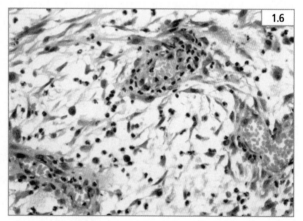

1.6

Fig. 1.5 Intestinal innate immunity. The small intestine is endowed with numerous innate immune defences, including peristaltic movement, an epithelial barrier, secreted antimicrobial substances, mucus production by goblet cells and the presence of intraepithelial T lymphocytes and phagocytic cells within the lamina propria.

Fig. 1.6 Acute inflammation. This section of canine skin displays acute inflammatory changes. There is vasodilation and tissue oedema with margination and egress of leucocytes (chiefly neutrophils) from vessels into the tissue. Those neutrophils distant from the vessel may be migrating along a chemotactic gradient towards the trigger of the inflammatory response (e.g. a local bacterial infection).

The **respiratory burst** involves assembly of the nicotinamide adenosine dinucleotide phosphate (NADPH) complex and uptake of oxygen by the neutrophil, which leads sequentially to the generation of large quantities of hydrogen peroxide (catalysed by superoxide dismutase) and then hypohalides such as OCl^-, when myeloperoxidase catalyses the reaction between H_2O_2 and halide ions such as Cl^- or SCN^-.

The second means by which a neutrophil can destroy the phagocytosed target involves the fusion of cytoplasmic granules (**lysosomes**) with the phagosome to form the **phagolysosome**. This process results in the release of lysosomal enzymes (e.g. lysozyme, proteases and acid hydrolases) and antimicrobial peptides (e.g. defensins) into the phagolysosome. The enzymes are able to digest the wall of the organism and the antimicrobial peptides act by inserting into and disrupting the structure of the cell wall of the target. Neutrophils are also able to release antimicrobial proteins into the extracellular environment (degranulation) in order to eliminate extracellular organisms.

Finally, neutrophils can destroy extracellular organisms by the release of **neutrophil extracellular traps** (**NETs**). NETs are composed of a core of DNA to which various proteins (including histone proteins, lactoferrin, cathepsins, myeloperoxidase and neutrophil elastase) are attached. NETs immobilize pathogens, which are subsequently destroyed by antimicrobial substances within the NET or are phagocytosed.

As suggested above, the acute inflammatory response takes place against the background of a complex network of soluble inflammatory mediators that are released at the site of inflammation. These include the initiating alarmins, **histamine** (derived from mast cells and a potent vasodilator), the **kinins** (such as bradykinin), chemokines (involved in the recruitment of leucocytes from the bloodstream) and cytokines (involved in recruitment and activation of leucocytes), molecules of the alternative pathway of **complement** (see Chapter 3), **coagulation factors** and the vasoactive lipids (collectively **eicosanoids**). Eicosanoids are derived from arachidonic acid released from phospholipids of damaged cell membranes by the action of phospholipases. Arachidonic acid may be converted to **leukotrienes** (e.g. leukotriene B_4) by the action of lipoxygenase, or to a range of **prostaglandins** (e.g. prostaglandin E_2), **thromboxanes** (e.g. thromboxane A_2) and **prostacyclins** (e.g. prostaglandin I_2) by the **cyclooxygenases** (COX) COX-1 and COX-2. Some of these molecules interact with nervous system sensors (pain receptors; nociceptors) and neuropeptides may be released from nerve endings within inflamed tissue.

The second stage of the inflammatory response (**chronic inflammation**) begins 24–48 hours after the initiating insult and is characterized by the recruitment of blood **monocytes** into the tissue. These cells differentiate into tissue **macrophages** and provide the second line of innate immune defence. While neutrophils are rapidly mobilized and effective phagocytic cells, they have a short life span and cannot undertake repeated phagocytosis and destruction of targets. Although macrophages are less rapidly recruited, they are more potent and long-lived phagocytes that are capable of multiple phagocytic events. Macrophages also have additional roles in activating adaptive immunity (see Chapter 7) and in tissue repair by removing neutrophils that have died by **apoptosis** (preventing inadvertent damage to tissue by viable enzymes within these cells) and necrotic tissue and by releasing enzymes capable of connective tissue remodelling.

Macrophages recognize and phagocytose target organisms in a similar fashion to neutrophils. One of the major enzymatic pathways of these cells involves the generation of **nitric oxide synthase** (NOS), which generates **nitric oxide** (NO) from arginine. NO in turn reacts with superoxide anions to produce substances such as nitrogen dioxide radicals that are highly toxic to phagocytosed organisms. Macrophages able to generate NO are known as **M1 cells** and are important in the chronic inflammatory response. A second subset of macrophages (**M2 cells**) uses arginase to convert arginine to ornithine. These cells are non-inflammatory, but they promote tissue repair and wound healing.

The chronic inflammatory response may be accompanied by systemic signs of illness in addition to local tissue inflammation. This effect largely relates to the release of a series of **pro-inflammatory cytokines** from activated macrophages. These include interleukin (IL)-1, IL-6 and tumour necrosis factor (TNF)-α (see Chapter 7). They interact directly with nerve cells in damaged tissue and are absorbed into the circulation where they are able to access the brain and bind to receptor molecules that mediate **pyrexia** (altering the hypothalamic body temperature set mechanism), **lethargy** (promoting sleep-inducing molecules) and **anorexia** (acting on the hypothalamic satiety centre). These circulating cytokines also stimulate the production of a collection of **acute phase proteins** by the liver. The acute phase proteins include molecules such as **C-reactive protein** (CRP), which may act as an opsonin promoting phagocytosis, **serum amyloid A** (SAA), which may act as a leucocyte chemoattractant and has some immunosuppressive function, and **haptoglobin**, which binds iron and thereby sequesters it from bacteria that have an obligate metabolic requirement for this element. The acute phase proteins may be detected in the blood and are useful indicators of the presence of inflammation.

The overall effect of the acute and chronic inflammatory responses, often in concert with adaptive immunity (see below), is to destroy and remove pathogens and promote tissue repair. There are, however, some initiators of inflammation that are very difficult to eliminate. These include intracellular pathogens able to subvert the protective mechanisms described above (e.g. *Mycobacterium bovis*), large structures (e.g. tissue migrating parasites) or inert irritants such as metal particles, suture materials or vaccine adjuvants. These substances tend to induce chronic and persistent inflammatory foci that become 'walled off' from normal tissue by formation of a **granuloma** (**Figure 1.7**). A granuloma may have a necrotic core, containing the foreign material with some neutrophils or eosinophils, that is surrounded by macrophages that may fuse together to form **multinucleate giant cells** (**Figure 1.8**). These cells are in turn surrounded by a zone of fibrous connective tissue. A 'sterile' granuloma (e.g. induced by suture material) has this typical composition, whereas an 'infectious' granuloma containing antigenic material may also include many lymphocytes.

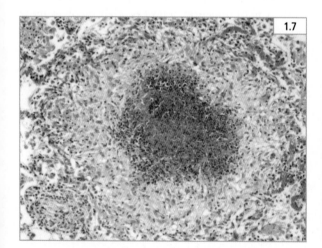

Fig. 1.7 Chronic inflammation. This is a section of lung from an alpaca with *Mycobacterium* infection. The lesion is a granuloma with a necrotic core, containing degenerate neutrophils and bacteria (not visible), that is walled-off by a layer of macrophages with scattered lymphocytes.

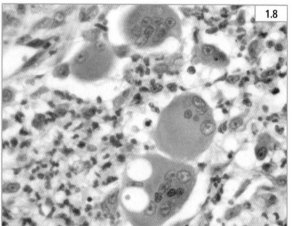

Fig. 1.8 Multinucleate giant cells. Section of skin from a cat with localized pyogranulomatous dermatitis. Within the inflammatory infiltrate there are multinucleate foreign body giant cells representing fused macrophages. The cell at the base of the image contains two large cytoplasmic vacuoles. No specific infectious cause for this reaction was identified and it may have been triggered by a penetrating foreign body.

The final stage of the inflammatory response is tissue repair, which may largely be regulated by M2 macrophages. These cells produce fibroblast and blood vessel growth factors (e.g. platelet-derived growth factor), and cytokines (e.g. **transforming growth factor** [TGF]-β), which promote the deposition of collagen and the growth of new vessels that replace areas of necrotic tissue. The fibrous repair (scar tissue) may be remodelled by **matrix metalloproteinases** (MMPs) derived from M2 macrophages. Scar tissue may be devoid of normal tissue elements in tissues that are incapable of regeneration (**Figure 1.9**). Other subtypes of M2 macrophages may have an immunosuppressive role via production of the cytokine IL-10.

The population of sentinel **dendritic cells** plays a key role in bridging the innate and adaptive immune response. As we shall see in Chapter 7, this class of cells has a pivotal role in **sampling foreign antigens** as they broach barrier defences and **transporting** them, via lymphatic vessels, from the site of infection to the closest area of organized lymphoid tissue. This antigen sampling and transport permits activation of the adaptive immune response so that the dendritic cell provides the link between these two halves of immunity.

Adaptive immunity

The **adaptive immune response** is younger than the innate immune response in evolutionary terms and is more **specific** and considerably more **potent** in its effects. The constituents of the adaptive immune response are the lymphoid cells. These include:

- The **T lymphocytes** and the cytokine and chemokine messenger proteins released by these cells, which direct and regulate the adaptive immune response.
- The **B lymphocytes**, which transform to the late-stage **plasma cells** that produce and secrete **antibody**.

The lymphoid cells of the adaptive immune response reside in, and circulate between, the various **lymphoid tissues** of the body (e.g. the **lymph nodes, spleen** and **mucosal lymphoid tissues**). In the adaptive immune response, antigen is first transported from a site of infection by a dendritic cell to the regional lymphoid tissue. That dendritic cell in turn activates antigen-specific T lymphocytes, which further activate antigen-specific B lymphocytes. These activated, antigen-specific lymphocytes must then be mobilized from the regional lymphoid tissue and sent to the site of infection, a process that involves these

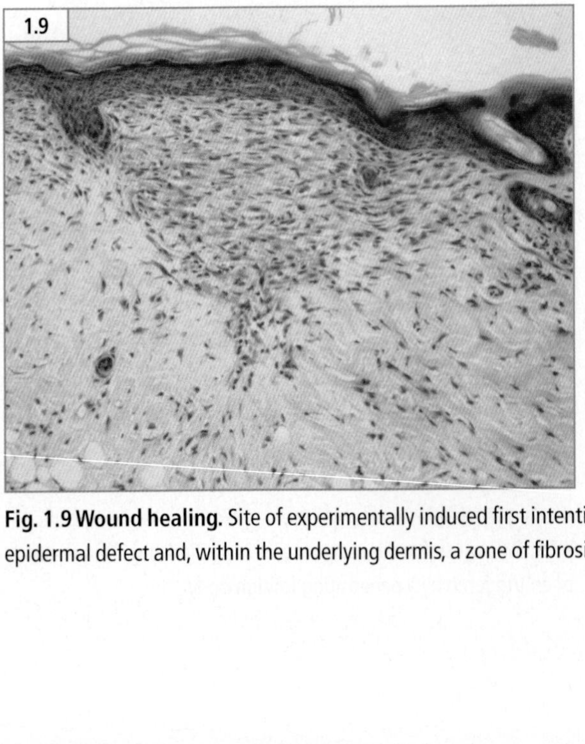

Fig. 1.9 Wound healing. Site of experimentally induced first intention wound healing in the skin of a mouse. There is repair of the epidermal defect and, within the underlying dermis, a zone of fibrosis that lacks hair follicles or glandular structures.

cells moving into the lymphatic and blood circulation and interacting with the endothelial lining of blood vessels. Once these cells reach the site of infection, they are able to mount a full-scale 'effector' response, which is considerably stronger than that permitted by innate immunity. As these processes take some time to occur (in the order of 4–7 days), there is a delay before adaptive immunity 'takes over' from the innate form of defence. This sequence of events will be discussed in more detail in Chapter 13. The final component of adaptive immunity is the development of a regulatory response that will switch off the system when it is no longer required (i.e. when the pathogen has been eliminated) so as not to cause damage to normal body tissue. However, once this is achieved, the immune system retains the memory of that immune response. Immunological memory is another key feature of

the adaptive immune response. Memory allows the generation of a much more effective secondary immune response if that same antigen is ever re-encountered, and this phenomenon underpins the application of vaccination in clinical medicine.

The military analogy is often used to explain these immunological phenomena and it may be helpful to consider the immune system as an army at war with invading pathogens (Figure 1.10). In this context, the innate immune system might be equated to the frontier defences of the body and the dendritic cells to messengers who may be dispatched from the frontier to the fort (regional lymphoid tissue), where the army of the adaptive immune response is marshalled. The messengers provide information that enables the army to select those troops best equipped to deal with the particular invader, to activate those troops

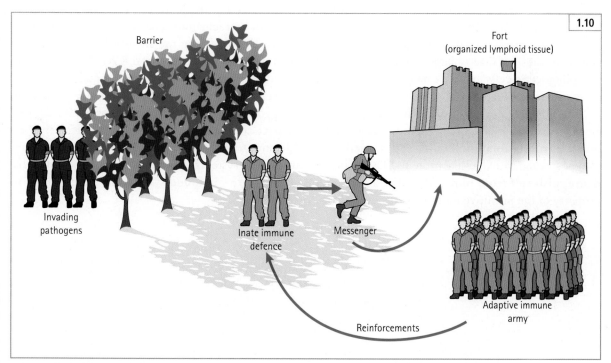

Fig. 1.10 The military analogy. The immune response is often likened to a war between invading pathogens and the army of the immune system. In this model the innate immune defence might be considered as a relatively weak frontier patrol surveying the outer reaches of the body. If an enemy invades this territory, a messenger is dispatched to the closest military fort, where a battalion of soldiers that is best equipped to deal with this type of enemy is mobilized and sent back to the place where the frontier has been breached. These reinforcements allow successful elimination of the enemy, following which the army is stood down when instructed by regulatory elements.

and dispatch them to the frontier, where they provide reinforcements to the innate system in the battle against the pathogen. These reinforcements may eliminate the invaders and then this adaptive army might be disbanded when instructed by regulatory cells that step in once the battle is won. This simplistic overview of the immune system will be expanded as we progress through the chapters of this book.

THE EVOLUTION OF THE IMMUNE SYSTEM

The evolution of the mammalian immune system has been widely studied. Even very primitive organisms have an **innate immune system** that functions to protect those organisms from potential pathogens. The innate immune system may have had its origins in the unicellular amoeba. These organisms move within their aquatic environment and engulf food particles that they encounter. The discrimination between food and another amoeba may be a receptor-mediated recognition process. These features of amoebae are similar to those of macrophages and it is suggested that **phagocytic cells** may have had their origin from these precursors.

The immune system of primitive species relies largely on the activity of a range of non-specific innate **antimicrobial molecules** and the action of phagocytes and cytokine-like proteins. The ability to **distinguish self from non-self** is also an ancestral property of the primitive immune system. Sponges, earthworms and starfish are all capable of 'graft rejection' when experimentally grafted with tissue from distinct species, but such rejection is mediated by the innate immune system. An excellent example of an ancestral immunological molecule that is relatively conserved throughout evolution is the **Toll-like receptor** (see Chapter 7). These molecules were first described in the fruit fly *Drosophila* and homologues are present in mammalian species and are thought to be active even in plants.

As organisms and the pathogens that target them co-evolved, there were continual requirements for the development of a more complex immune system. The development of **adaptive immunity** has been described as the **immunological 'big bang'** and is thought to have occurred in an ancestor of the jawed fish. The key feature of adaptive immunity is the ability to generate **diversity in antigen receptor molecules**. The event that led to development of this ability is thought to relate to integration of a circle of extrachromosomal DNA (a 'transposable element') containing the ancestral **recombination activating genes** (*RAG-1* and *RAG-2*) into a region of the genome encoding an ancestor gene encoding a molecule similar to a T- or B-cell receptor. In parallel, the process of **gene duplication**, as discussed with respect to the immunoglobulin superfamily (see Chapters 6 and 8), allowed creation of a wide diversity in immune system molecules. The broad evolutionary stages of the immune system are summarized in *Table 1.2*.

TABLE 1.2. EVOLUTION OF THE IMMUNE SYSTEM

	Phagocytic cells and TLRs	NK cells	Ig	MHC	T and B lymphocytes	Lymph nodes
Invertebrates						
Protozoa	+	-	-	-	-	-
Sponges	+	-	-	-	-	-
Annelids	+	+	-	-	-	-
Arthropods	+	-	-	-	-	-
Vertebrates						
Elasmobrachs (sharks, skates, rays)	+	+	+	-	+	-
Teleost fish	+	+	+	+ (some)	+	-
Amphibians	+	+	+	+ (some)	+	-
Reptiles	+	+	+	+	+	-
Birds	+	+	+	+	+	+ (some)
Mammals	+	+	+	+	+	+

TLR, Toll-like receptor; NK, natural killer; Ig, immunoglobulin; MHC, major histocompatibility complex. (Adapted from Abbas AK, Lichtman AH (2003) *Cellular and Molecular Immunology*, 5th edn. WB Saunders, Philadelphia, p. 7.)

KEY POINTS

- The two halves of the immune response are innate and adaptive immunity.
- Innate immunity is evolutionarily older, simple, fast-acting and non-specific.
- Innate immunity is important at the mucosal and cutaneous sites most likely to encounter pathogens.
- Acute and chronic inflammation mediate the initial response to tissue damage or infection.
- Acute inflammation involves a series of vasoactive events allowing recruitment of neutrophils into affected tissue.
- Chronic inflammation involves the subsequent recruitment of macrophages into affected tissue.
- Both neutrophils and macrophages are phagocytic cells, but they achieve this effect through different mechanisms.
- The systemic signs of chronic inflammation are mediated by pro-inflammatory cytokines interacting with central nervous system centres regulating physiological function.
- The synthesis of acute phase proteins by the liver may be detected in the blood and used to monitor inflammation.

- The sequela to inflammation is tissue repair.
- Some initiators of inflammation are persistent and lead to the formation of granulomas.
- The dendritic cell is the link between innate and adaptive immunity.
- The adaptive immune response is made in organized lymphoid tissue.
- The adaptive immune response is slower, but more potent and specific, than the innate response.
- A regulatory system is required to switch off the immune response when no longer required.
- The adaptive immune system retains memory of previous antigenic exposure.
- The memory (secondary) immune response is more potent that the initial (primary) response.
- Early life forms have a simple innate immune system.
- The immunological 'big bang' occurred in an ancestor of the jawed fish and led to evolution of the adaptive immune response through the ability to develop diversity in receptor molecules.

CHAPTER 2

Antigens and Antibodies

OBJECTIVES

At the end of this chapter you should be able to:
- Understand what makes one substance more antigenic than another.
- Define 'epitope', 'immunodominant' and 'hapten'.
- Describe how adjuvants enhance the immune response.
- Describe the basic structure of the immunoglobulin molecule.

- List the five classes of immunoglobulin and describe the structure and function of each.
- Describe how an antigenic epitope binds to an antibody.
- Define 'affinity' and 'avidity' as they relate to antigen binding by antibody.

INTRODUCTION

This chapter reviews two very basic elements of the immune response (antigens and antibodies) and the means by which these molecules interact *in vivo* and *in vitro*. An understanding of the core concepts presented here underpins much of the remainder of the material covered in this book.

ANTIGENS

An antigen may be simply defined as a substance that binds to a lymphocyte receptor. In associating with the receptor the antigen may or may not initiate an immune response. Classically, an antigenic molecule is defined by its ability to be bound by a specific antibody (see below), but some antigens fail to stimulate antibody production as part of the immune response. The related term **immunogen** refers to a substance that induces an immune response when injected into an individual. Antigens may be one of several diverse classes of molecules that interact with the immune system. The majority of antigens are foreign to the body and may enter a host via a range of possible routes (e.g. percutaneous absorption, injection, ingestion, inhalation or sexual contact). These are referred to as **heteroantigens** and include infectious agents (e.g. viruses, bacteria, fungi, protozoa or helminths), environmental substances (e.g. pollens or pollutants) and chemicals (e.g. drugs). Other classes of antigen arise from tissues or cells. These include **alloantigens** carried by foreign cells or tissue from a genetically dissimilar member of the same species that is grafted into an individual (i.e. during transplantation), or **xenoantigens** present on graft tissue derived from a different species (e.g. the transplantation of porcine heart valves into a human being). Finally, in some circumstances it is possible for the immune system to recognize components of the host's own body (**autoantigens or 'self-antigens'**) a situation that might give rise to **autoimmune disease**.

There are certain properties of an antigen that determine the potency of the immune response made to that antigen; this is referred to as the **antigenicity** of the substance. The most effective antigens:

- Are foreign to the host.
- Are of molecular mass >10 kD.
- Are particulate or aggregated (small soluble molecules are poorly antigenic).
- Have a complex (tertiary) molecular structure.
- Carry a charge.
- Are chemically complex.
- Are biologically active.

The latter property means that infectious agents are generally excellent antigens, although some organisms have developed the ability to evade the host immune response and induce chronic persistent infection (see Chapter 1).

Given that the majority of antigens are structurally complex, there are often numerous distinct regions within the antigen that are individually capable of interacting with the immune system. One antigen may therefore comprise multiple **epitopes** or **determinants**, each of which may be bound by a specific antibody or cellular receptor molecule (**Figures 2.1a–d**). Some epitopes within an antigen

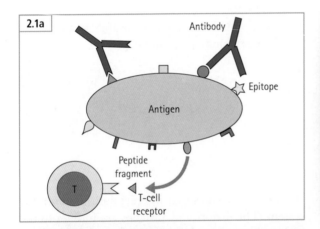

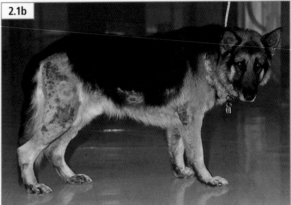

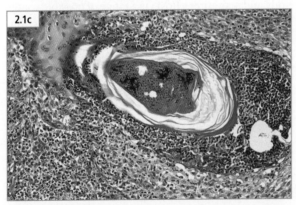

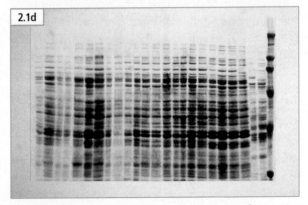

Figs. 2.1a–d Antigenic epitopes. (a) A complex antigen may be composed of numerous individual epitopes each capable of interacting with the host immune system. The most potent of these epitopes are considered immunodominant. **(b, c)** This German shepherd dog has staphylococcal infection of the hair follicles (deep pyoderma) and colonies of staphylococci are seen within the follicular lumen on biopsy. **(d)** Each individual *Staphylococcus* may be considered an antigen composed of multiple epitopes capable of inducing an antibody response. In this experiment, staphylococci have been disrupted and the component epitopes separated by molecular mass through polyacrylamide gel electrophoresis. The epitopes have been electophoretically transferred to an inert membrane and demonstrated by use of an antiserum in the technique of western blotting.

may be more effective at inducing an immune response (as they incorporate more of the properties listed above) and these are known as the **immunodominant** epitopes.

A discussion of antigens must include mention of a **hapten**, defined as a small chemical group which, by itself, cannot elicit an immune response but, when bound to a larger **carrier protein**, is capable of generating an antibody or cellular immune response (**Figure 2.2**). The clinical relevance of this phenomenon lies in the fact that some drugs may bind carrier proteins and inappropriately stimulate a **drug reaction** (**Figures 2.3a, b**).

The science of immunology most often involves the study of the interaction of antigens with the immune system. These investigations are often performed experimentally by exposing an animal to an antigen and documenting the ensuing immune response. In such an experimental context we have learnt that the potency of the immune response generated can be determined by a number of factors. These lessons have direct clinical relevance where an immune response is artificially induced in an animal through **vaccination**. The factors that determine the efficacy of an immune response include:

- The method of preparing the antigen.
- The species and genetic background of the recipient.
- The dose of antigen administered.
- The route of administration.
- The use of an adjuvant.

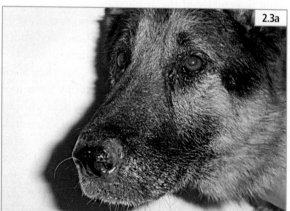

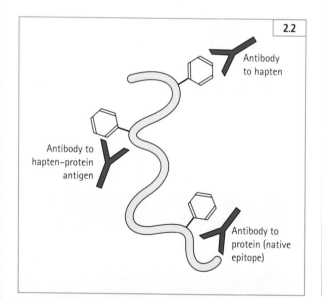

Fig. 2.2 Hapten. This small chemical group is non-immunogenic unless it is conjugated to a large carrier protein. The combined hapten–carrier may trigger an immune response (represented by antibody) to the hapten alone, the carrier protein alone or a novel antigen formed of both the hapten and carrier.

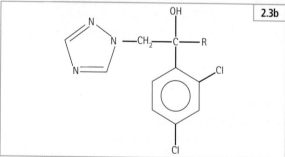

Figs. 2.3a, b Drug reaction. This German shepherd dog (a) was being treated with the systemic antifungal drug ketoconazole (chemical formula shown, b) and subsequently developed lesions affecting the planum nasale and periorbital skin. In this instance the drug may be acting as a hapten by binding to dermal protein and triggering a local immune response. Such reactions may spontaneously resolve once administration of the drug is halted.

An **adjuvant** is a substance which, when combined with antigen, non-specifically enhances the ensuing immune response to that antigen. Adjuvants additionally lead to general enhancement of immune function. Classical adjuvants such as **Freund's adjuvant** (an oil in water emulsion), **Freund's complete adjuvant** (incorporating killed mycobacteria into the emulsion) or **peanut oil** are highly irritant substances that induce a local inflammatory response and stimulate **antigen presentation** (see Chapter 7). Adjuvants such as these may also produce a **depot effect** whereby small quantities of antigen are slowly released from the antigen–adjuvant amalgam to maintain a more prolonged antigenic stimulation. Many of the non-infectious vaccines currently used in veterinary and human medicine are adjuvanted to increase the immunogenicity of the antigenic component of the vaccine (see Chapter 20). Vaccine adjuvants must be considerably safer than the selection described above and the most commonly employed is **alum** (aluminium hydroxide or aluminium phosphate). Another form of adjuvant is the **liposome** or **iscom** (immune stimulatory complex) in which antigen is held within a minute vesicle made up of lipid membrane. The search for more effective and safer adjuvants is an active area of research. The latest generation of adjuvants may have a more targeted effect, enhancing particular aspects of immunity. Small fragments of bacterial DNA rich in cytosine and guanidine (**CpG motifs**) or recombinant immunomodulatory **cytokines** (see Chapter 7 and Chapter 20) are such substances. They are collectively referred to as **molecular adjuvants**.

ANTIBODIES

The fraction of blood that remains fluid after clotting represents the **serum** (i.e. plasma without fibrinogen); it may be electrophoretically separated into constituent proteins including albumin and the alpha, beta and gamma globulins (**Figure 2.4**). The gamma globulins comprise chiefly the immune globulins (**immunoglobulins**), also known as **antibodies**.

The basic molecular structure of a single immunoglobulin molecule is well characterized (**Figure 2.5**). It is comprised of four glycoslyated protein chains held together by interchain disulphide

bonds in a Y-shaped conformation. Two of the chains are of higher molecular mass (**heavy chains**, approximately 50 kD) and two chains are smaller in size (**light chains**, approximately 25 kD). In terms of structure and amino acid sequence, the two heavy chains in any one immunoglobulin are identical to each other, as are the two light chains. This means that the two 'halves' of the molecule are essentially mirror images of each other. Although we commonly depict immunoglobulins diagrammatically as linear structures, these molecules have a complex tertiary structure. Each chain is formed of a series of **domains**, which have a roughly globular structure that is created by the presence of intrachain disulphide bonds. A further basic feature of an immunoglobulin is that the structure and amino acid sequence towards the C-terminal end of the molecule are relatively uniform (conserved) from one molecule to another, while the structure towards the N-terminal end has considerable variation between immunoglobulins. Within each of the four chains this gives rise to the presence of an N-terminal **variable region** and a series of **constant regions** towards the C terminus. Therefore, each light chain is composed of two domains, a variable region of the light chain (V_L) and a constant region of the light chain (C_L). Similarly, each heavy chain is comprised of a variable region of the heavy chain (V_H) and a series

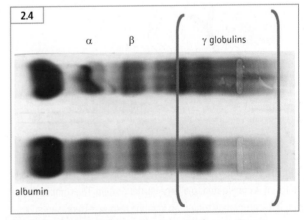

Fig. 2.4 Serum protein electrophoresis. The constituent proteins of serum include albumin and the alpha, beta and gamma globulins. The latter are equivalent to antibody molecules or immunoglobulins.

of constant region domains named C_{H1}, C_{H2} and C_{H3}. The variable regions contain further sub-areas in which there is the greatest degree of variation in amino acid sequence between different immunoglobulins. These sub-areas are known as the **hypervariable regions** or **complementarity determining regions** (CDRs). Most immunoglobulins have a distinct region between the C_{H1} and C_{H2} domains, involving an interchain disulphide bond known as the **hinge region**. This confers on the molecule the ability of the short arms of the Y-shaped structure to move through approximately 180°.

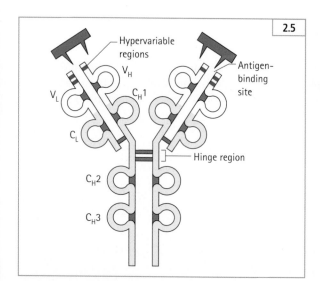

Fig. 2.5 Immunoglobulin structure. The basic Y-shaped structure of an immunoglobulin is composed of two identical heavy chains and two identical light chains linked together by interchain disulphide bonds. Intrachain disulphide bonds confer a globular domain structure to each chain. The N-terminal domains (V_L and V_H) show greatest variation in amino acid sequence between immunoglobulins and represent the site of antigen binding, particularly through the hypervariable regions. The C-terminal domains (V_H, C_{H1} to C_{H3}) have conserved amino acid sequence and undertake functions including complement fixation and receptor binding. The hinge region between C_{H1} and C_{H2} allows mobility of the short arms of the molecule. The enzyme papain cleaves the molecule on the N-terminal side of the hinge, creating a single Fc and two Fab fragments. The enzyme pepsin cleaves the molecule on the C-terminal side of the hinge, creating one Fc and one Fab'$_2$ fragment.

The globular domains of the immunoglobulin molecule have distinct functional attributes. The structure formed by the variable regions (V_L and V_H) is that portion of the molecule that binds to an antigenic epitope (the **antigen-binding site**). The C_{H2} domains are involved in activation of the complement pathway (see Chapter 3) and the C_{H3} domains in binding of the molecule to cellular immunoglobulin receptors called **Fc receptors** (see Chapter 3).

Early immunological research characterized the way in which the Y-shaped immunoglobulin molecule may be fragmented by incubation with particular proteolytic enzymes (**Figure 2.5**). The enzyme **papain** cleaves the molecule on the N-terminal side of the hinge region, creating three fragments: the joined C-terminal heavy chains (the 'body' of the Y shape), known as the **Fc region** (for 'fragment crystallizable'), and the joined N-terminal heavy chains and light chains (the 'arms' of the Y shape), each known as a **Fab** fragment ('fragment antigen-binding'). In contrast, the enzyme **pepsin** cleaves the molecule on the C-terminal side of the hinge region, creating two fragments: an Fc region and both Fab fragments still joined through the intact hinge region disulphide bond (the **Fab'$_2$**).

IMMUNOGLOBULIN CLASSES

At the simplest level, there are five distinct forms of immunoglobulin heavy chain, named by the Greek letters α (alpha), δ (delta), ε (epsilon), γ (gamma) and μ (mu). Similarly, there are two distinct forms of light chain named κ (kappa) and λ (lambda). As will be discussed in Chapter 9, this situation arises from the fact that there is a series of genes that encode these distinct protein molecules. Given that one Y-shaped immunoglobulin is composed of two identical heavy and two identical light chains, a single immunoglobulin must therefore consist of a pair of one of the five types of heavy chains, coupled to a pair of either κ or λ light chains. Therefore, there are ten possible ways in which these chains may combine to form an antibody molecule. Five **immunoglobulin (Ig) classes** are defined by usage of these heavy chain molecules: **IgA** (α chain), **IgD** (δ chain), **IgE** (ε chain), **IgG** (γ chain) and **IgM** (μ chain). For IgG and IgA, further diversity amongst the genes encoding the heavy chains means that there are **subclasses** of immunoglobulin that have subtle differences between the amino acid sequence and the structure of the constant regions.

The best characterized immunoglobulins and immunoglobulin genes are those of humans and experimental rodents. However, readers should be aware that while extrapolations may be made to domestic animal species, distinct species differences exist. Domestic animal species share the same basic five immunoglobulin classes, but there is variation in the range of IgG and IgA subclasses and some unique species-specific modifications in immunoglobulin structure exist (*Table 2.1*). For example, four IgG subclasses (IgG1–IgG4) are recognized in humans and dogs, while there are seven in the horse (IgG1–IgG7).

TABLE 2.1. IgG, IgA AND IgM IN MAN AND ANIMALS

Species	IgG subclasses	Serum IgG concentration (mg/ml)	IgA subclasses[1]	Serum IgA concentration (mg/ml)	Serum IgM concentration[2] (mg/ml)
Man	G1, G2, G3, G4	7.5–22.0	A1, A2	0.5–3.4	0.2–2.8
Dog	G1, G2, G3, G4	10.0–20.0	Four allelic variants in hinge region	0.2–1.6	1.0–2.0
Cat	G1, G2, G3	5.0–20.0	Not recognized	0.3–2.0	0.2–1.5
Horse	G1, G2, G3, G4, G5, G6, G7	11.5–21.0	Not recognized	1.0–4.0	1.0–3.0
Cow	G1, G2, G3	17–27	Not recognized	0.1–0.5	2.5–4.0
Sheep	G1, G2, G3	18–24	Three allelic variants in hinge region	0.1–1.0	0.8–1.8
Pig	G1, G2a, G2b, G3, G4	9.0–24.0	Two allelic variants in hinge region	0.5–1.2	1.9–3.9
Mouse	G1, G2a, G2b, G3	2.0–5.0	Two allelic variants in hinge region	1.0–3.2	0.8–6.5

[1] Two *IGHA* genes are recognized in man, but only one in other species.

[2] Subclasses of IgM are not recognized.

Humans have two IgA subclasses encoded by distinct IgA heavy chain (*IGHA*) genes and rabbits have 13 such genes, most of which produce functional protein. In contrast, other domestic animals have a single *IGHA* gene, but genetic variation in the hinge region of the IgA heavy chain gene has been identified in pigs, sheep and dogs, which may translate into functionally distinct IgA proteins. In addition to standard four-chain IgG, camelid species produce homodimeric IgG made up of two heavy chains and no light chain. Chickens have a major immunoglobulin known as IgY, a four-chain molecule not dissimilar to mammalian IgG in structure. The heavy chain of IgY (υ or upsilon chain) has one variable and four constant domains, but lacks a hinge region. Some avian species also have a truncated version of IgY with heavy chains of only two constant domains. As this molecule does not have an Fc region, it is known as IgY(ΔFc) and is of unknown function.

IgG

The IgG molecule comprises a single Y-shaped unit with a molecular structure as described above. IgG consists of paired γ heavy chains with either paired κ or λ light chains. The molecule has two N-terminal antigen-binding sites and is therefore said to have an antigen-binding **valence** of two. IgG is the dominant form of immunoglobulin found in the serum, and where IgG subclasses are defined, the relative serum concentrations of these may vary. The molecular mass of IgG (approximately 150 kD) means that it is readily able to leave the circulation and enter the extracellular tissue space when there is increased permeability of the vascular endothelium (for example in an inflammatory response), but some IgG is normally found in this environment and may be actively transported there from the blood. The functional properties of IgG include complement fixation, immunoglobulin Fc receptor binding and opsonization (see Chapter 3). IgG molecules effectively bind and neutralize toxins and are the dominant immunoglobulin in the **secondary immune response** (see Chapter 9).

IgM

The IgM molecule is the largest of the immunoglobulins and consists of a pentamer of five basic Y-shaped immunoglobulin units linked together by a **joining (J) chain** and additional disulphide bonds between the C-terminal domains (**Figure 2.6**). Each of the component units comprises paired μ heavy chains and each of these carries an additional C-terminal C_{H4} **domain**. The IgM molecule **lacks a distinct hinge region**, but there is mobility at the level of C_{H2} to C_{H3}. The large molecular mass of IgM means that this immunoglobulin is mainly found in the circulation, as it would not readily diffuse between vascular endothelia to enter the tissue space. For this reason,

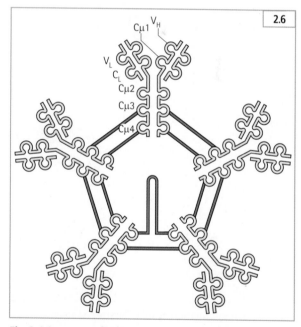

Fig. 2.6 Structure of IgM. IgM is a pentamer of five basic immunoglobulin units linked together by a joining chain and additional disulphide bonds between the C_{H3} and additional C_{H4} domains present in the μ heavy chain.

IgM plays an important role in the immune response to infections of the blood (e.g. bacteraemia). IgM is able to fix complement (see Chapter 3) and because of its antigen-binding valence of 10, it is able to attach to and draw together multiple particulate antigens in a process known as **agglutination (Figures 2.7a, b)**. IgM is of greatest importance in the **primary immune response** (see Chapter 9).

IgA

The IgA molecule may be found as a **monomer** of a single Y-shaped immunoglobulin (utilizing α heavy chains) or as a **dimer** of two such units linked together by a J chain (**Figure 2.8**). These variants have an antigen-binding valence of 2 or 4, respectively. The occurrence of monomeric versus dimeric IgA is dependent on the species and anatomical location. Relatively small quantities of IgA may be found within the circulation as a monomer in humans and as a dimer in most domestic animal species. The highest concentration of IgA is found in the secretions bathing the **mucosal surfaces** of the body (i.e. the gastrointestinal, respiratory and urogenital tracts, the eye and the mammary glands) or in secretions related to these surfaces (e.g. bile, tears, colostrum or milk). This distribution reflects the fact that the majority of IgA in the body is produced at mucosal surfaces and plays a key role in the immune defence of those surfaces, particularly in preventing colonization by pathogenic bacteria by inhibiting receptor-mediated attachment of such organisms to the mucosal surface (**Figures 2.9a, b**). The IgA molecule is also able to neutralize toxins, but is a relatively weak opsonin (see Chapter 3).

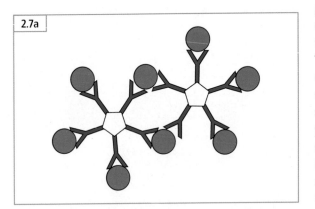

2.7a

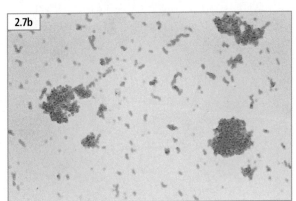

2.7b

Figs. 2.7a, b Agglutination by IgM. The size and antigen-binding valence (10) of IgM makes this molecule particularly effective at binding and drawing together particulate antigens in the process of agglutination. A clinical example of this phenomenon occurs in immune-mediated haemolytic anaemia (IMHA) in which IgM autoantibodies cause aggregation and destruction of erythrocytes within the circulating blood. (a) IgM molecules bind to different erythrocytes to form an agglutinate. (b) A drop of blood from a dog with IMHA shows the presence of large agglutinates of red blood cells.

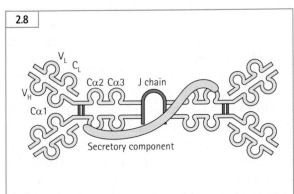

2.8

Fig. 2.8 Structure of IgA. Dimeric IgA comprises two Y-shaped immunoglobulin units with α heavy chains linked by a J chain. Where secreted onto mucosal surfaces the molecule also carries a secretory component that wraps around the C-terminal ends of the immunoglobulin units to protect the IgA from proteolytic degradation.

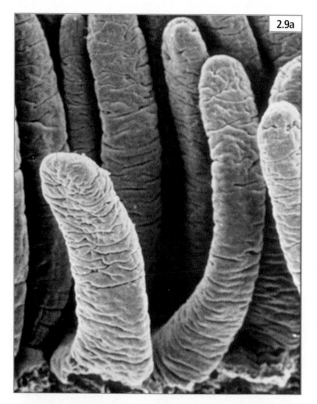

This secreted form of IgA is dimeric in all species and in those species with distinct IgA subclasses there may be regional preferences for the secretion of those subclasses to mucosal surfaces. As mucosal surfaces are rich in proteolytic enzymes, secreted dimeric IgA has one further modification that protects it from enzymatic degradation once secreted. This modification is the presence of a **secretory component**, which wraps around the C-terminal ends of the subunits and is attached to the C_{H2} domains by disulphide bonds. The pathway of mucosal IgA secretion has been defined (**Figure 2.10**). As for all immunoglobulins, the dimeric IgA molecule is secreted by a **plasma cell** (see Chapters 5 and 9) within the lamina propria underlying the mucosal epithelium. This molecule is bound by the **polymeric immunoglobulin receptor (pIgR)** on the basolateral surfaces of the epithelial lining cell (in the intestine the epithelial cells at the base of the crypts express pIgR) and the complex of pIgR and IgA dimer is internalized into the cytoplasm of the epithelial cell. The complex

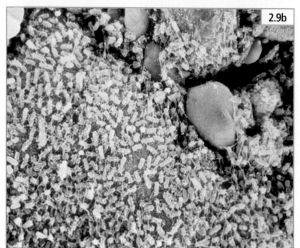

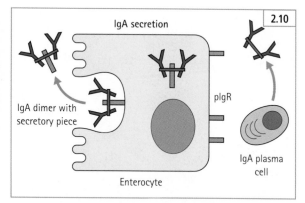

Figs. 2.9a, b Function of IgA. (a) This scanning electron microscope image shows the normal finger-like villi of the small intestine. (b) A higher magnification showing intestine from a different animal with diarrhoea caused by *Escherichia coli* infection. There is a carpet of rod-shaped bacteria over the mucosal surface. Attachment of such pathogens to mucosae would normally be inhibited by secreted IgA that blocks receptor-mediated attachment. (Images courtesy G. Hall)

Fig. 2.10 Secretion of IgA. Most IgA is produced at mucosal surfaces and secreted across the lining epithelium as a dimeric molecule. During this transition the secreted IgA molecule acquires a protective secretory component that is formed from a portion of the polymeric immunoglobulin receptor that mediates its transition across the epithelial barrier.

translocates through the cytoplasm and is re-expressed on the mucosal surface of the cell, where the IgA is released from the surface, carrying a portion of the pIgR that becomes the secretory component.

IgD

The IgD molecule is a single Y-shaped immunoglobulin unit comprising two δ heavy chains and with an antigen-binding valence of 2. IgD has a very limited distribution in the body and is restricted to being expressed on the surface of naïve B lymphocytes (see Chapter 9). There are numerous species differences in the structure of this immunoglobulin. Murine IgD has two constant region domains and an extended hinge region, making it susceptible to proteolysis. IgD of domestic animals, man and primates has three constant region domains. In most of these species (except the pig) the hinge region is also long relative to that of other immunoglobulin classes.

IgE

The IgE molecule is a single Y-shaped immunoglobulin unit composed of two ε heavy chains and has a valence of 2. Similar to IgM, the IgE molecule has an additional C_{H4} **domain** and an **indistinct hinge** region. IgE is found at low concentration free in the circulation of humans, but at proportionally higher concentration in the blood of most domestic animal species. This is thought to relate to the relatively greater level of endogenous parasitism of domestic animals, as one of the major beneficial roles of IgE is as a participant in the immune response to endoparasites (see Chapter 13). IgE may also be found attached to specific Fcε receptors on the surface of tissue mast cells (**Figure 2.11**) and circulating basophils, and it is intrinsic to the immunological phenomenon known as **type I hypersensitivity** (see Chapter 12). Related to this mechanism is the key role of IgE in mediating a range of **allergic diseases** (e.g. asthma, atopic dermatitis [AD], flea allergy dermatitis) of major significance in human and animal populations (see Chapter 17) (**Figure 2.12**).

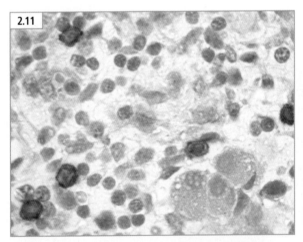

Fig. 2.11 IgE associates with mast cells. Section of intestinal mucosa from a foal labelled immunohistochemically to show the presence of IgE (red colour). IgE molecules are expressed only by mast cells and not by other leucocytes or epithelial cells.

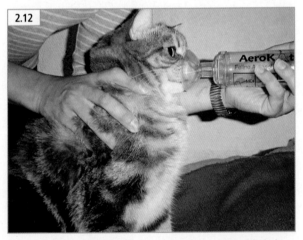

Fig. 2.12 IgE in allergic disease. This cat is receiving inhaled medication through a purpose-designed delivery system for the treatment of asthma. Asthma is an immune-mediated disease involving the excessive production of IgE antibodies specific for environmental antigens.

ANTIGEN–ANTIBODY INTERACTION

The interaction between antigens and antibodies specifically involves the recognition of an antigenic epitope by the N-terminal variable (Fab) regions of the antibody molecule. In three dimensions, the V_L and V_H domains form a **cleft or groove**, lined by the hypervariable regions (or CDRs) of amino acid sequence, into which the epitope slots or, alternatively, these domains flatten out to form a planar area of interaction that permits a larger area of contact with the antigen. This interaction is exquisitely precise and there are specific points of interaction (**contact residues**) between the epitope and antigen-binding site (**Figures 2.13a, b**). Some antigenic epitopes will have perfect match for the antigen-binding site of immunoglobulin and interact like a 'lock and key' to produce a **high-affinity** binding. Antibody affinity refers to the strength of binding of one Fab of an antibody to one antigenic epitope (**Figure 2.14**).

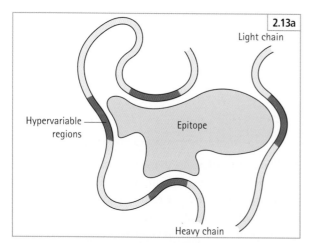

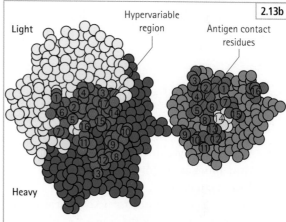

Figs. 2.13a, b **Antigen–antibody binding.** (a) The antigenic epitope sits within a cleft or groove formed by the variable domains of the heavy and light chains and lined by hypervariable regions (or complementarity determining regions) that form the contact residues between the two molecules. (b) Depicted more three dimensionally, the red hypervariable regions of the yellow light and blue heavy chain variable regions provide contact residues with the corresponding red epitope of the green antigen. The green antigen in this model would move through 90° to sit on top of the Fab region shown.

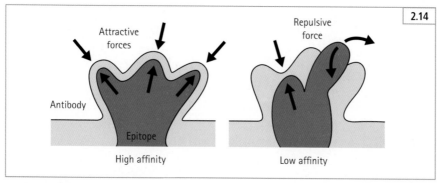

Fig. 2.14 **Antigen antibody binding affinity.** Affinity is the sum of attractive and repulsive forces between the antigenic epitope and the Fab antigen-binding site of the antibody. High- and low-affinity interactions are demonstrated.

In this situation the antigen is held tightly in place by interactions involving the formation of van der Waal's forces, hydrogen bonds, electrostatic forces and hydrophobic forces. Other antigenic epitopes will interact with antigen-binding sites with **low affinity** or display no interaction at all. A second term used to describe the strength of interaction between antigen and antibody is avidity. **Avidity** refers to the strength of overall binding of the two molecules, such that a low-avidity interaction might involve the binding of one Fab within an immunoglobulin to one epitope on an antigen, whereas an interaction of higher avidity would involve multiple Fab–epitope binding (**Figure 2.15**).

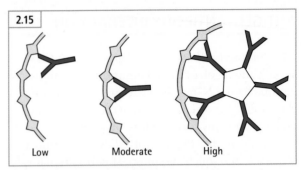

Fig. 2.15 Antigen–antibody binding avidity. The interaction between an antigen comprised of repeating units of an epitope and specific antibodies is shown. The greater the number of interactions the higher is the avidity of binding.

KEY POINTS

- Antigens initiate the immune response.
- Most antigens are foreign to the body (heteroantigens).
- The most potent antigens are chemically complex and biologically active.
- Antigens may have multiple epitopes, some of which are immunodominant.
- Adjuvants may be mixed with antigen to non-specifically enhance the immune response.
- Antibodies are Y-shaped units composed of two identical heavy and two identical light chains.

- The chains of an antibody molecule have globular domain structure with distinct function ascribed to each domain.
- Antibodies bind antigenic epitopes, activate complement and bind cellular receptors.
- The five classes of antibody (IgG, IgM, IgA, IgD and IgE) have a distinct structure, anatomical distribution and function.

CHAPTER 3

The Complement System

OBJECTIVES

At the end of this chapter you should be able to:
- Give a definition of complement.
- Briefly describe the classical, lectin, alternative and terminal pathways and the trigger factors that initiate each of these pathways.
- Understand why it is necessary to regulate the complement pathways and give examples of mechanisms involved in such control.

- Describe how the complement pathways lead to cytolysis.
- Discuss the role of complement in inflammation.
- Define chemotaxis as it relates to complement.
- Define opsonization and immune adherence.
- Describe how complement function may be measured *in vitro*.

INTRODUCTION

Complement is a collective noun that describes a series of approximately 30 plasma proteins. When activated they interact sequentially, forming a self-assembling enzymatic cascade and generating biologically active molecules mediating a range of end processes that are significant in the immune and inflammatory response. The basic principle of this cascade system is depicted in **Figure 3.1** and in general terms this is similar to the coagulation pathways involved in secondary haemostasis. Intrinsic in such pathways is the presence of a regulatory system that can switch off the cascade when no longer required in order to avoid inappropriate damage to normal tissue.

There are four complement pathways (**Figure 3.2**), known as the **classical**, **lectin**, **alternative** and **terminal** pathways. The first three share a common end-point, which in turn is the start of the shared terminal pathway. Complement components generated by the activation of these pathways mediate

the four key biological effects of the system, which will be described below. Complement is recognized in all animal species and the constituent components are relatively conserved. These components are mostly described using the abbreviation 'C' (for complement), with a number to indicate the specific component (e.g. C4) and a lower case letter to indicate a subfraction of that component (e.g. C4a and C4b). The numbering of the components does not always follow a logical sequence, as each component was numbered in the order in which it was discovered rather than by the position it holds in the hierarchy of the system. Some components and regulatory proteins do not conform to the 'C' nomenclature. To add further confusion, there is traditionally some minor difference in nomenclature used in North America and Europe (for example, the classical pathway C3 convertase is C4bC2b in Europe and C4bC2a in North America) and readers of other texts should be aware of this, as the European system is presented here.

THE CLASSICAL AND LECTIN PATHWAYS

The classical pathway, so called as it was the first discovered, is triggered by the binding of the first component of complement (C1) to the surface of an antigen (e.g. a pathogen). In the case of some bacteria, this binding might be directly to a cell wall structural component (e.g. lipoteichoic acid of the wall of gram-positive bacteria), or C1 may bind C-reactive protein, which is in turn attached to a bacterial polysaccharide. Most often, C1 attaches to an immune complex of **antigen and antibody** (IgG or IgM) by binding to a specific area of the immunoglobulin component of the complex (e.g. to the C_{H2} domain of IgG). It is also possible for C1 to bind to an aggregate of antibody molecules in the absence of antigen (**Figure 3.3**). The antigen in these situations is generally relatively large (e.g. a cell or microbe) and provides a surface area onto which the complement molecules deposit as they are activated. **C1** is comprised of three subunits, **C1q**, **C1r** and **C1s**. C1q attaches to the antigen or immunoglobulin molecule, causing a conformational change in the associated C1r–C1s complex. This in turn stimulates the enzymatic activity of C1r, which subsequently activates the C1s enzyme.

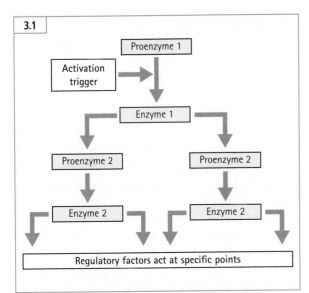

Fig. 3.1 An enzymatic cascade system. The complement pathways are enzymatic cascade systems similar to the coagulation pathways of haemostasis. Such cascades require an initiating trigger, which causes the conversion of the first proenzyme in the series to active enzyme. Active enzyme 1 subsequently acts on two molecules of proenzyme 2, converting these to active enzyme 2 and so on. At each stage of the reaction there is an amplification effect as more active enzyme molecules are generated. Intrinsic to such systems must be a means of controlling the cascade so that it might be stopped when no longer required in order to avoid any possible pathological consequences of inappropriate activation.

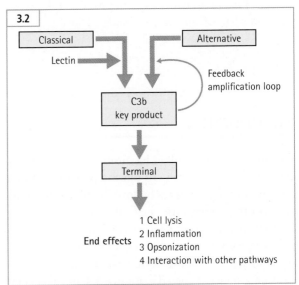

Fig. 3.2 The complement pathways. The four complement pathways interact as depicted in this diagram. The end-point of the classical and alternative pathways is the generation of the key molecule, complement factor C3b. The lectin pathway shares elements of the classical system. A variant unique to the alternative pathway is the feedback amplification loop. The common terminal pathway begins with factor C3b. Complement factors generated during activation of these pathways mediate the four key biological end effects shown.

C1s then acts on the next component in the sequence, **C4**, and splits this into two subunits, C4a and C4b. The C4b fraction attaches to the surface of the antigen and binds **C2**, which is also cleaved by C1s to C2a and C2b. The C2b fragment remains associated with the C4b fraction and this complex has

now become the classical pathway '**C3 convertase**'. As this name suggests, the next stage of the sequence is that the C4bC2b (C3 convertase) acts on **C3** to split this molecule into C3a and C3b. C3a has a major biological role (see below), but it does not affix to the surface of the antigen. In contrast, C3b deposits adjacent to the C4bC2b complex to form a new complex of C4bC2bC3b, which becomes a '**C5 convertase**'. The generation of this C5 convertase is the final stage in the classical pathway.

As for all complement pathways, a system of **regulatory control** is built into the classical pathway to inactivate the system when no longer required. The first means of control is relatively simple and relates to the fact that these complement components have a short half-life when generated. Moreover, complement molecules are highly susceptible to heat and, *in vitro*, the molecules may be inactivated by heating a sample of serum (containing the molecules) to 56°C for a short period of time (a process known as 'heat-inactivation' of complement). Additional means of controlling the classical pathway relate to the presence of a series of specific inhibitory factors that act at different points of the pathway. The **C1 inhibitor** cleaves C1r from C1s, thereby disrupting the activity of this complex. The **C4-binding protein** displaces C2b from C4b and works in combination with **Factor I**, which subsequently cleaves C4b into two inactive subfractions, C4c and C4d. Factor I is also able to cleave C3b into the inactive subfractions C3c and C3d.

As these complement molecules have high biological potency, there must be a means of protecting normal cells that lie in the immediate vicinity of the activated classical pathway and may be potentially susceptible to complement fragments that diffuse away from the site of activation. In fact, normal cells have an in-built protective mechanism, as their cell membrane includes a series of constitutively expressed proteins that are able to disrupt the C3 convertase should it form on their surface. These proteins include the decay accelerating factor (**DAF**), complement receptor 1 (**CR1**) and membrane co-factor protein (**MCP**).

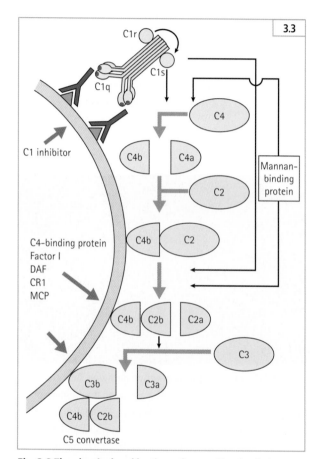

Fig. 3.3 The classical and lectin pathways. The classical pathway of complement is usually triggered by the binding of antibody to antigen and proceeds through the stages shown (from top to bottom) to generate the membrane-associated C5 convertase. This sequential deposition of complement components occurs on the surface of the antigen. The points of control of the system are indicated to the left of the diagram with solid red arrows. The related lectin pathway is initiated by the action of serum mannan-binding protein, which generates C3 convertase through activation of MASP-2.

The **lectin pathway** of complement was the most recently discovered and shares elements of the classical pathway (**Figure 3.3**). The serum mannan-binding lectin (**MBL**) is a C1q-like molecule associated with the enzymes MBL-associated serine protease (MASP)-1 and MASP-2. MBL initially associates with a bacterial surface carbohydrate (i.e. mannose and some other sugars) and is then able to activate the MASPs. Activated MASP-2 replicates the effects of C1s by activating C4 and C2 to form the C3 convertase complex.

THE ALTERNATIVE PATHWAY

The **alternative pathway** of the complement system is older in evolutionary terms than the classical pathway and as it does not require the presence of antibody to be activated, it may be considered part of the **innate immune system** (see Chapters 1 and 13). The alternative pathway has two distinct phases. The first of these continually cycles at a low level in clinically normal animals and is often referred to as the **'tick over' phase**. The key feature of the tick over phase is that it occurs within the extracellular fluid space and is not associated with the surface of cells. The second phase reflects full activation of the system and requires the presence of an appropriate trigger factor, which in the case of the alternative pathway is the presence of a **'trigger surface'** that permits deposition of molecules of the enzymatic cascade. Such trigger surfaces are provided by microbes (particularly bacteria or yeast), by abnormal tissue cells (e.g. virally infected or neoplastic cells), by aggregates of immunoglobulin or by foreign material (e.g. asbestos) (**Figure 3.4**). The molecules on trigger surfaces responsible for activation of the alternative pathway and the molecules that activate the lectin and classical pathways in the absence of antibody are all examples of classes of molecules known as pathogen-associated molecular patterns (PAMPs) or damage-associated molecular patterns (DAMPs), which will be discussed in Chapter 7.

The tick over phase (**Figure 3.5**) is initiated by **C3** in the extracellular fluid, which undergoes spontaneous hydrolysis to form **C3i**. In the presence of Mg^{+2}, some C3i is bound by **Factor B** to form a complex of **C3iB**. Bound Factor B is acted upon by **Factor D**, which fragments the molecule to Bb and Ba. Bb remains associated with C3i to form a **C3 convertase**, which in turn splits further C3 molecules in the fluid phase to C3a and C3b. In the tick over pathway, the majority of the C3b that is generated undergoes spontaneous hydrolysis and inactivation. Should any C3b deposit onto the surface of adjacent normal cells, it will be inactivated by the combination of MCP, DAF, CR1, Factor H and Factor I.

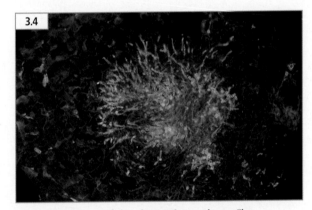

Fig. 3.4 Activation of the alternative pathway. The alternative pathway becomes fully activated in the presence of an appropriate trigger surface that allows sequential deposition of the constituent complement molecules. Microbial surfaces provide an ideal trigger for this pathway. This is a colony of *Aspergillus* fungi growing within the pancreas of a German shepherd dog with disseminated *Aspergillus* infection. The fungi appear green as they have been specifically labelled with an antiserum conjugated to fluorescein. The antiserum detects complement C3 deposition on the surface of the hyphae. (From Day MJ, Penhale WJ (1991) An immunohistochemical study of canine disseminated aspergillosis. *Australian Veterinary Journal* **68**, 383–386, with permission)

Exactly the same initiating sequence occurs in the fully activated phase of the alternative pathway, but in this instance an adjacent trigger surface permits the deposition of these molecules onto that surface (**Figure 3.6**). Once the alternative pathway C3 convertase (C3bBb) has been deposited, it then becomes associated with the molecule **properdin** (P),

which stabilizes the complex as **PC3bBb**. This stable C3 convertase initiates the **feedback amplification loop**, which generates further C3b that deposits on the trigger surface. The final step in the activation phase of the alternative pathway is the addition of further C3b to the C3 convertase (**PC3bBbC3b**) to form the alternative pathway **C5 convertase**.

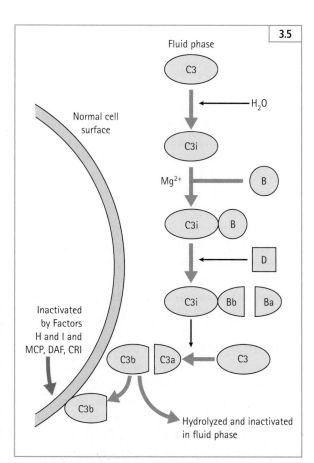

Fig. 3.5 Alternative pathway 'tick over' phase. This complement pathway continually cycles at a low level in the extracellular tissue fluid of clinically normal individuals. Any C3b that is generated is either degraded and inactivated in the fluid phase or inactivated by the range of membrane protective molecules found in normal tissue cells.

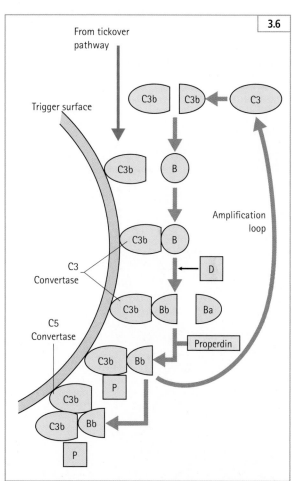

Fig. 3.6 Alternative pathway activation phase. The presence of an appropriate trigger surface permits deposition of the C3b generated from the tick over phase. This then complexes with Factor B, and is acted on by Factor D, to become a C3 convertase, which in turn becomes stabilized by properdin to activate the feedback amplification loop. The end-point of the pathway is the formation of the PC3bBbC3b complex, which is a C5 convertase.

THE TERMINAL PATHWAY

In contrast to the pathways described above, the **terminal pathway** is relatively straightforward and benefits from the fact that the constituent molecules are named in correct numerical sequence (**Figure 3.7**). Accordingly, the pathway is initiated by C5 convertase splitting **C5** to the subfractions C5a and C5b. C5a has potent biological activity similar to that of C3a, but has its effect distant to the surface of the cell that is the target of complement activation. Activated C5b recruits C6 and C7 to form a complex of **C5bC6C7,** which associates with the membrane of the target cell. This complex in turn binds **C8**, which penetrates the cell membrane and recruits a number of **C9** molecules that insert into the membrane to form a 'doughnut-like' transmembrane pore known as the **membrane attack complex** (MAC). The formation of the MAC represents the end-point of the terminal pathway.

BIOLOGICAL CONSEQUENCES OF COMPLEMENT ACTIVATION

Cytolysis

Once the terminal complement pathway is activated, in reality not one but thousands of MACs are generated within the membrane of the cell that is the target of complement activation (**Figures 3.8a, b**). The surface of this target cell becomes riddled with holes and an **osmotic imbalance** between the cell cytoplasm and extracellular fluid is established such that there is a net influx of water into the cell. The cell swells and subsequently bursts in a phenomenon known as **'osmotic lysis'**. If that target cell is a bacterium or an abnormal tissue cell, then clearly this mechanism of cellular lysis (cytolysis) is beneficial to the host and is a valuable part of the protective immune response. Antibody-mediated (classical pathway) complement cytolysis is the basis for the **type II hypersensitivity** reaction that will be discussed in Chapter 12.

Generation of bioactive substances

The second major consequence of complement activation is the generation of those fragments of complement that do not associate with the membrane of target cells. The two most important of these are **C3a** and **C5a**. C5a is more potent than C3a, but much larger quantities of C3a are generated. These molecules are sometimes known as **anaphylatoxins** or **chemoattractants** after the fundamental effects that they mediate.

C3a and C5a have key roles in the tissue inflammatory response via a number of mechanisms (**Figure 3.9**). These molecules mediate **vasodilation** of small vessels within the tissue in which they are generated. Dilated vessels with leaky endothelial cell junctions permit the egress of fluid, protein and cells

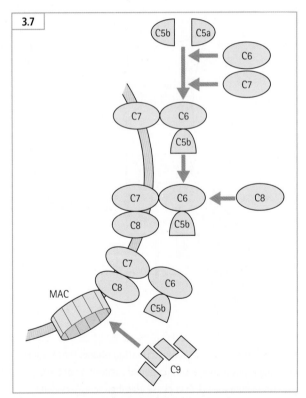

Fig. 3.7 The terminal pathway. The terminal pathway is initiated when C5 convertase splits C5 into C5a and C5b. C5b recruits C6 and C7 and this complex associates with the membrane of the cell that is the target of the complement system. Subsequent recruitment of C8 and several molecules of C9 leads to the formation of a transmembrane pore known as the membrane attack complex (MAC).

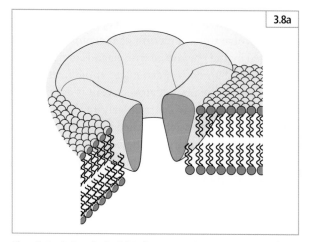

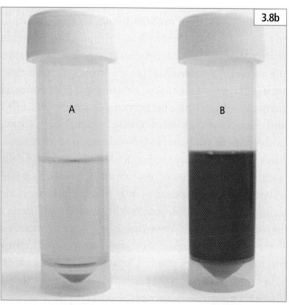

Figs. 3.8a, b Cytolysis. (a) A diagrammatic representation of the lipid bilayer of the membrane of a cell that has been targeted by the complement system. Numerous MACs insert through the membrane, establishing an osmotic imbalance with a net influx of water into the cell cytoplasm. The target cell will swell and burst. (b) This phenomenon is readily seen when erythrocytes become the target of complement-mediated cytolysis, as rupture of RBCs leads to release of free haemoglobin. These two test tubes contain erythrocytes that were suspended in saline. In tube A the normal red cells have settled to the base of the tube, leaving clear saline above. In tube B the action of antibody and complement (mixed with the saline) on the cells has led to release of free haemoglobin that colours the saline red; there is also an absence of a significant pellet of erythrocytes at the base of the tube.

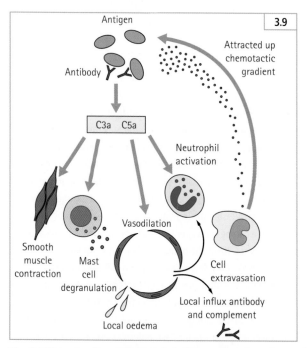

Fig. 3.9 The role of complement in inflammation. Complement fragments C3a and C5a have profound effects on the local tissue inflammatory response. These molecules mediate vasodilation with associated tissue oedema and egress of leucocytes and plasma proteins into tissue. These events may be amplified through mast cell degranulation, which may also be directly mediated by C3a and C5a. These complement fragments may further activate the recruited leucocytes and form chemotactic gradients that direct these cells to the location of infectious agents or damaged cells within the tissue.

from the circulation into the tissue. If the generation of C3a and C5a has resulted from infection or damage within that tissue, this process has a clear benefit to the animal. Vascular fluid loss leads to **tissue oedema**, which may be important in diluting locally produced toxins. Leakage of blood proteins (immunoglobulins and complement molecules) may be beneficial if these molecules participate in a local immune response. Migration of leucocytes, particularly phagocytic cells such as neutrophils and macrophages, is likely to be of benefit in the removal of infectious agents or tissue debris. C3a and C5a may additionally have direct activating effects on neutrophils in order to enhance their phagocytic function and release of further inflammatory mediators. The **chemotactic** role of C3a and C5a may further enhance the value of local tissue recruitment of leucocytes. After migrating from the circulation into tissue, phagocytic cells may be directed towards the location of pathogens or damaged cells by moving up a **'chemotactic gradient'**. This gradient is formed by complement molecules that are at highest concentration at the point at which they were generated and at progressively lower concentration the further away from that source they are within that tissue.

In some circumstances the actions of C3a and C5a may cross the border between a useful role in local inflammation and induction of a pathological inflammatory response. Both molecules may act on tissue **mast cells** to cause them to **degranulate** and further expand the tissue inflammatory response (see Chapter 12). In the respiratory tract this may result in contraction of bronchiolar smooth muscle (**bronchoconstriction**).

Removal of particulate antigen or immune complexes

The third biological consequence of complement activation is enhancing the removal and destruction of particulate antigen or complexes of antigen and antibody by phagocytic cells such as neutrophils and macrophages (**Figure 3.10**). A phagocyte might encounter such antigen within the tissue space by random encounter as it migrates through the tissue space. In this instance the phagocytic cell might

internalize and destroy the particle and this process might involve the interaction of receptor molecules expressed by the phagocyte with ligands found on the target (see Chapter 7). Particulate antigen would be more likely to be phagocytosed were it aggregated together by antibody (particularly IgM antibody), making it a 'larger target' for the phagocytic cell. The interaction between target antigen and phagocyte can also be enhanced by the complement system by the processes of opsonization and immune adherence.

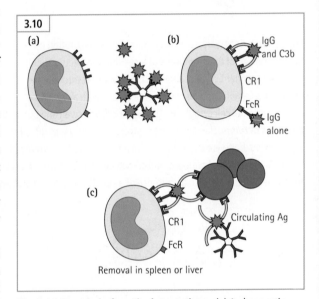

Fig. 3.10 Removal of particulate antigen. (a) A phagocytic cell such as a neutrophil or macrophage may randomly encounter particulate antigen as it migrates through tissue spaces and engulfs that antigen for destruction. This process may be a receptor-mediated event. Antigen that is aggregated by immunoglobulin provides a larger target and is more likely to be phagocytosed. (b) The interaction between antigen and phagocyte can be greatly enhanced if the antigen is pre-coated with IgG and C3b, as the phagocyte bears membrane receptors for these molecules. This process is known as opsonization. (c) Circulating erythrocytes bear CR1 receptors that permit binding of particulate antigen within the bloodstream that is coated by C3b. This antigen may be transferred to macrophages in the liver or spleen via the CR1 molecules expressed by these cells and subsequently destroyed by the phagocyte. This process of immune adherence is important in the removal of such material from the circulation.

The phenomenon of **opsonization** arises because phagocytic cells express on their membrane receptors for IgG (the **Fcγ receptor**) and a series of receptors for the complement molecule C3b and its proteolytic derivatives (**complement receptors [CR]1–CR4**). CR1, which binds C3b, is the best characterized of these receptors. Simply put, if a particulate antigen is already coated with IgG, it is more likely to be phagocytosed due to the enhanced contact with that cell mediated through the IgG–FcR interaction. Even better is if the antigen is also coated with C3b so that there is dual interaction involving IgG–FcR and C3b–CR1 binding (**Figures 3.11a, b**). 'Opsonization' comes from the Greek 'to make tasty for the table' and the analogy is often used that coating a target antigen with IgG and C3b is akin to covering dinner with gravy!

A related event is that of **immune adherence**, a process that is of great importance in clearing particulate antigen from the bloodstream. Immune adherence arises from the fact that erythrocytes express CR1 (but not FcR), and this permits circulating antigen that is coated with C3b (with or without antibody) to attach to the surface membrane of red cells. As these antigen-laden red cells pass through the hepatic sinusoids and spleen, they encounter phagocytic cells resident in those tissues that bind the antigen via their own CRs and remove the antigen from the red cells for internalization and destruction.

Interaction with other inflammatory pathways

As discussed above, the complement pathways have key roles in the inflammatory and immune responses. During inflammation a series of biochemical pathways is activated in parallel within the same tissue (see Chapter 1), so it is not surprising that there may be molecular interactions between the mediators within the different pathways. Complement molecules may have a range of effects on the kinin, coagulation and fibrinolytic pathways, the fine details of which are beyond the scope of this discussion.

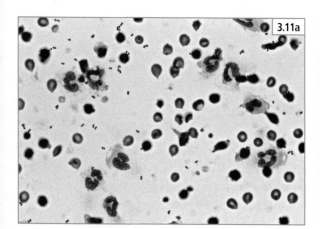 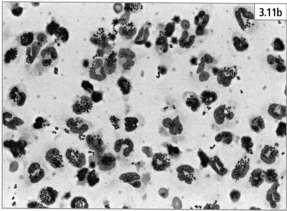

Figs. 3.11a, b Opsonization. This experiment demonstrates the effect of opsonization. Neutrophils were isolated from the blood of a dog and placed into two tubes. A suspension of staphylococcal bacteria was placed into tube A (left) and a suspension of bacteria that had been previously incubated with dog serum was placed into tube B (right). Most of the neutrophils in tube B have numerous bacteria within their cytoplasm, but only low numbers of organisms are present in the cytoplasm of some neutrophils in tube A. The bacteria in tube B had been opsonized by coating with antibody and complement present in the dog's serum, and this has led to much more efficient phagocytosis of these targets.

TESTS OF COMPLEMENT FUNCTION

The complement pathways have been defined in most domestic animal species and, although rarely performed, it is possible to test for complement function. Complement molecules are very heat-labile (and may be destroyed by heating a serum sample to 56°C for 30 minutes), so such assays require freshly collected serum frozen rapidly to –70°C to preserve the components. The **total haemolytic complement assay** (CH$_{50}$) tests for the overall function of the classical and terminal pathways. Essentially, this test (**Figure 3.12**) involves incubating patient serum with an indicator system of antibody-coated RBCs. Complement present within the serum will cause lysis of these erythrocytes. A titration of the serum sample

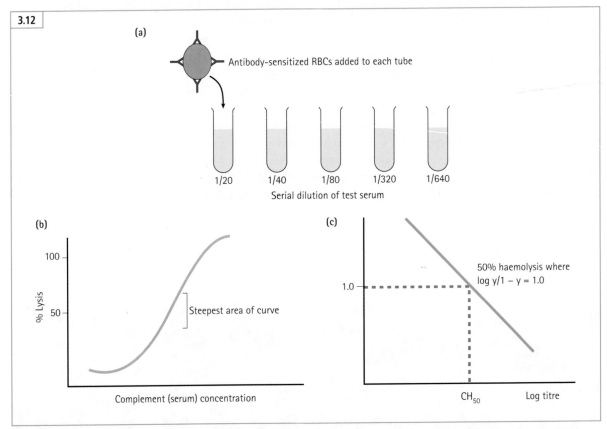

Fig. 3.12 Total haemolytic complement assay. (a) In this assay, serial dilutions of test serum are prepared and incubated with a standard volume of antibody-coated RBCs. The amount of lysis in each tube is determined by the concentration of complement present and may be measured by spectrophotometrically detecting the release of haemoglobin. The amount of haemolysis in each tube can be related to a 0% control (buffer only) or a 100% haemolysis control (water). Plotting serum concentration versus % lysis generates a sigmoidal curve, and 50% lysis generally falls within the steepest area of this curve. (b) The % lysis for each serum dilution is calculated using the formula:

$$\% = \frac{\text{absorbance test} - \text{absorbance (0\% control)}}{\text{absorbance (100\% control)} - \text{absorbance (0\% control)}} \times 100$$

and the value y/1 – y is calculated for serum dilutions in which y is between 10 and 90%. (c) This value is then plotted against the CH$_{50}$ titre on a log–log scale and the titre of the sample that intersects the curve at the value y/1 – y = 1.0 is the CH$_{50}$ for that serum sample.

is performed and the CH_{50} value for the sample is defined as the reciprocal of the serum dilution that gives 50% haemolysis. An alternative to the tube-based CH_{50} assay is to perform the test by adding serum to wells cut in an agarose gel containing the sensitized erythrocytes. After appropriate incubations, haemolysis in such plates is indicated by the formation of a clear zone around the well. The diameter of this cleared ring is proportional to the log of the concentration of complement in the serum sample. Finally, it is also possible to measure the concentration of individual complement components using single radial immunodiffusion (SRID) (see Chapter 4) or a haemolytic assay in which an excess of all complement components, except the one being tested, is provided such that the missing component derives from the test sample.

KEY POINTS

- Complement is a self-assembling enzymatic cascade.
- The end effects of the cascade are important components of the immune and inflammatory responses.
- The cascade requires regulation to prevent damage to normal tissue.
- The classical, lectin and alternative pathways of complement feed into a common terminal pathway.
- The terminal pathway leads to cytolysis by formation of multiple MACs in the target cell.

- C3a and C5a act as anaphylatoxins and chemoattractants.
- Coating of particulate antigen by IgG and C3b leads to enhanced phagocytosis by interacting with FcR and CR1 on the surface of phagocytic cells. This process is called opsonization.
- Immune adherence is important in the removal of particulate antigen from the bloodstream.

CHAPTER 4

Serological Testing

OBJECTIVES

At the end of this chapter you should be able to:
- Define 'serology'.
- Understand the role of serological testing in clinical veterinary medicine.
- Describe the production of an antiserum.
- Define 'sensitivity', 'specificity', 'positive predictive value' and 'negative predictive value'.
- Understand the concept of false-positive and false-negative test results.

- Briefly describe the principle of agglutination, precipitation, the complement fixation test, the haemagglutination inhibition test, the virus neutralization test, the immunofluorescent antibody test, the enzyme-linked immunosorbent assay, immunochromatography and western blotting.

INTRODUCTION

Serology is the study of **antigen–antibody binding** *in vitro* and has major significance in clinical medicine. Most practising veterinarians will employ diagnostic serological testing at least once every day. One of the most common applications of serology is in the **diagnosis of infectious disease**. Serological tests may be used to detect minute quantities of microbial antigen in a sample or, more commonly, look for evidence of antibody specific for that organism as confirmation that the animal has been exposed to that agent. More refined serological tests may be used to quantify the amount of antibody present and by collecting paired samples from a patient (e.g. 2 weeks apart) one can determine whether the amount of antibody might be increasing (as in an active progressing infection) or decreasing (as in recovery). Some serological tests are designed to **detect either IgG or IgM** antibody and the relative proportions

of these may indicate the **stage of the infection**. Serological tests are most commonly performed on blood samples or the serum fraction of blood, but they have equal applicability to a range of other body fluids.

The level of specific antibody activity present in a sample is defined as the **titre** of that antibody. The titre is defined as the reciprocal of the highest serum dilution giving an unequivocally positive reaction in a serological test. The principle of titre is explained in **Figure 4.1.** All serological tests involve the interaction *in vitro* of an antigen and an antibody. In some tests the antigens are large and particulate, allowing direct visualization of the reaction when mixed with antibody, but in many tests both components (antigen and antibody) are soluble and determination of their interaction requires a **secondary indicator system**. A range of such systems has been developed, but most of these require the use of an **antiserum** able to detect and bind to the antibody component of the reaction.

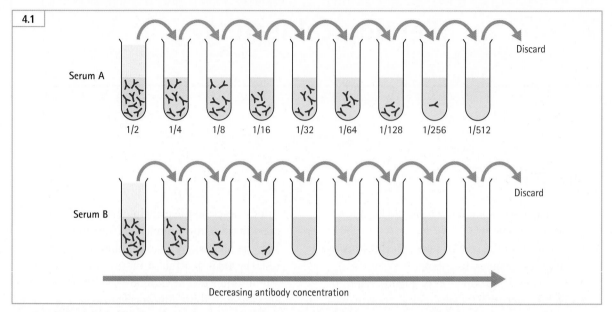

Fig. 4.1 Antibody titre. This diagram explains the principle of antibody titre. Serum samples are taken from two animals, A and B. Both animals have been exposed to the same antigen, but the serum from animal A contains more antibodies than that of animal B. In this serological experiment, a series of test tubes is set up for each serum sample. One volume of serum is added to the first tube in the series and one equal volume of a diluent (e.g. saline) is added to each of the remaining tubes. One equal volume of diluent is added to the first tube, which will dilute the number of antibody molecules by a factor of 2. One volume is now removed from the first tube and transferred to the second. When mixed, the original number of antibody molecules is now diluted by a factor of 4. This process is repeated along the line of test tubes to produce a 'doubling dilution series' in which the final tube has a 1/512 dilution of the original sample. The final volume taken from the last tube is discarded. The content of each test tube is now used in a serological test that is sensitive enough to detect a single antibody molecule (in this example). For the serum from animal A the test will be positive up to and including the tube containing the 1/256 dilution of serum. For serum from animal B the test will be positive up to and including the tube containing the 1/16 dilution of serum. The titre of each sample is expressed as the reciprocal of the last positive serum dilution (i.e. a titre of 256 for animal A and 16 for animal B). The higher titred serum contains the larger number of antibody molecules. It should be remembered that the titre is not an absolute number, but represents a range. For example, a titre of 256 indicates that the titre is not less than 128 and not more than 512, so there may be very little difference between a titre of 256 and one of 512.

An **antiserum** is serum collected from an animal that has been exposed to a particular antigen and therefore contains antibodies to that antigen. For most serological tests the antiserum is produced artificially by deliberately immunizing an animal (most commonly a mouse, rabbit, sheep or goat) with the antigen of interest and subsequently collecting blood (serum) from that immunized animal (**Figure 4.2**). Where the immunizing antigen carries a number of epitopes it is likely that the responding animal will generate antibodies against several of these epitopes. Such an antiserum is said to be **polyclonal** in nature.

It is also possible to generate antibody of a single specificity and the production of such **monoclonal** antibodies will be discussed in Chapter 9.

SEROLOGICAL TESTS

A range of serological tests is currently used for diagnosis in veterinary medicine. Many of these are tests used by diagnostic laboratories, but there is a good range of commercially available, simple serological test kits designed for in-practice or patient-side use. Serological tests vary in their complexity. Some tests

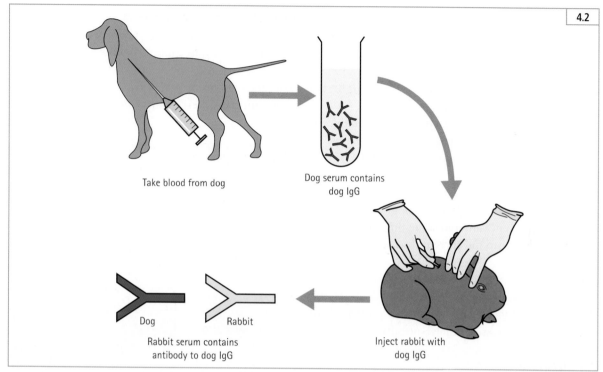

Fig. 4.2 Production of antiserum. To produce an antiserum that is able to bind to dog IgG, blood is taken from a dog, the IgG is biochemically extracted from the serum and the IgG is then injected into a rabbit. Once the rabbit has mounted an immune response to the foreign dog protein, serum taken from the rabbit will contain rabbit antibodies specific for dog IgG. The immunized rabbit serum is a rabbit anti-dog IgG antiserum.

are very simple and based on principles that were first defined over a century ago. Other procedures are only decades old and their increased sophistication generally means that they have greater sensitivity and specificity. The serological tests that will be considered in this chapter include:

- Agglutination.
- Precipitation.
- Complement fixation test (CFT).
- Haemagglutination inhibition (HAI).
- Virus neutralization (VN).
- Immunofluorescent antibody test (IFA).
- Enzyme-linked immunosorbent assay (ELISA).
- Immunochromatography.
- Western blotting.

As for any laboratory diagnostic procedure, veterinarians should always be aware of the sensitivity and specificity of the test that they are using. **Sensitivity** is defined as the probability that a given test

will correctly identify those animals with the disease, whereas **specificity** is the probability that a given test will identify those animals that do not have the disease under consideration. The **positive predictive value** of a diagnostic test is the probability that an animal with a positive test result actually has the condition for which the test was conducted, and the **negative predictive value** is the probability that an animal with a negative test result is actually free of the condition for which the test was conducted. Serological tests may produce both **false-positive** and **false-negative** results. For example, a test designed to detect serum antibody as evidence of exposure to a specific antigen might be falsely negative if:

- The animal has a very low titred antibody and the test is insufficiently sensitive to detect this level of antibody.
- The animal is tested too soon after exposure to the antigen when there has not been sufficient time to develop serum antibody.

- The animal is incapable of making an antibody response because it is neonatal, immunodeficient or immunosuppressed.

A false-positive result in such a test might be obtained if:
- The animal has a cross-reactive antibody induced in response to an unrelated antigen that shares some epitopes with the antigen of interest.
- The animal has been vaccinated with an attenuated version of a pathogen.
- The animal has a persistent serological response to an antigen encountered some time ago, but no longer relevant to the current disease state.

Interpretation of serological tests should always be made in light of the age, vaccination history and clinical status of the animal, which may provide clear reasons for false-positive or false-negative results.

Agglutination

Agglutination is a simple procedure that may be performed when the antigen of interest is **particulate** (e.g. RBCs, bacteria) or when soluble antigen is coated onto particles such as tiny latex beads. Particulate antigen is mixed in optimum proportions with antibody and if the antigen bears appropriate epitopes, the antibody may bind these and cross-link different antigens to form an **agglutinate**. The agglutinate may be visible to the naked eye or require light microscopic examination. A number of commonly employed veterinary immunodiagnostic procedures are based on the phenomenon of agglutination and one example is presented in **Figure 4.3**.

Precipitation

This test relies on the ability of antibodies to precipitate antigen within solution or an agar gel matrix. Although an historical technique, the method is still used in veterinary diagnosis for some infectious diseases (**Figure 4.4**). The formation of precipitates depends on the two reactants (antigen and antibody) being present at optimum concentration, where they are able to form a classical 'lattice-like' structure.

Complement fixation test

The CFT is used in the diagnosis of infectious disease (e.g. to determine whether cattle may have been exposed to *Brucella* antigens). Antigen is added to a tube containing serum from the test animal and if the animal is seropositive, an antigen–antibody

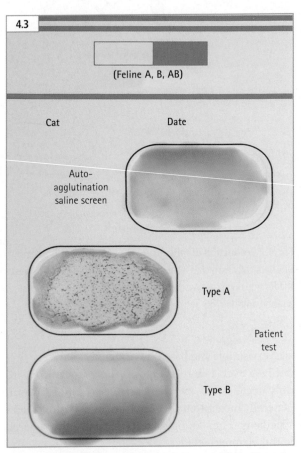

Fig. 4.3 Agglutination. This commercially available test is used to determine the blood group of a cat and is designed for rapid in-practice use where an emergency blood transfusion might be required. The three 'wells' in the card are first activated by the addition of diluent. A drop of blood from the cat is added to each well and mixed with a spatula. The top well contains no antiserum and serves as a control to ensure that the erythrocytes in the blood sample are not spontaneously agglutinating. The second well is impregnated with antiserum able to detect the feline blood group A antigen and the third well with reagent able to detect the feline B blood group antigen. In this test, the cat's red cells express A, but not B, as seen by the clumping (agglutination) of red cells in the second well after incubation. The cat is therefore of blood group A.

complex will form. A source of complement (e.g. fresh plasma) is added to the tube and where an antigen–antibody complex is present, the complement will be activated and integrated into the complex. If the animal is seronegative, the complement will remain intact as the free antigen does not activate it. As all of these interactions are invisible to the eye, a secondary indicator system is employed made up of a second antigen–antibody complex. This system utilizes

erythrocytes (often conveniently obtained from a sheep) that are pre-coated with anti-erythrocyte antiserum. The antibody-coated erythrocytes are added to the CFT tube. In a test from a seronegative animal, the free complement within the tube will be activated by the indicator system and result in haemolysis of the indicator erythrocytes. Lack of haemolysis in this test indicates a positive reaction (**Figure 4.5**).

Haemagglutination inhibition

The HAI test is commonly used in virology and relies on the ability of **virus particles to cause agglutination of erythrocytes** from particular animal species. If a patient has serum antibody specific for virus,

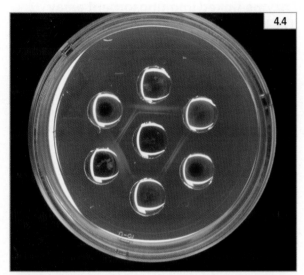

Fig. 4.4 Precipitation. Precipitation with an agar gel is still routinely used in the diagnosis of some infectious diseases, particularly fungal infections. An agar gel is formed within a petri dish and a series of holes punched in the agar. Shown is a gel designed to detect serum antibody to the fungus *Aspergillus fumigatus* in dogs with presumptive nasal aspergillosis. *Aspergillus* antigen is loaded into the central well and appropriately diluted serum from different dogs is loaded into the surrounding wells. The gel is incubated for 24 hours and during that time antigen diffuses from the central well and antibody (if present) from the peripheral wells. A white line of precipitation forms in the gel where the antigen and antibody meet in optimum proportion. This technique is known as agar gel diffusion (AGD) or the Ouchterlony technique after its discoverer. Four of the dogs in this experiment have serum antibody to *Aspergillus* and in each case there are at least two distinct precipitin lines consistent with two antibodies to each of two distinct epitopes. Where the precipitin line is continuous between two patients (a 'line of identity') the antigen–antibody interaction is identical, but crossed lines indicate non or partial identity.

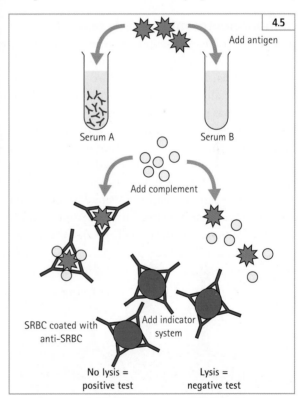

Fig. 4.5 Complement fixation test. During the first stage of the test, serum is incubated with the antigen of interest and an immune complex will form where that animal is seropositive. A source of complement is subsequently added, but will only be utilized where an antigen–antibody complex is present. Finally, a secondary indicator system of antibody-coated erythrocytes is added. Where the animal is seronegative, complement is still available to lyse the erythrocytes, providing a visual read out for the test. SRBC, sheep red blood cell.

pre-incubation of virus particles with antibody will inhibit the ability of the virus to subsequently cause haemagglutination when incubated with erythrocytes.

Virus neutralization

The VN test is also used to detect the presence of serum antibody specific for a virus in an animal. Test serum is incubated with live virus particles that are subsequently incubated with a monolayer of cells capable of being infected by the virus. The 'read out' for the test is the observation of **cytopathic effect** (cell damage and destruction) in the monolayer. In a positive test, serum antibody will neutralize the virus, thereby preventing infection *in vitro* and preserving the structure of the target cells.

Immunofluoresent antibody test

The IFA test has wide application in the diagnosis of a number of infectious diseases of animals (**Figures 4.6a, b**). In this procedure the infectious agent (either alone or associated with cultured cells in which it has grown) is spread over the surface of a sectored glass microscope slide and fixed *in situ*. Serum from the patient (in appropriate dilution) is added to that region of the slide and if the animal is seropositive, antibody will bind to the antigen. This primary interaction requires a secondary detection system. In the IFA test, a secondary antiserum designed to detect immunoglobulin (usually IgG) of the species

of interest is subsequently layered over that region of the slide. The secondary antibody is chemically **conjugated to a fluorochrome**. When the slide is examined at a particular wavelength of light under a fluorescence microscope, the fluorochrome becomes excited and the antibody-labelled organism becomes visible. The most commonly used fluorochrome for this purpose is fluorescein isothiocyanate, which emits an apple-green fluorescence under ultraviolet light.

Enzyme-linked immunosorbent assay

The ELISA is the basis of probably the majority of serological tests currently used in veterinary diagnosis and forms the foundation from which newer modalities (e.g. immunochromatography, western blotting) were developed. There are two fundamental types of ELISA. The first is designed to **detect the presence of antibody** specific for a particular antigen as evidence that the animal has been previously exposed to that antigen. The second is designed to **detect and quantify antigen**, perhaps as evidence that antigen from an infectious agent is currently circulating in an animal with active infection.

ELISA for detection of antibody

In a laboratory setting, the ELISA is most often performed in a 96-well microtitration plate with flat-bottomed wells. Examples of the use of ELISA to detect serum antibody are presented in **Figures 4.7a–d**

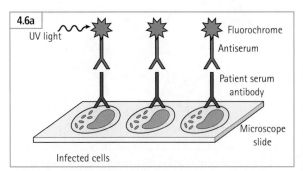

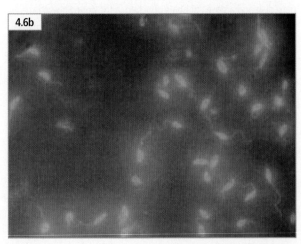

Figs. 4.6a, b Immunofluorescent antibody test. This test is widely used in the diagnosis of infectious disease; for example, infection with the sand fly-transmitted protozoal pathogen *Leishmania infantum*. (**a**) *Leishmania* organisms are cultured within an appropriate cell line and infected cells are fixed to the surface of a microscope slide. Patient serum is overlaid onto the slide and any binding of serum antibody and antigen is subsequently detected by the use of a secondary antiserum chemically conjugated to a fluorochrome. (**b**) When excited by light of an appropriate wavelength under a fluorescence microscope, the labelled organisms give apple-green fluorescence on a black background.

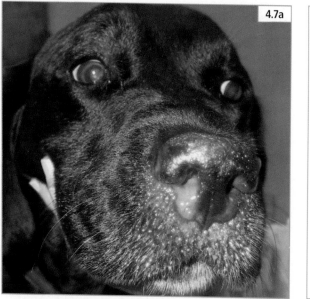

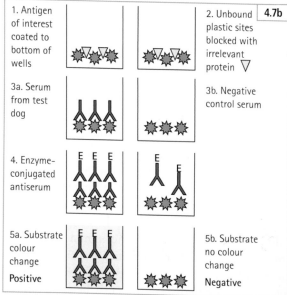

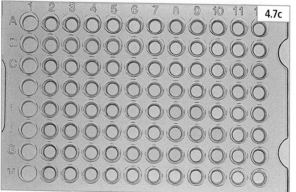

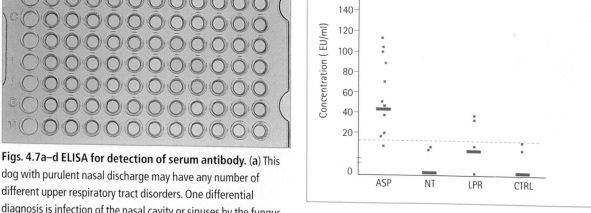

Figs. 4.7a–d ELISA for detection of serum antibody. (a) This dog with purulent nasal discharge may have any number of different upper respiratory tract disorders. One differential diagnosis is infection of the nasal cavity or sinuses by the fungus *Aspergillus fumigatus*. One of the diagnostic procedures used to determine if this infection is present is the detection of serum antibody to *Aspergillus*. **(b)** In the ELISA technique, *Aspergillus* antigen is coated onto the wells of microtitration trays and areas of the plastic well not coated by antigen are 'blocked' with an irrelevant protein. Serum from the patient (at an appropriate dilution) is added to the wells and incubated. After washing out unbound serum protein, rabbit antiserum specific for dog IgG that is chemically conjugated to the enzyme alkaline phosphatase is added to each well for a second period of incubation. Unbound antiserum is washed from the wells, and an appropriate substrate added to produce a colour change (yellow) in positive wells. **(c)** An ELISA plate at the completion of an assay. Wells with yellow colouration represent a positive reaction. An ELISA plate reader is used to determine spectrophotometrically the absorbance (optical density) at a specific wavelength of light. **(d)** In this study, sera from normal dogs (CTRL) and dogs with nasal aspergillosis (ASP), nasal tumours (NT) or idiopathic lymphoplasmacytic rhinitis (LPR) were tested in an ELISA. It is clear that this ELISA has good specificity and sensitivity for the diagnosis of canine nasal aspergillosis. (Data from Billen F *et al.* (2008) Comparison of the value of measurement of serum galactomannan and *Aspergillus*-specific antibodies in the diagnosis of canine sino-nasal aspergillosis. *Veterinary Microbiology*, **133**, 358–365.)

and **Figures 4.8a, b**. The antigen of interest is first coated onto the bottom of the wells of the plate and a second unrelated protein may be used to block any areas of 'free plastic' that are not coated by antigen. Appropriately diluted serum from the patient animal is added to one well and positive and negative control sera may also be employed. If the test serum contains relevant antibodies, these will bind to the antigen in the primary phase of the reaction. As the antigen and antibody are not visible to the eye, a secondary detection system is required to determine whether such binding has occurred. In this instance, after unbound antibody is washed from the wells, an appropriately diluted antiserum specific for the immunoglobulin of interest (e.g. IgG) from the patient species is added. In an ELISA this antibody is chemically conjugated to an enzyme. A range of enzymes may be used, but the most commonly employed is **alkaline phosphatase**. If the patient serum contains antibodies specific to the antigen of interest, the enzyme-linked antiserum will detect and bind to that patient immunoglobulin (which is in turn bound to the antigen). After washing to remove any unbound conjugated secondary antiserum, an appropriate **substrate** is added to each well to initiate a **colour change**, which is measured spectrophotometrically at a particular time point when the enzyme–substrate reaction may be deliberately stopped. The same colour change would occur in wells incubated with positive control serum, but no colour would develop in negative controls. The optimum conditions for performance of an ELISA (e.g. dilutions of antigen, serum and antiserum, time and temperature of incubations) must first be determined experimentally.

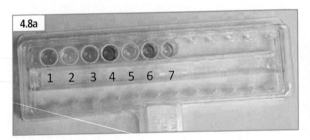

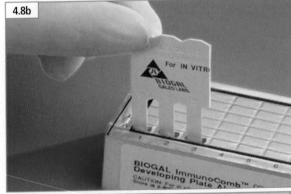

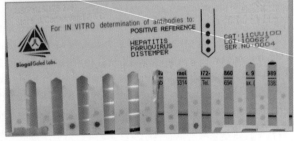

Figs. 4.8a, b ELISA for detection of serum antibody. An important practice-based application of the ELISA is in testing to ensure that dogs have been protected by vaccination. There is a strong correlation between the presence of serum antibody specific for canine distemper virus (CDV), canine adenovirus (CAV) and canine parvovirus (CPV) and protection from these diseases. These two commercial tests can rapidly determine whether a dog is protected or whether it may require revaccination. (**a**) The first test kit (Titrechek®, Zoetis) utilizes a well-based ELISA as described in **Figure 4.7** to test for the presence or absence of CDV and CPV antibodies. Shown is a CDV test. Well 1 is a positive control (blue) and well 2 is a negative control (clear). Wells 3 to 7 test serum samples from individual dogs. Only dog 5 is seronegative and requires revaccination. (**b**) The second test kit (Vaccicheck®, Biogal Laboratories) uses a system in which viral antigens are impregnated into a 'spot' on the 'teeth' of a 'comb'. The 'dot-ELISA' is performed by sequentially dipping the comb into a series of wells containing diluted dog serum, enzyme-linked antiserum and substrate. Each 'tooth' presents four dots – the top dot represents the positive control and beneath this are the reactions for CAV, CPV and CDV. A grey colouration represents a positive reaction that can be scored semiquantitatively against a colour scale. These test kits provide a major advance in rapidly determining, in the practice, the vaccine requirements of individual dogs.

ELISA for detection of antigen

ELISAs may also be used for the detection and quantification of antigen within a fluid sample (**Figures 4.9a, b**). The antigen may be derived from an infectious agent or be a host molecule (e.g. immunoglobulin or cytokine). This form of ELISA is known as a 'capture' system. In a **capture ELISA**, the wells of the microtitration tray are coated with an antibody (antiserum) specific for the antigen of interest. The test sample is subsequently added to the well and if antigen is present, it will be 'captured' and bound by the antiserum. Unbound antigen is then washed from the well. As this primary interaction remains invisible, a secondary detection system is required. In this ELISA a second antibody, also specific for the antigen of interest, but usually designed to interact with a separate epitope, will bind to antigen molecules that have previously been captured by the primary antiserum. The second antibody may be chemically conjugated to enzyme and after this incubation and further washing, the appropriate substrate is added to cause colour change in any positive well. In some ELISAs (of either type) it is sometimes better (or necessary due to commercial availability) to utilize a more complex detection process involving a secondary antiserum, followed by a **tertiary antiserum** that carries the enzyme.

In-practice serological test kits

The principle of the ELISA has been exploited in many of the rapid, in-house, serodiagnostic tests that have been produced for veterinarians. One variant of

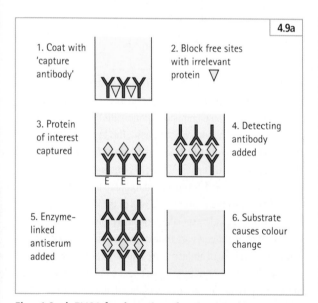

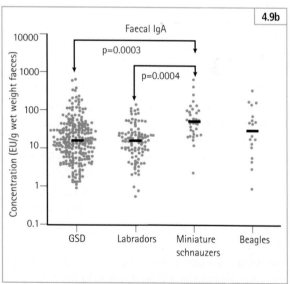

Figs. 4.9a, b ELISA for detection of antigen. In this experiment we wish to determine whether dogs of different breeds have any difference in the concentration of IgA in faeces. (**a**) Wells of the microtitre plate are initially coated with antiserum specific for canine IgA (**1**). Unbound plastic sites are blocked with irrelevant protein (**2**). An extract prepared from faecal samples of different dogs in standard fashion is added to each well. IgA in the faecal extract is 'captured' by the antiserum (**3**). The wells are washed to remove unbound faecal protein. Captured IgA is subsequently detected using a secondary antiserum (**4**) and then a tertiary antiserum chemically conjugated to enzyme (**5**). After washing to remove unbound secondary antiserum, substrate is added to produce a colour change that is measured spectrophotometrically (**6**). (**b**) This graph presents the faecal IgA measurement from a large number of dogs of several different breeds. Miniature schnauzers have significantly more faecal IgA than German shepherd dogs, Labradors or beagles. (Data from Peters IR, Calvert EL, Hall EJ *et al.* (2004) Measurement of immunoglobulin concentrations in the feces of healthy dogs. *Clinical and Diagnostic Laboratory Immunology* 11:841–848.)

this type of test is SNAP® technology produced by Idexx (**Figure 4.10**). The **rapid immunomigration** or **immunochromatographic** system is another widely used test system (**Figure 4.11**).

Western blotting

A further refinement of the ELISA is the process of western blotting, which provides specific information concerning the specific proteins to which patient

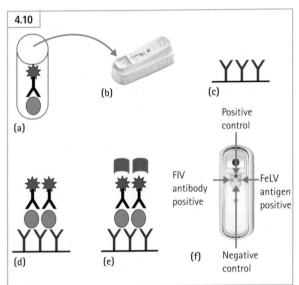

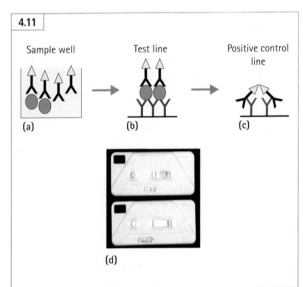

Fig. 4.10 In-practice serological test kits. The principle of the ELISA is used in numerous test kits designed for in-practice use as rapid patient-side diagnostics. These tests can be used to detect circulating antigen from infectious agents or serum antibody against infectious agents (blood samples) or antigen present within faecal samples. One of the most commonly used technologies is the Idexx SNAP® test. In the example shown, circulating feline leukaemia virus (FeLV) antigen is detected by specific antibody conjugated to enzyme (star symbol) when serum and conjugated antibody are mixed in a sample tube (**a**). The content of the sample tube is added to the sample well of the kit (**b**). The sample passes over a matrix containing capture antibodies specific for the antigen of interest (**c**). The 'snap' technology of the kit permits the sample to flow bidirectionally over the capture antibodies to enhance binding of the antigen and associated antibody conjugate (**d**). After a washing step to remove unbound components of the sample, the exposure to enzyme substrate allows development of a colour reaction (**e**). Pictured is a dual test kit that permits the detection of FIV antibody and FeLV antigen concurrently (**f**). This cat is positive for both retrovirus infections.

Fig. 4.11 In-practice serological test kits. An alternative technology for detection of molecules of interest (e.g. antigens or antibodies) is the rapid immunomigration (RIM®) methodology, also known as immunochromatography. This test modality is the basis of the Zoetis WITNESS® test system. The example shown is a test for detection of the p27 antigen of the feline leukaemia virus (FeLV). Sample (serum containing FeLV antigen) and buffer are added to the sample well of the kit. If antigen is present, it is bound by specific antibody within the sample well (**a**). These antibodies are conjugated to gold particles. The immune complexes of antigen and conjugated antibody then migrate along the matrix strip in the direction of the arrows. At the first position in the window of the kit, the complexes encounter a zone of further antibody to the antigen, which binds and immobilizes the antigen, forming a visible line in the window (**b**). Non-complexed conjugate continues to migrate along the strip until it encounters a second zone of the strip containing antibody specific for the primary antibody molecules. This forms a second reaction line, which is the positive control for the test (**c**). In the two tests shown, the top example is positive for FeLV antigen and the lower test is negative (**d**).

antibodies bind (**Figure 4.12**). This has particular relevance in infectious disease and can be used to distinguish between vaccinal antibody and antibody produced through field exposure to pathogen. In western blotting the antigenic mixture under question is electrophoretically separated (by molecular weight) in an acrylamide gel and the separated proteins are subsequently transferred ('blotted') onto a membrane (e.g. nitrocellulose). The membrane may be cut into small strips, and each strip is incubated (after a blocking step) with appropriately diluted patient serum. Serum antibody binds selectively to specific antigenic determinants, and this binding is visualized by the use of a secondary antiserum that is conjugated to an enzyme, as for an ELISA. The reaction is finally demonstrated via either a colour change or emission of light (chemiluminescence).

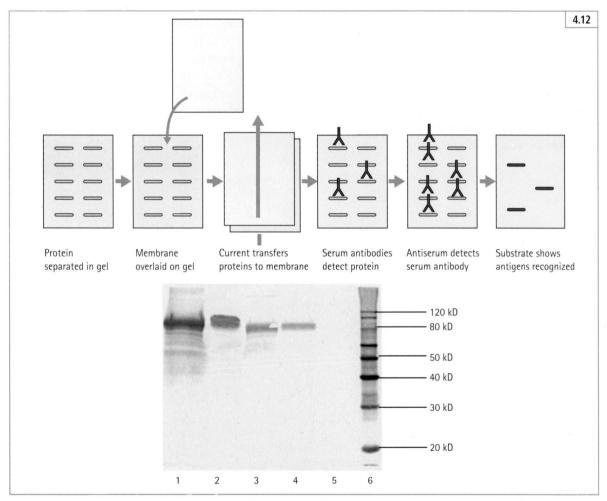

| Protein separated in gel | Membrane overlaid on gel | Current transfers proteins to membrane | Serum antibodies detect protein | Antiserum detects serum antibody | Substrate shows antigens recognized |

120 kD
80 kD
50 kD
40 kD
30 kD
20 kD

1 2 3 4 5 6

Fig. 4.12 Western blotting. This experiment aims to determine whether canine IgA is associated with a secretory component. Initially, a series of proteins is electrophoretically separated by molecular mass in an acrylamide gel. The numbered lanes in the gel contain the following samples: (**1**) purified human secretory component, (**2**) purified human secretory IgA, (**3**) canine bile, (**4**) canine saliva, (**5**) canine serum and (**6**) molecular mass marker proteins. The separated proteins are then electrophoretically transferred to a membrane. After a blocking stage, the membrane is probed with an antiserum specific for the human secretory component and then a secondary antiserum conjugated to alkaline phosphatase. Binding of primary antiserum is recognized by addition of substrate that produces a colour change at that site on the membrane. The results of this experiment show that antiserum to human secretory component cross-reacts with the equivalent canine molecule, and that dog salivary and biliary IgA has a secretory component that is not present in circulating (serum) IgA.

KEY POINTS

- Serology is the study of antigen–antibody binding *in vitro*.
- Serology is widely used in clinical veterinary practice.
- Titre is a measure of the amount of antibody in a (serum) sample.
- Many serological tests require the use of an antiserum.
- Antiserum is made by immunizing an animal with the antigen of interest and subsequently collecting serum (containing antibody) from that animal.
- Sensitivity is the probability that a diagnostic test will correctly identify animals with the disease being tested for.
- Specificity is the probability that a diagnostic test will correctly identify animals that do not have the disease being tested for.
- False-positive and false-negative results may occur in serological tests.
- Agglutination and precipitation involve direct interaction of antigen and antibody that may be observed visually.
- The CFT, HAI test, VN test, IFA test, ELISA, immunochromatography and western blotting all require the use of an indicator system to visualize the primary antigen–antibody interaction.

CHAPTER 5

Cells and Tissues of the Immune System

OBJECTIVES

At the end of this chapter you should be able to:
- Understand the difference between primary and secondary lymphoid tissue and give examples of each.
- Describe the genesis of T and B lymphocytes.
- Describe the microanatomical structure of a lymph node.
- Understand the difference between a small lymphocyte and a lymphoblast.
- Give some criteria by which T and B lymphocytes might be differentiated.

- Describe the pathway of lymphocyte recirculation.
- Define Burnett's clonal selection theory.
- Understand why lymphocyte recirculation is essential to the immune system.
- Define 'high endothelial venule', 'vascular addressin' and 'homing receptor'.
- Discuss why it is important that lymphocytes activated at one mucosal surface are able to recirculate to multiple mucosal surfaces.

INTRODUCTION

The preceding chapters have described some of the important soluble protein mediators of the immune response (antibodies and complement) and we must next turn our attention to the cellular elements of immunity and the lymphoid tissues in which they largely reside. This chapter will discuss the key cells of the adaptive immune system (**T and B lymphocytes** and **plasma cells**) and the **primary** and **secondary** lymphoid tissues. Primary lymphoid tissues are the sites where the lymphoid cells are formed and undergo initial maturation, whereas secondary lymphoid tissue comprises fully developed lymphoid cells that are capable of participating in immune responses.

PRIMARY LYMPHOID TISSUE

The first of the primary lymphoid tissues is the **bone marrow** (**Figure 5.1**). Within the marrow is a population of primordial **stem cells**. These give rise to committed stem cells responsible for production of the various haemopoietic lineages (erythroid, platelet, myeloid), including the lymphoid cells. The earliest forms of both T and B lymphocytes are recognized within the bone marrow, but in most species both immature cell types are exported from the marrow to undergo final maturation in further primary lymphoid tissues elsewhere in the body. In birds, maturation of B cells takes place in the **bursa of Fabricius**, a lymphoepithelial organ located near the cloaca. In an early immunological experiment, it was noted that bursectomy (surgical removal of the bursa) in chicks led to failure of B-cell development and an inability to produce antibody in adults. In fact, this observation led to the naming of B lymphocytes (bursa-derived lymphocytes). In other domestic animals and man (group I mammals) this process of B-cell maturation is thought to occur within the intestinal tract, particularly in the very developed B-cell enriched **ileal Peyer's patches** found in ruminants, pigs and dogs. These patches are the major site of B-cell development in sheep, in which the bone marrow contains fewer lymphocytes than that of mice. Surgical removal of the ileal Peyer's patch in a lamb leads to a transient deficiency in B cells and antibody production. The ileal Peyer's patch is of maximum size before birth. It disappears over the first 15 months of the lamb's life and is not detectable in adults. Although pigs also have a well-developed ileal Peyer's patch, surgical removal

of this tissue in piglets does not affect the development of B or T lymphocytes. This suggests that the bone marrow, rather than the ileal Peyer's patch, may be the primary lymphoid organ for B-cell development in the pig. Horses have multiple smaller ileal lymphoid patches rather than a single Peyer's patch and in people there is a concentration of Peyer's patch tissue in the distal ileum. In contrast, rabbits and rodents (group II mammals) lack an ileal Peyer's patch and B-cell development occurs within the bone marrow and in the appendix of rabbits. These species have multiple ileal Peyer's patches, as found in the jejunum of all animals including humans. The jejunal Peyer's patches are as described below with interfollicular T cells. The stages of B-cell development will be further described in Chapter 9, but at this point one should recall that B lymphocytes are involved in the production of antibody, which comprises the **humoral immune response**.

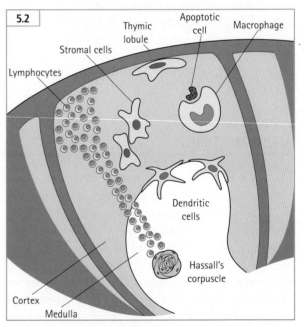

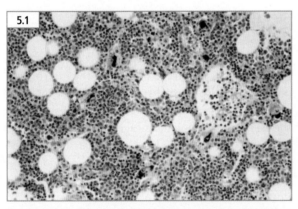

Fig. 5.1 Bone marrow. Normal canine bone marrow comprises a mixture of haemopoietic elements and adipose tissue. The large multinucleate cells are megakaryocytes. Both T and B lymphocytes arise in the bone marrow from committed stem cell precursors.

Fig. 5.2 Thymic structure. The thymus is an encapsulated primary lymphoid tissue divided into lobules by connective tissue septa. There is an outermost cortex and inner medulla, both densely packed with actively dividing and apoptotic T lymphocytes. Interspersed with the lymphocytes are the thymic epithelial cells, dendritic cells and macrophages that phagocytose debris from apoptotic lymphocytes. The squamous epithelial Hassall's corpuscles produce cytokines, which influence T-cell development.

Another primary lymphoid tissue is the **thymus**, an organ found in the mediastinum of the thoracic cavity just anterior to the heart. Immature T lymphocytes are exported from the bone marrow to the thymus for their final maturation. They are therefore named T lymphocytes because of this thymic stage of development, which will be fully discussed in Chapter 8. The thymus is an intriguing organ that is of maximal size at birth and involutes (shrinks) during puberty to become virtually impossible to see grossly in adult animals. Two observations led to an understanding of the role of the thymus in T-cell development. Surgical removal of this organ (thymectomy) in neonatal animals leads to an absence of T cells in adults and an inability to mount **cell-mediated immunity** (CMI), for which T cells are responsible. Similar observations were made in congenitally athymic animals (i.e. animals born without a thymus). Interestingly, this genetic mutation is often associated with an inherited inability to form a hair coat, typified by inbred laboratory strains of 'nude' athymic rats and mice. At least one of the hairless canine breeds (the Mexican hairless dog) is also known to have impaired thymic development (see Chapter 19).

Histologically, the thymus is an **encapsulated** organ consisting of a series of lobules each of which has a distinct **cortex** and **medulla** (**Figures 5.2–5.4**). The majority of thymic tissue is composed of a closely packed population of T lymphocytes, with fewer interspersed **thymic epithelial cells** and **dendritic cells**, which are almost impossible to identify in a standard microscopic section. Within the medulla is a series of **Hassall's corpuscles**, which are made up of modified squamous epithelium and are thought to produce growth factors that influence T-cell development. As will be discussed in Chapter 8, there is an incredible turnover of thymic T cells, with numerous cells dying by apoptosis and the cellular debris subsequently being phagocytosed by macrophages.

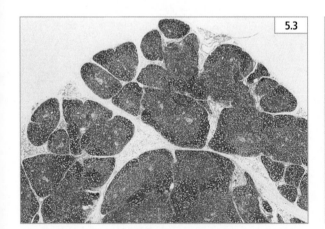

Fig. 5.3 Thymic histology. Low-power view of the canine thymus showing the lobulated structure of the organ and the presence of a darker cortical region and paler medullary area within each lobule.

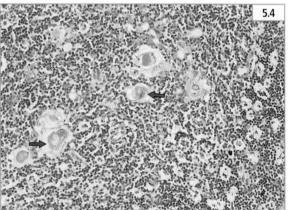

Fig. 5.4 Thymic histology. Higher magnification of the canine thymus showing the junction between cortex and medulla. The Hassall's corpuscles of the medulla are arrowed. Clear spaces within the cortex represent sites where apoptotic debris has been phagocytosed by a macrophage.

SECONDARY LYMPHOID TISSUE

The secondary lymphoid tissues may be broadly divided into those that are **encapsulated** (the lymph nodes and spleen) and those that are **unencapsulated** (the mucosal lymphoid aggregates). A network of **lymph nodes** is present throughout the peripheral and visceral areas of the body (**Figure 5.5**). Lymph fluid containing assorted cells from the local tissues drains into the lymph node via the **afferent lymphatic vessels**. This fluid first enters the **subcapsular sinus** and then percolates through the nodal tissue to the large **medullary sinus** from where it leaves the node in the **efferent lymphatic vessel**. Lymph nodes have an arterial and venous blood supply, which provides an alternative point of entry and exit for lymphoid cells. The **cortical area** of the lymph node is composed of a closely packed population of lymphocytes arranged as spherical **follicles** within a surrounding **paracortex** (**Figure 5.6**). These two regions contain distinct subpopulations of lymphocytes. The follicles are principally composed of B cells and the paracortex of T cells. This **compartmentalization** of the major lymphoid populations can be readily demonstrated

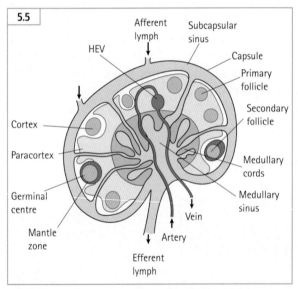

Fig. 5.5 Lymph node structure. The lymph node is an encapsulated organ with a cortex and a medulla. Afferent lymph flows into the node from local tissues and carries lymphocytes, antigen presenting cells and antigen. Lymph enters the subcapsular sinus and then percolates through the node to the medullary sinus before leaving in the efferent lymphatic vessel. The lymph node has an arterial and venous blood supply and lymphocytes may enter the node through the high endothelial venules (HEVs). The cortex of the lymph node comprises follicular aggregates of B lymphocytes surrounded by the paracortical T-cell zone. Follicles may be primary or secondary, with a mantle zone surrounding a germinal centre. The medullary cords provide a framework for the medullary sinus and also contain lymphoid cells.

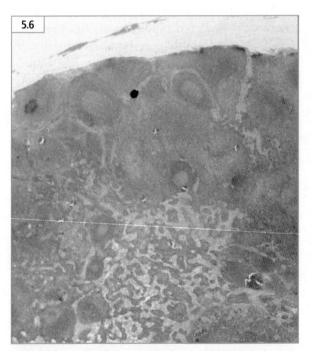

Fig. 5.6 Lymph node histology. Low-power view of a canine lymph node showing cortical follicles surrounded by paracortex and a central medullary sinus crossed by interlacing medullary cords.

by immunohistochemical labelling (**Figures 5.7a, b**). The follicles may take one of two histological forms. **Primary follicles** are smaller and consist of a dense aggregate of small inactive lymphocytes. **Secondary follicles** are larger, and have a distinct **mantle zone** of small lymphocytes surrounding an innermost **germinal centre** of larger, actively dividing B lymphocytes (**Figure 5.8**). The germinal centre classically includes both a **dark zone** and a **light zone** defined by the staining affinity of the lymphoid cells. The medullary sinus of the lymph node is given structure by a network of **medullary cords** that act as a framework holding the sinus open. These cords are also packed with lymphoid cells, particularly **plasma cells**. The pig has an 'inside-out' lymph node composed of multiple nodules with an innermost cortex and peripheral medulla. Afferent lymph flows into the centre of each nodule and percolates through closely packed cells (rather than medullary sinuses) to the peripheral medullary areas to reach the efferent flow. This structure means that lymphocytes rarely leave the node in efferent lymph, but migrate directly into the bloodstream via paracortical high endothelial venules (HEVs) (see below).

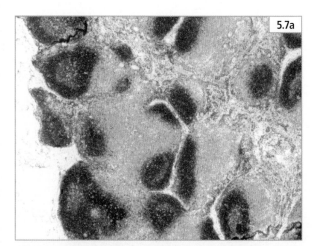
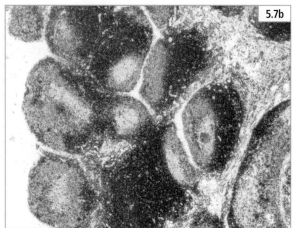

Figs. 5.7a, b Compartmentalization of the lymph node. These two images represent serial sections of the same lymph node immunohistochemically labelled to show the position of follicular B cells (**a**) and paracortical T cells (**b**). Some T cells are present within the follicles and are directly involved in B-cell activation.

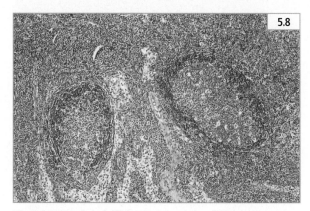

Fig. 5.8 Secondary follicles. Two secondary follicles are present at the junction of the cortex and the medulla. The follicles have a pale germinal centre surrounded by a dark mantle zone. Surrounding paracortex is to the top of the image and the medullary sinus and cords to the bottom.

The **spleen** is a visceral organ that has arterial and venous blood supply, but no lymphatic drainage (**Figure 5.9**). The spleen is encapsulated and, contiguous with the capsular connective tissue, is a network of **trabeculae** that create a framework for the splenic structure. Between the trabeculae the splenic substance comprises a mixture of red and white pulp. The **red pulp** is a reservoir of blood and the **white pulp** represents the splenic lymphoid tissue (**Figures 5.10a, b**). As in the lymph node, this tissue is compartmentalized into T- and B-cell zones. The splenic T cells are closely associated with arteriolar blood vessels and form a cylindrical surround to such vessels (akin to the 'lagging' on a water pipe). This T-cell region is known descriptively as the **periarteriolar lymphoid sheath** (PALS). Splenic B cells are also found within primary or secondary **follicles** adjacent to the PALS and both structures are surrounded by a narrow **marginal zone** that includes a mixture of cell types. The marginal zone is not readily seen on light microscopy, but immunohistochemical labelling can clearly identify the T- and B-cell areas.

The secondary unencapsulated lymphoid tissue is largely scattered throughout the **mucosal surfaces**

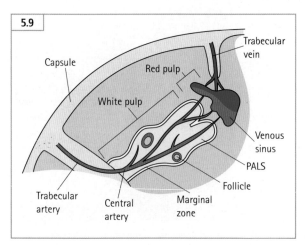

Fig. 5.9 Structure of the spleen. The spleen is an encapsulated organ given structure by a network of connective tissue trabeculae. Lymphoid tissue is localized to the white pulp that lies within the surrounding red pulp. The red pulp consists of blood, which in some animal species (e.g. the dog) is contained by endothelial-lined vascular sinuses. In other species (e.g. the cat) the spleen is non-sinusal. The spleen does not have lymphatic drainage, but is considered part of the blood vascular circulation. White pulp lymphoid tissue is compartmentalized. T cells reside in the periarteriolar lymphoid sheath (PALS) and B cells within follicles. A narrow marginal zone delineates the periphery of the white pulp.

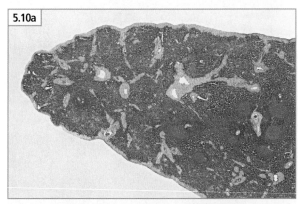

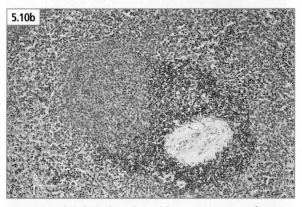

Figs. 5.10a, b Splenic histology. (a) Low-power view of canine spleen showing the outermost capsule, which is continuous with the network of connective tissue trabeculae. The regions of white pulp are seen throughout the surrounding red pulp. **(b)** Higher magnification of an area of white pulp reveals the periarteriolar lymphoid sheath encircling a central arteriole with an adjacent follicular aggregate. The narrow marginal zone is not readily discerned by routine light microscopy.

of the body and represents a significant proportion of the total lymphoid tissue. For example, the largest proportion of lymphoid tissue is to be found in the intestinal mucosa. These **mucosa-associated lymphoid tissues (MALT)** include gastrointestinal-associated lymphoid tissue (**GALT**), bronchial-associated lymphoid tissue (**BALT**), nasal-associated lymphoid tissue (**NALT**) and conjunctiva-associated lymphoid tissue (**CALT**). The best characterized of these tissues is GALT (**Figure 5.11**). GALT comprises the **inductive** sites of the intestinal immune system (i.e. where alimentary immune responses are induced) and the **effector** sites (where the end effects of alimentary immune responses take place [e.g. IgA production]). The inductive sites of GALT are the organized Peyer's patches of the small intestine and solitary lymphoid follicles (which are most prominent in the stomach and large intestine). The Peyer's patch is an unencapsulated lymphoid aggregate comprising a series of B-cell follicles (often with secondary structure) surrounded by an intervening zone of predominantly T cells (**Figure 5.12**).

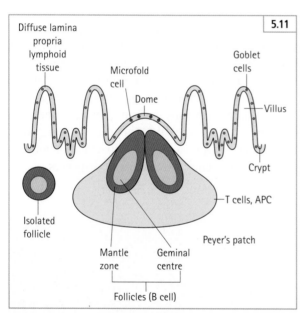

Fig. 5.11 Unencapsulated mucosal lymphoid tissue. The lamina propria of most mucosal tissues has a diffuse population of lymphoid cells with a specific lymphoid population localized to the surface epithelium (effector sites of mucosal immunity). Scattered individual lymphoid follicles and organized structures such as in the intestinal Peyer's patch are considered the inductive sites of mucosal immunity. Peyer's patches include B-cell follicles surrounded by a mixed zone of T cells and antigen presenting cells (APCs). There is modification of the overlying mucosa such that villi are replaced by a broader dome-shaped region. Microfold cells within the epithelium of the dome serve to sample antigen from the intestinal lumen and transfer it to the underlying lymphoid tissue.

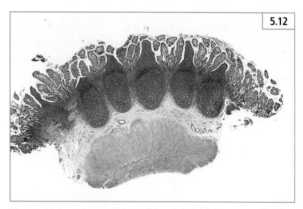

Figs. 5.12 Peyer's patch histology. A full-thickness sample of canine intestine showing the mucosa, submucosa and muscularis propria. The position of a Peyer's patch in the mucosa–submucosa is clear.

These mucosal lymphoid structures are accompanied by an alteration to the microanatomy of the overlying epithelium and lamina propria, which forms a broad-based **dome** rather than having villous microarchitecture (**Figures 5.13a, b**). Within the epithelium covering the Peyer's patch is a specialized population of **microfold cells** (M cells), which sample antigen from the intestinal lumen and transfer this to the underlying lymphoid tissue. The Peyer's patches are linked to the draining **mesenteric lymph nodes** by the mesenteric afferent lymphatic vessels. Although intestinal immune responses may be amplified in the associated mesenteric lymph nodes, these are not considered part of GALT as they do not directly sample mucosal antigen.

The effector sites of mucosal immunity consist of the diffusely scattered lymphocytes and plasma cells of the lamina propria and the specialized compartment of IELs that reside in the epithelial layer lining the mucosal surfaces.

LYMPHOCYTES

In this chapter we consider the T and B lymphocytes and associated plasma cells that are the core components of the adaptive immune response. Antigen presenting cells (APCs) are considered in Chapter 7 and NK cells in Chapter 8. Other leucocytes (neutrophils, eosinophils, basophils and mast cells) have ancillary roles in many immune responses. The developmental lineages of these cells are summarized in **Figure 5.14**.

The lymphocytes within lymphoid tissue, blood and lymphatic fluid may be broadly divided morphologically into small and large lymphocytes (lymphoblasts) and plasma cells. **Small lymphocytes** are in the order of 6–9 μm in diameter and have a large, round nucleus with condensed chromatin and a minimal amount of surrounding cytoplasm with few organelles (**Figures 5.15, 5.16**). Small lymphocytes might be either T or B cells and functionally may be either **naïve** (**virgin**) or **memory** cells. A naïve lymphocyte has not been previously exposed to the antigenic epitope it is pre-programmed to recognize via its specific receptor. In contrast, a memory cell has previously participated in an immune response and retains the memory of that event.

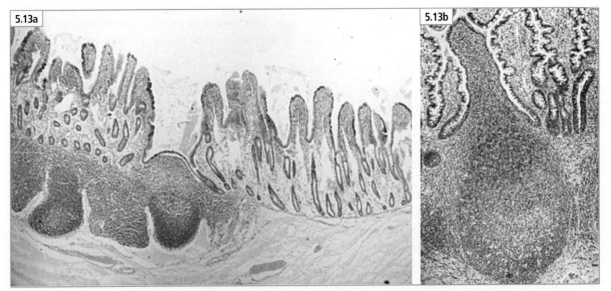

Figs. 5.13a, b Peyer's patch dome. Peyer's patches from a pig (**a**) and a dog (**b**) showing modification of the overlying small intestinal villous structure to form a broad-based dome filled by lymphoid cells. (Image **5.13a** courtesy G. Hall)

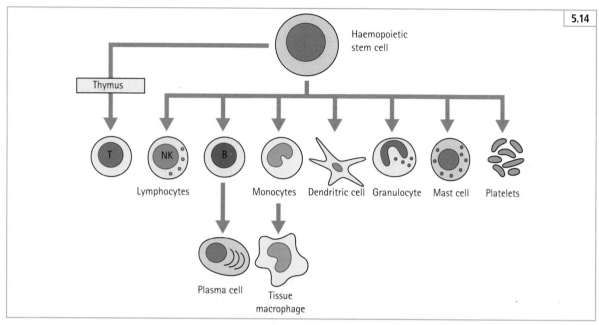

Fig. 5.14 Developmental lineages of immune and haemopoietic cells. All the cells of the immune system arise from the primordial bone marrow stem cells, which in turn give rise to separate developmental lineages through committed stem cells. Plasma cells are a late maturation stage of B lymphocytes and tissue macrophages derive from blood monocytes.

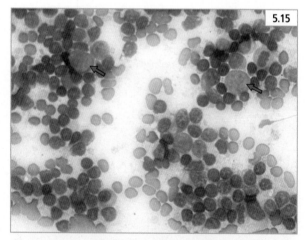

Fig. 5.15 Small and large lymphocytes. A fine-needle aspirate from a canine lymph node. The majority of cells in this field are small lymphocytes, which are only marginally larger than the erythrocytes in the background. These cells have a large, round nucleus with dense chromatin and a narrow, pale blue cytoplasmic rim. Several large lymphocytes or lymphoblasts are also present (arrows). These cells are 2–4 times larger than the small lymphocyte, with a pale nucleus and proportionally more cytoplasm.

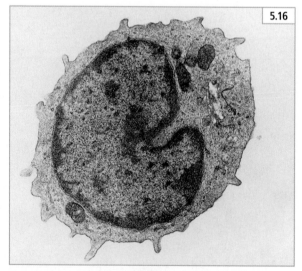

Fig. 5.16 Lymphocyte ultrastructure. Transmission electronmicrograph of a single small lymphocyte. The nucleus of this cell is cleaved and there is marginal condensation of chromatin. The cytoplasm contains few organelles. Note the characteristic ruffling of the cell surface.

Large lymphocytes or **lymphoblasts** are morphologically larger cells of 12–15 μm diameter (**Figure 5.15**) that have proportionally more cytoplasm with a greater number of organelles than a small lymphocyte. Lymphoblasts also have less condensed nuclear chromatin. Lymphoblasts are active cells that have been recently stimulated by antigen and are participating in a current immune response. The cells within lymphoid follicular germinal centres are lymphoblastic.

Plasma cells are a late stage of development of B lymphocytes. Although B lymphocytes can synthesize immunoglobulin and display this on their cell membrane, only plasma cells can secrete immunoglobulin in high concentration. Plasma cells have a more oval shape, with a round nucleus placed to one side of the cell (an 'eccentric' nucleus) (**Figure 5.17**). The nucleus has characteristic linear condensation of chromatin and this is sometimes referred to as 'clock face' or 'bicycle wheel' chromatin.

The cytoplasm of a plasma cell is packed with the machinery of protein production (endoplasmic reticulum and Golgi apparatus) and, even at the light microscopical level, a distinct perinuclear pale region (the 'Golgi zone') may be observed (**Figure 5.18**). Immunohistochemical labelling can be used to demonstrate the cytoplasmic immunoglobulin within a plasma cell.

DISTINGUISHING BETWEEN IMMUNE CELLS

In examining small or large lymphocytes in a blood smear or histological section it is not possible to determine unequivocally whether any one individual cell might be a T or a B cell. In the case of a tissue section, the microanatomical location is suggestive of identity (i.e. most follicular lymphocytes are B cells and most paracortical or PALS lymphocytes are T cells). In order to identify more precisely these cells

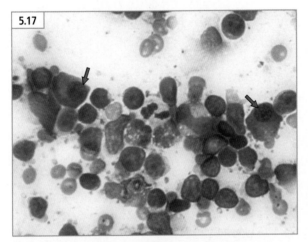

Fig. 5.17 Plasma cells. Fine-needle aspirate from the lymph node of a dog. A variety of cells are present including background erythrocytes, small lymphocytes and two central eosinophils. Plasma cells are arrowed. These are oval cells with plentiful cytoplasm and a round nucleus located to one side of the cell. A perinuclear Golgi zone is seen as a pale area within the cytoplasm.

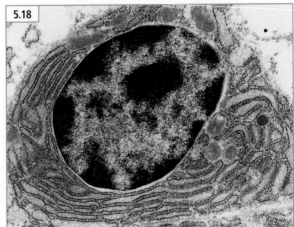

Fig. 5.18 Plasma cell ultrastructure. Transmission electronmicrograph of a single plasma cell. The nucleus contains condensed chromatin and sits within abundant cytoplasm containing a large amount of endoplasmic reticulum.

in suspension or tissue section, immunologists have developed a range of techniques that underpin much experimental research in cellular immunology.

These techniques are based on the fact that T and B cells express a series of unique molecules on their surface membrane and that these molecules might be identified by the use of antisera (see Chapter 4) or monoclonal antibodies (see Chapter 9). For example, only T cells express a surface **T-cell receptor** (TCR) and only B cells carry surface immunoglobulin as the **B-cell receptor** (BCR). Other molecules restricted to T cells include CD3, CD4 and CD8, and the molecules restricted to B cells are CD21 and surface Fc and CR1 receptors (**Figure 5.19**). In reality, there

are now several hundred surface membrane molecules expressed by different leucocytes and defined by specific antisera. These molecules are conveniently classified by the CD (**cluster of differentiation**) numbering system and, as we progress through this book, a number of CD molecules will be discussed.

Antisera or monoclonal antibodies specific for surface membrane molecules may be used to tag specific subpopulations of leucocyte while held in liquid suspensions of cells. At the simplest level, the antiserum or monoclonal antibody is chemically conjugated to a fluorochrome (see Chapter 4) and when added to the cell suspension it will selectively bind the cells of interest (**Figure 5.20**). Labelled cells may then

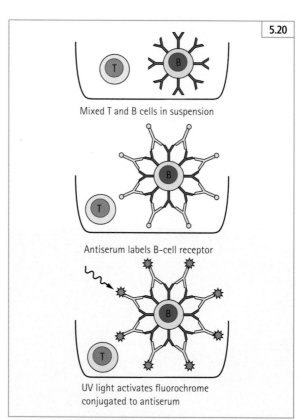

Fig. 5.20 Distinction between T and B cells. T and B cells within a suspension (e.g. blood) may be differentiated by the use of an antiserum or monoclonal antibody raised to one of the molecules depicted in this diagram. Such reagents may be conjugated to a fluorochrome so that when the labelled cell suspension is examined at an appropriate wavelength of light using an ultraviolet microscope, the tagged cells emit fluorescent light.

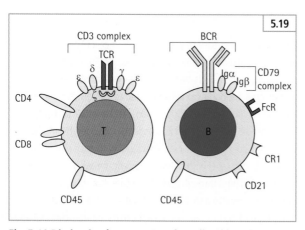

Fig. 5.19 Distinction between T and B cells. Although small and large T and B lymphocytes cannot be distinguished by light microscopy, the expression of surface molecules unique to each cell type allows detection by immunological means. Some molecules (e.g. CD45) are shared by both cells. Some of the key molecules that permit phenotyping of T and B cells are depicted.

be viewed with a fluorescence microscope that emits light of a wavelength able to excite the fluorochrome (**Figure 5.21**). In a more refined procedure, labelled cells may be passed through a **flow cytometer**, which separates the cell suspension into droplets containing individual cells that are 'interrogated' by a laser beam to determine whether fluorescence is emitted. Each fluorescent cell is counted by the machine, which will determine the proportion of labelled cells within the suspension (**Figure 5.22**). Flow cytometers are now able to measure light emitted by multiple fluorochromes conjugated to multiple antisera or monoclonal antibodies, and this enables individual cells to be characterized for their expression of a number of surface membrane or cytoplasmic molecules. Some flow cytometers are also able to sort differentially labelled cells into separate test tubes, which permits subsequent experimental studies of the function of those subpopulations.

A similar immunolabelling process may be used to identify cells within tissue sections. Fluorochrome-labelled antisera or monoclonal antibodies may be overlaid onto tissue sections on a microscope slide and will selectively bind to target molecules expressed by specific cell types (**Figure 5.23**). When viewed with a fluorescence microscope, these cells appear coloured on a black background (the colour determined by the type of fluorochrome used) (**Figure 5.24**). As for flow cytometry, several different antisera or monoclonal

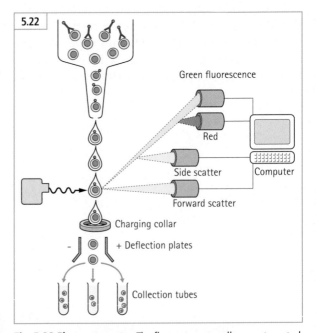

Fig. 5.22 Flow cytometry. The flow cytometer allows automated analysis of mixed populations of lymphocytes in suspension. In this example the cells have been incubated with two separate monoclonal antibodies, one conjugated to a fluorochrome that emits green fluorescence (fluorescein), and another to a different fluorochrome that emits red fluorescence (phycoerythrin). The population contains some cells that label with each reagent and some cells that label with neither. The cells are taken up into the machine and pass through a vibrating chamber, which releases individual cells into a sheath of buffer fluid. Each cell is then 'interrogated' by laser beams (specific to each fluorochrome) and will emit a pulse of light if labelled by the relevant antiserum. The burst of light is recorded and after 10,000 cells are examined, the proportion of the population comprising red or green fluorescent cells is calculated. Some flow cytometers subsequently allow the different populations to become electrically charged as a means of sorting the cells into purified populations that may then be used experimentally.

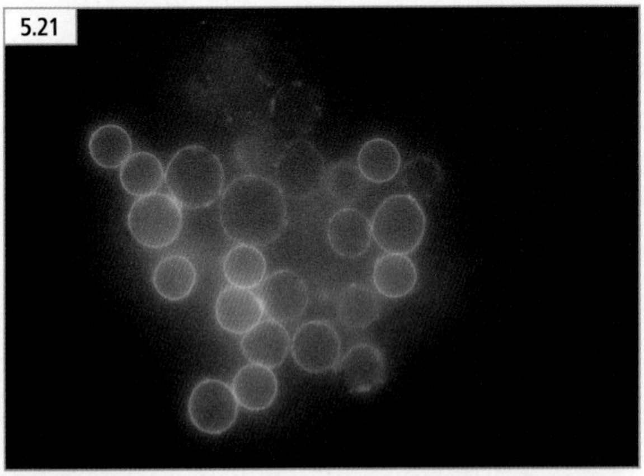

Fig. 5.21 Distinction between T and B cells. The lymphocytes in this image have been labelled with an antiserum specific for a T-cell surface molecule that is conjugated to fluorescein. The image is taken with a camera attached to a microscope that emits light at a wavelength capable of exciting the fluorescein to emit this characteristic apple-green fluorescence.

antibodies conjugated to different fluorochromes may be applied to any one tissue section. An alternative to this technique (known as **immunofluorescence** microscopy) is **immunohistochemical** methodology (**Figure 5.25**). In this method the antiserum or monoclonal antibody is conjugated to an enzyme such that when substrate is added to the section in the presence of a chromogen, there is colour (often brown, blue or red) deposited at the position the cell occupies in the tissue (**Figure 5.26**). Immunohistochemistry allows better understanding of the relationship of labelled cells to the tissue, as the background may be counterstained and the section examined with a standard light microscope.

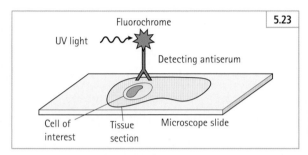

Fig. 5.23 Immunofluorescence microscopy. This technique permits the identification of specific cells or molecules within a histological section of tissue. The section is overlaid with an antiserum or monoclonal antibody specific for the molecule of interest. The reagent is conjugated to a fluorochrome such that when the section is examined under an appropriate wavelength of light there will be localized emission of fluorescent light.

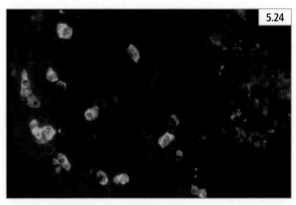

Fig. 5.24 Immunofluorescence microscopy. This section of dog tissue is labelled with a fluorescein-conjugated antiserum specific for IgA. Examination under an ultraviolet microscope reveals the presence of plasma cells containing cytoplasmic IgA within the tissue.

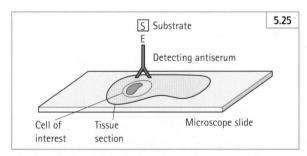

Fig. 5.25 Immunohistochemistry. This technique is as described in **Figure 5.23** for immunofluorescence except that the antiserum is conjugated to an enzyme rather than a fluorochrome. Addition of an appropriate substrate and a chromogen leads to deposition of colour at the site of antibody binding. In this technique the surrounding tissue can be counterstained to evaluate the morphology and the section examined with a standard light microscope.

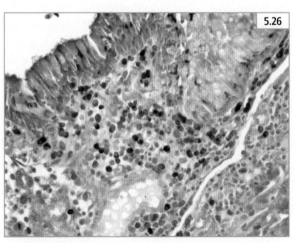

Fig. 5.26 Immunohistochemistry. A section of bronchial mucosa from a dog with allergic respiratory disease labelled for IgA by immunohistochemistry. Numerous plasma cells within the lamina propria have cytoplasmic IgA, and secreted IgA is present on the surface of the overlying epithelial cells.

LYMPHOCYTE RECIRCULATION

The lymphocytes within the body are not static cells that remain in fixed locations in particular areas of lymphoid tissue. In fact, lymphoid cells and other leucocytes move on a very large scale using the pathway shown in **Figure 5.27**. Lymphoid cells may move from tissue to lymph nodes via the **afferent lymph** and may subsequently leave that lymph node in the **efferent lymphatic** vessel. The efferent lymphatic vessel discharges into the common **thoracic duct**, which in turn drains into the blood circulation. The lymphocyte may continue its journey through the closed loop of the blood circulation and may detour through the spleen. Circulating lymphocytes may migrate from the blood into tissue or another lymph node via the mechanisms discussed below. This pathway of movement is referred to as **lymphocyte recirculation**. To give an idea of the scale of this recirculation, in rats 4×10^7 lymphocytes enter the blood from the thoracic duct every hour, such that the entire blood lymphocyte count can be replaced 10–20 times per day.

The question arises as to why it is necessary for lymphocytes to continually undergo this elaborate migratory cycle. In order to address this question it is first necessary to understand a fundamental premise in immunology – the '**clonal selection theory**' first proposed by Macfarlane Burnett in 1957. This theory is based on the concept that although there are vast numbers of lymphocytes within the immune system, each of these cells is virtually unique in terms of its specificity for antigen (i.e. each lymphocyte bears an antigen-specific TCR or BCR that is genetically pre-programmed to interact with one specific antigenic epitope). This model therefore suggests that each individual is endowed with a set of lymphocytes at birth that provides the capacity to cover any potential antigenic insult that an individual might receive throughout his/her lifetime. This is sometimes referred to as the '**repertoire**' of the lymphocytes of the immune system. A corollary of this is that each individual must also carry within the repertoire numerous lymphocytes bearing receptors that may

never be required by that individual. In a nutshell, the clonal selection theory states that when an antigen (that may bear many epitopes) enters the body, the adaptive immune system must select from its repertoire those lymphocytes bearing receptors pre-programmed to interact with those epitopes. As the number of these cells may be relatively low, the second phase of the process involves cloning the activated lymphocytes (one cell division gives rise to two identical daughter cells that in turn each give rise to two further identical cells and so forth) such that a very large number of antigen-specific cells are generated to take part in

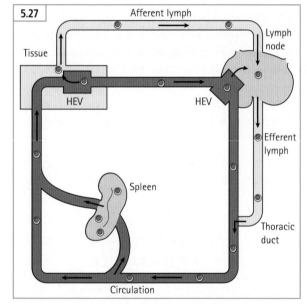

Fig. 5.27 Lymphocyte recirculation. This diagram summarizes the routes by which lymphocytes may move throughout the body. Lymphocytes may leave tissue in afferent lymph and arrive in the regional draining lymph node. The cells may then leave that node via the efferent lymphatic vessel, which connects to the common thoracic duct and then into the blood circulation. While circulating in the blood, the lymphocytes may detour through the spleen or leave to re-enter tissue or lymphoid tissue through specialized high endothelial venules (HEVs).

the immune response to the inciting antigen. Every lymphocyte within the cloned population is identical to the original cell and bears the same antigen receptor molecule (**Figure 5.28**). We shall return to the clonal selection theory in Chapter 8.

Having this knowledge, it is now possible to see that the simple reason why lymphocyte recirculation is required is to maximize the likelihood of those relatively few antigen-specific lymphocytes coming in contact with the antigen that their receptors are designed to interact with (the cognate antigen).

A clinical example can be used to illustrate this point. The puppy shown in **Figure 5.29** has swollen paws due to a local staphylococcal infection (pyoderma). If those lymphocytes with specificity for staphylococcal antigen had permanent residence in the spleen, there would be little chance of contact between antigen and lymphocyte and little hope that the puppy would mount an adaptive immune response. In reality, bacterial antigen is carried to the draining axillary lymph node by APCs (see Chapter 7), which maximizes the opportunity for that

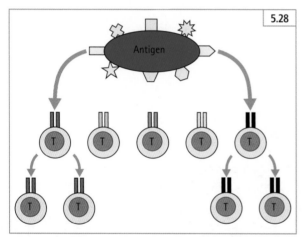

Fig. 5.28 The clonal selection theory. The clonal selection theory proposes that each lymphocyte in the body has unique antigen specificity conferred upon it by expression of a genetically encoded antigen-specific receptor. When a foreign antigen enters the body, the immune system must select from its repertoire those lymphocytes that bear receptors able to interact with epitopes on the antigen. The lymphocytes that are selected must then be clonally expanded by repeated division in order to generate large numbers of identical lymphocytes relevant to that particular antigen.

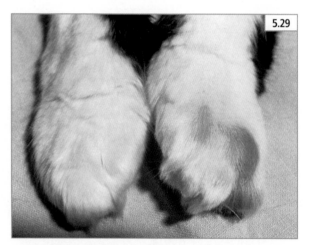

Fig. 5.29 The need for lymphocyte recirculation. This puppy has bacterial infection (pyoderma) of the skin of the digits. Bacterial antigen is carried to the draining axillary lymph node by APCs in order to stimulate those lymphocytes in the immune system repertoire that are pre-programmed to express receptors specific for the organism. These lymphocytes patrol the body in search of antigen and must enter the axillary node in order to initiate the adaptive immune response. If these cells were not mobile and were permanently resident elsewhere (e.g. in the popliteal lymph node), the immune response could never take place.

antigen to encounter different lymphocytes as they migrate through that node (**Figure 5.30**). It may still seem remarkable that such interactions occur, but protective immune responses could not otherwise take place. As discussed in Chapter 1, following antigen stimulation, the cloned army of antigen-specific lymphocytes travels back to the site of infection using the lymphatic–vascular migratory pathway.

This example raises a further question related to lymphocyte recirculation. In the puppy described above, how is it possible that the activated antigen-specific lymphocytes circulating in the blood know that they should leave the circulation through the wall of a blood vessel located in the dermis of the infected foot, and not at any other point within the circulation? The answer to this question lies in the phenomenon of lymphocyte homing.

Lymphocyte homing involves the interaction between two sets of molecules: **homing receptors** expressed on the surface of leucocytes (such as antigen-specific lymphocytes) and **vascular addressins** expressed on the surface of endothelial cells (**Figure 5.31**). These designations (homing receptor and vascular addressin) are simplifications that cover numerous different molecules and their ligands. Vascular addressins literally give the 'address' of the particular portion of the blood circulation that expresses those molecules. Vascular addressins are generally found on the luminal surface of a group of modified cuboidal endothelial cells that protrude into the lumen of the vessel. These cells are known as **high endothelial venules** (HEVs). HEVs may be found throughout the circulation and act a little like stations along a railway track, providing a gateway

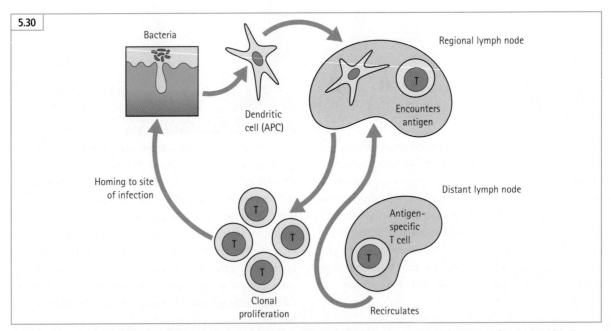

Fig. 5.30 Immune surveillance. This diagram depicts the sequence of events described in **Figure 5.29**. Bacterial antigen within the skin is taken to the regional lymph node by an APC. A lymphocyte able to respond to an epitope on that antigen is currently located within a distant lymph node, but during the course of its subsequent migration it travels through the node of interest and meets the antigen. The adaptive immune response is stimulated and the clonally expanded lymphocytes are sent via lymph and blood back to the tissue site where they are required to fight the infection.

from blood into tissue for circulating leucocytes. In normal individuals, HEVs are often found associated with lymphoid tissue and HEVs may be induced at sites of inflammation such as the skin of the puppy described above. An example of expression of a vascular addressin is shown in **Figure 5.32**.

The ligands for vascular addressins are the homing receptors. Therefore, as an antigen-specific lymphocyte travels through the bloodstream it encounters numerous HEVs. As the HEVs protrude into the flowing blood, they establish local turbulence in blood flow, and this encourages the circulating lymphocytes to bump up against the surface of the HEVs and test whether their homing receptors might be able to bind those vascular addressins. When such an interaction occurs, the circulating lymphocyte slows down and rolls along the endothelial surface as it makes and breaks these molecular bonds. Eventually, the lymphocyte will be halted and it then has the opportunity to squeeze between adjacent endothelial cells (**diapedesis**) or, less commonly, through endothelial cells (**transcellular migration**)

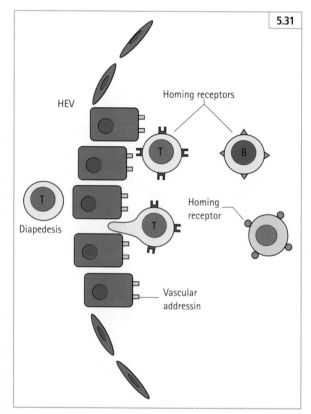

Fig. 5.31 Lymphocyte recirculation. Lymphocytes recirculating within the bloodstream must have the ability to know their location within the circulation and know how to exit the blood for tissue at a specific point where they may be required. Along the length of the circulation are focal regions where the lining endothelial cells take on a cuboidal morphology and protrude into the vessel lumen, creating a region of turbulent flow. These HEVs are also endowed with a series of surface molecules collectively called vascular addressins. Vascular addressins differ between HEVs. Vessels within lymphoid tissue normally express HEVs and these may be induced in tissue undergoing an inflammatory response. Circulating lymphocytes bear ligands for vascular addressins, collectively referred to as homing receptors. Only a lymphocyte bearing a homing receptor for a specific vascular addressin will be able to bind to the HEV and diapedese between endothelial cells into the tissue.

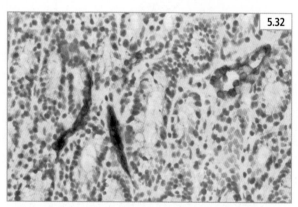

Fig. 5.32 Vascular addressin. This section of canine intestinal mucosa is labelled to show the expression of a vascular addressin molecule by capillary endothelial cells. The 'mucosal addressin cell adhesion molecule' (MAdCAM) is expressed by endothelia at mucosal sites of the body, but not in other tissues, and permits circulating lymphocytes that express the appropriate homing receptor ($\alpha_4\beta_7$) to exit the blood and enter these tissues.

into the tissue matrix (**Figure 5.33**). In this fashion, the lymphocyte might be considered to carry a ticket, which allows it to exit from only one station along the vascular railway.

This model allows us to postulate how lymphocytes might migrate within the body at different stages of their life (**Figure 5.34**). A naïve (virgin) lymphocyte searching for its cognate antigen would want to patrol

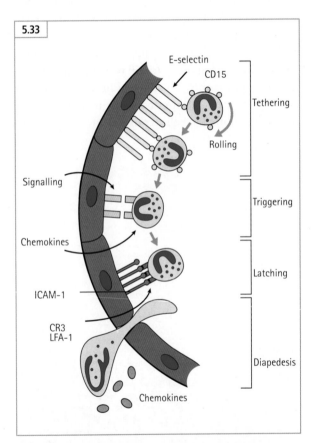

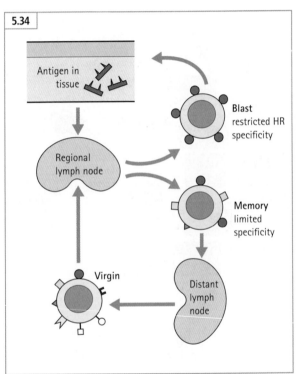

Fig. 5.33 Leucocyte adhesion. The interaction between endothelial cells and leucocytes (including lymphocytes) progresses through several stages. Initially, the leucocyte is 'tethered' loosely by molecular interactions (e.g. E-selectin and CD15) and rolls along the surface of the vessel, making and breaking contact as it slows. Once the cell has stopped rolling, it is activated and then makes a firm attachment ('latching') through interactions with molecules such as ICAM-1 (intercellular adhesion molecule-1). Further molecular interactions allow the leucocyte to diapedese between endothelial cells and enter the tissue. The recruitment of cells from blood to tissue may also involve the action of chemotactic cytokines (chemokines). LFA-1, leucocyte function-associated antigen-1.

Fig. 5.34 Lymphocyte migration during the immune response. This diagram proposes a model that might account for differential mobility of lymphocytes at different stages of their life cycle. A naïve (virgin) lymphocyte that had not previously encountered antigen might have a wide range of homing receptors (HRs), allowing it to access numerous body sites during immune surveillance. Once antigen is encountered, the activated lymphocyte would have HR expression restricted to the tissue in which the antigen is located. This change in HR expression would occur during the process of activation of the adaptive immune response within the regional lymphoid tissue. The memory lymphocytes that persist once the immune response is completed may have a more limited HR expression, permitting the memory cells to access areas that are most likely to be sites of re-encounter with that antigen.

widely throughout the body as it would not know which sites were likely to allow entry of that antigen. Such cells might be considered to hold numerous tickets allowing access to numerous tissue stations. Once the lymphocyte has been activated as part of an adaptive immune response, it may be allowed to carry only a single ticket on its journey from the lymph node in which it encountered antigen. This would ensure that the cell arrived back into the tissue where it was required to mediate an effector immune response. It is believed that this specificity is 'imprinted' on the lymphocyte during the process of activation within the lymphoid tissue draining that specific anatomical site. Finally, after the immune response has finished, the population of residual memory lymphocytes might be allowed to carry a more restricted set of tickets, as these cells might only wish to access those tissues in which they know they are most likely to re-encounter their cognate antigen.

MUCOSAL LYMPHOCYTE RECIRCULATION

One particular example of selective lymphocyte recirculation is that related to the mucosal immune system. Although there is clear specificity in recirculation of lymphocytes activated by mucosal antigen (e.g. cells induced in GALT by exposure to enteric antigen will preferentially recirculate to the effector sites of the intestinal lamina propria), it is also possible for activated cells to migrate to other mucosal sites of the body. In order for this to be possible, there must be sharing of some common vascular addressins, thereby permitting a lymphocyte activated in the context of one mucosal site (e.g. in response to an enteric infection with *Escherichia coli*) to access not only the intestinal tissue where the effector response is required, but also the mucosae of the respiratory tract, urogenital tract, eye and mammary gland (**Figure 5.35**). For domestic animals this system has very particular relevance, as it permits lymphocytes with memory of enteric and respiratory pathogens to localize in the mammary gland and play a role in the generation of antibodies in milk, which mediate protection of the neonate from infectious disease (see Chapter 18).

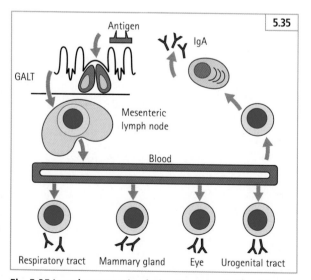

Fig. 5.35 Lymphocyte recirculation to mucosal sites. A lymphocyte activated by an enteric pathogen within the inductive site of GALT would be expected to recirculate to the intestine to participate in the effector immune response (e.g. IgA production). However, some of these antigen-specific cells might also enter other mucosal tissues. The greatest relevance of this pathway is to permit antigen-specific cells from the gut and respiratory tract to enter the mammary gland and contribute to the passive transfer of immunity to vulnerable neonates.

KEY POINTS

- All lymphocytes arise from the bone marrow stem cell.
- B-cell maturation occurs in the avian bursa of Fabricius and in other anatomical locations in mammals.
- T-cell maturation occurs in the thymus.
- B cells mediate humoral immunity.
- T cells undertake CMI.
- T and B cells compartmentalize in lymphoid tissue.
- The spleen has no lymphatic drainage, but is continuous with the blood circulation.
- T and B cells may be morphologically small lymphocytes (naïve or memory cells) or lymphoblasts (active).
- Plasma cells are a terminal stage of B-cell differentiation.
- Plasma cells secrete immunoglobulin.
- T and B cells carry unique surface molecules that allow their detection with antisera by flow cytometry, tissue immunofluorescence or immunohistochemistry.

- Lymphocytes continually recirculate throughout the body via lymphatic and blood vessels.
- The clonal selection theory suggests that lymphocytes have genetically determined antigen specificity and must be selected for clonal expansion when required.
- Lymphocyte recirculation allows immune surveillance of the body for antigen.
- Lymphocytes know their location in the blood circulation because of the expression of vascular addressins by HEVs that interact with lymphocyte homing receptors.
- Recirculation of antigen-specific lymphocytes from the gut and respiratory tract to the mammary gland contributes to the development of passively acquired immunity for neonatal animals.

The Major Histocompatibility Complex

INTRODUCTION

This chapter introduces a key set of immunological molecules encoded by a linked set of genes known as the **major histocompatibility complex**. The primary importance of these molecules is in the phenomenon of **antigen presentation**, which will be discussed in Chapter 7. Here we consider the biology of the molecules and their encoding genes, the important role of these molecules in tissue transplantation and their association with phenotypic traits such as disease susceptibility.

GRAFT REJECTION

Transplantation of organs (e.g. kidney, liver, heart, heart and lungs) or cells (e.g. bone marrow) has had huge impact on medical science over the past decades. Tissue transplantation may take one of several forms. **Autografts** (e.g. transplantation of skin from one area of the body to another) and **isografts** (transplantation between genetically identical individuals) are generally very successful as there is perfect matching between the donor and recipient. The most widely practised form of transplantation is **allografting** in which cells or tissue from a closely matched, but still genetically dissimilar, donor are transplanted into a recipient. The success of allografting is increased by obtaining the closest possible match between the tissues of donor and recipient. It is for this reason that national or international registers are kept to allow rapid shipment of organs as they become available. Rejection of allografts may also be controlled by treatment of recipients with potent immunosuppressive medical protocols. The use of **xenografts** (transplantation of cells or tissue from one species into another) is widely investigated, particularly the potential for the use of pigs as donors. Reservations about cross-species transmission of uncharacterized infectious agents (e.g. retroviruses) have slowed development in this area.

Although much of the basis for human transplantation surgery was first defined experimentally in porcine and canine models, this procedure has limited application in modern veterinary medicine. Canine and feline kidney transplantation is carried out in some US centres and bone marrow transplantation has been performed in individual cases. However, questions of ethics have limited such practices in other countries. Despite this, an understanding of the process of graft rejection is important, as this is an immunological event that has bearing on knowledge of fundamental aspects of immunology. What determines the 'tissue type' in a transplant and what mediates the immunological rejection of incompatible donor tissue is a group of molecules known collectively as **major histocompatibility antigens**. It is these molecules that must be closely matched for a successful donor–recipient pairing but, more than this, these histocompatibility molecules are of prime importance in the generation of the adaptive immune response.

The basis for graft rejection is summarized in **Figure 6.1**. Any tissue or organ will contain a resident population of **'passenger' leucocytes** of donor origin that are very difficult to remove entirely from that tissue. After transplantation, donor leucocytes may migrate out of the donor tissue into afferent lymphatics and thus to regional lymph nodes. Either these leucocytes or recipient APCs that have taken up shed donor antigen will activate alloreactive

lymphocytes within that lymphoid tissue. Activated **alloreactive T and B lymphocytes** leave the lymph node in efferent lymph and home to the site of the transplanted tissue, where they may mediate graft rejection. A variety of immunological factors, including antibody, complement and cytotoxic T and NK cells, are involved in this process. The alloreactive immune response may target the graft vasculature (leading to **ischaemic necrosis** of the graft) or result in **cytotoxic destruction** of grafted cells. Graft rejection may be **peracute** (in an immunologically sensitized individual), **acute** (days to weeks) or **chronic** (months to years) in nature.

In a **recipient who is highly immunosuppressed** it is also possible for the reverse scenario to occur – the donor leucocytes may attack the defenceless tissue of the recipient in a process known as **graft-versus-host disease (GVHD)**. GVHD may arise when donor lymphocytes in transplanted bone marrow infiltrate a range of recipient tissues. GVHD is recognized in some immunosuppressed dogs following bone marrow transplantation, where it manifests clinically as erythematous and exudative skin lesions, mucous membrane inflammation, jaundice, diarrhoea and Coombs-positive haemolytic anaemia.

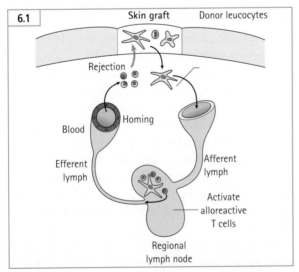

Fig. 6.1 Graft rejection. Passenger leucocytes within a graft or donor histocompatibility antigens enter afferent lymphatics and travel to regional lymphoid tissue where alloreactive T and B lymphocytes are activated. These cells home to the site of the graft and mediate graft rejection by attacking the vascular supply to the graft tissue (causing ischaemic necrosis) or infiltrating the graft, leading to cytotoxic destruction of graft cells.

MAJOR HISTOCOMPATIBILITY ANTIGENS

The major histocompatibility antigens responsible for the events described above are very well characterized and in broad terms fall into one of two classes. These antigens are transmembrane molecules, which are expressed on the cell surface, anchoring into the cell membrane with a cytoplasmic tail (**Figure 6.2**). **Class I** histocompatibility antigens have two chains – a longer **α chain** paired with a short chain known as the **β_2 microglobulin**. The α chain has three extracellular domains known as α_1, α_2 and α_3. Class I histocompatibility molecules are expressed on all **nucleated cells** of the body. **Class II** histocompatibility antigens comprise two transmembrane chains, an **α chain** with two extracellular domains (α_1 and α_2) and a **β chain** with two similar domains (β_1 and β_2). Class II antigens have a more restricted cellular distribution, being normally located on the surface of **immune cells**, including macrophages, dendritic cells and lymphocytes (particularly B cells), but they are inducible on the surface of an array of epithelial and stromal cells. The β_2 microglobulin and α_3 domain of class I molecules and the α_2 and β_2 domains of class II molecules have a relatively **conserved amino acid**

sequence from one class I or II molecule to another. In contrast, the α_1 and α_2 domains of class I, and the α_1 and β_1 domains of class II molecules have much greater **variation in their amino acid sequence**. This basic structural arrangement is very similar to that described in Chapter 2 for the heavy and light chains of immunoglobulin. In fact, the constant domains of immunoglobulins, histocompatibility antigens and a number of other key immune molecules are all related to each other, and these molecules are considered part of the '**immunoglobulin superfamily**'. As discussed in Chapter 1, this relatedness in immune molecules arose during evolution through the process of gene duplication.

THE MAJOR HISTOCOMPATIBILITY COMPLEX

The genes encoding the protein histocompatibility antigens are clustered together in one area of the genome known as the **major histocompatibility complex**. Every species has an MHC, although it is located in different chromosomal regions in different species. As histocompatibility antigens were initially characterized on leucocytes, the MHC is also

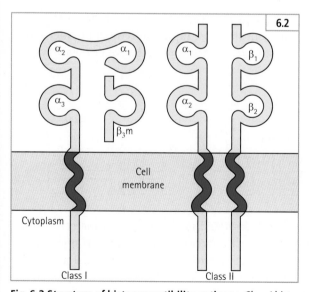

Fig. 6.2 Structure of histocompatibility antigens. Class I histocompatibility antigens comprise an α chain with three globular domains (α_1, α_2 and α_3) and an associated β_2 microglobulin. Class II histocompatibility antigens consist of an α and β chain each having two globular domains.

known as the **'leucocyte antigen' system** and this nomenclature is used to describe the MHC of different species as the human leucocyte antigen (HLA) system, dog leucocyte antigen (DLA) system, feline leucocyte antigen (FLA) system, equine leucocyte antigen (ELA) system, bovine leucocyte antigen (BoLA) system, ovine leucocyte antigen (OLA) system, swine leucocyte antigen (SLA) system and so on.

The HLA and murine (H2) systems are best characterized and genetic maps that show the arrangement of the genes within the complex are available (**Figure 6.3**). Maps of animal MHC regions are now emerging and reveal a high level of conservation with some species differences. There are three regions of the MHC described in most species. The centromeric **class II region** encodes the class II histocompatibility antigen α and β chains. These genes are described as 'D region' genes and are named by the suffix 'D'. For example, in the dog, the key class II genes recognized to date are *DLA-DRB1*, *DLA-DQA1* and *DLA-DQB1*. There are two further nonfunctional pseudogenes in this area, *DLA-DQB2* and *DLA-DRB2*. Of comparative interest is that the cat stands alone in having a deletion of the DQ region. The telomeric **class I region** encodes the class I genes. The most important of these in humans are known as A, B and C. In contrast, there are four canine class I genes recognized (*DLA 1-12*, *DLA 1-64*, *DLA 1-79* and *DLA 1-88*). Sandwiched between the class I and class II regions is a series of **class III region** genes.

These genes do not encode classical histocompatibility antigens, but an array of **other immunologically relevant molecules** including some complement factors (C2, C4 and Factor B) and the cytokine tumour necrosis factor (TNF). Their inclusion within the MHC is again probably a quirk of evolution whereby a genetic recombination event led to incorporation of this set of genes in this chromosomal region. Similarly, the presence of a number of class I and class II genes within the complex probably reflects a series of gene duplication events throughout evolution, mediated by pressure to develop greater complexity within the immune system (see Chapter 1).

A unique feature of the canine (DLA) and feline (FLA) MHC is that the gene complex is split between two chromosomal areas. In the dog, class I, II and III genes are located on chromosome 12, with the remainder of the MHC on chromosome 35. Feline class I, II and III genes are on the long arm of chromosome B2, while the remainder of the complex lies on the short arm of chromosome 2. That part of the MHC on distant chromosomes includes a segment of DNA encoding some of the *TRIM* (tripartite motif) genes through to genes encoding olfactory receptors. This genetic event must have occurred before the evolutionary divergence of dogs and cats 55 million years ago.

A particular feature of MHC genes is that they represent the most **highly polymorphic** loci within the genome. That is to say, it is possible for a very large

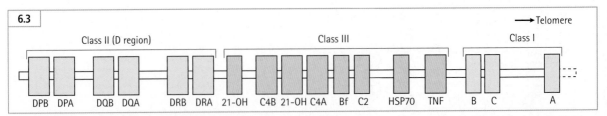

Fig. 6.3 The major histocompatibility complex. A simple genetic map of the human MHC is shown and the arrangement is likely to be similar in most animal species. The D region genes encode α and β chains of class II molecules, whereas the A, B and C genes encode class I molecules. Caught up between these areas of the MHC are the class III genes that encode a range of immunological molecules not directly related to tissue type. The inclusion of this group of genes probably represents a genetic recombination event during evolution.

number of different alleles to be encoded by any one locus to give the allotype of any individual human or animal. To give an approximate idea of this genetic diversity, for human class I genes there may be 50–200 possible alleles and for class II Dβ genes in the order of 20–70 alleles are recognized. In the dog, the current degree of polymorphism recognized amongst class II genes is 31 *DLA-DQA1* alleles, 90 *DLA-DQB1* alleles and 144 *DLA-DRB1* alleles. Again, the development of increasing polymorphism of each locus throughout evolution conferred an advantage on the evolving species in the ability of those species to successfully mount immune responses to evolving pathogens.

THE INHERITANCE OF MHC

Each individual human or animal has two complete sets of MHC molecules (**haplotypes**), one on each of the paternally and maternally derived chromosomes. The MHC genes are **co-dominantly expressed** such that no one gene is dominant or recessive to another. Therefore, in each individual human there are six MHC class I genes (an A, B and C on each chromosome) and each of these genes is transcribed such that any nucleated cell carries six different class I antigens, each one of a single allotype (**Figure 6.4**). In the case of class II genes, greater diversity is possible as different α and β chains may pair to give distinct class II products. Coupled with the knowledge that only one of a relatively large number of alleles is present at any one locus, it is possible to see that the range of MHC genes inherited by any one individual is almost unique and explains the difficulty in tissue matching between individuals in a population.

The stretches of chromosomal DNA containing the MHC are **usually inherited in their entirety** ('*en bloc*') such that a complete haplotype passes to the offspring from the maternal and paternal MHC (**Figure 6.5**). Rarely, minor **recombination events** may occur between the paternal and maternal

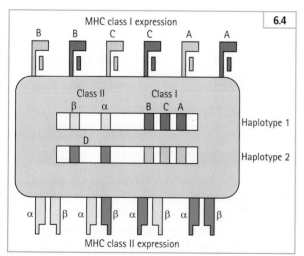

Fig. 6.4 Expression of histocompatibility antigens. Each individual has two sets of MHC genes (haplotypes) inherited on the paternal and maternal chromosomes. Products from these genes are co-dominantly expressed. In the example shown, this cell expresses six different MHC class I proteins and several different class II molecules created by differential combination of D region α and β genes.

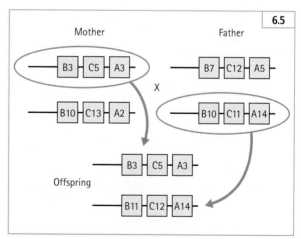

Fig. 6.5 Inheritance of MHC genes. In most individuals, MHC genes are inherited in *en bloc* fashion. In this example the three human class I genes are shown for simplicity. The offspring inherits one set of genes from each parental haplotype.

chromosomes before inheritance and this can create further diversity in the MHC (**Figure 6.6**). Because of the *en bloc* inheritance of the MHC, these molecules are inherited within a family by simple **Mendelian genetics (Figure 6.7)**. This means that within a family there is a theoretical one in four chance that two siblings might share MHC type and therefore be an appropriate donor–recipient pairing in the context of transplantation.

A useful analogy for thinking about the inheritance of these gene products is to consider the MHC as a pack of 52 playing cards with four separate loci correlating to the four suits. Each number or picture card within a suit represents a possible allele at that locus. In compiling the MHC haplotype of an individual, a single card (allele) is selected from each suit (locus) and the final hand of cards represents the MHC type of that individual. The large number of

possible permutations and combinations in this model is consistent with that which occurs within the MHC (**Figures 6.8a, b**).

Although the concepts surrounding the MHC are complex, a clear understanding of this area is important. Here we have focussed on the role of these molecules in mediating graft rejection, but they play a much more fundamental and important role in immunity and this will be discussed in Chapter 7.

MHC–DISEASE ASSOCIATIONS

In human medicine it was recognized many years ago that individuals who inherited particular MHC allotypes appeared to have a greater risk of developing particular immune-mediated or infectious diseases. When the inheritance of combinations of alleles (haplotypes) is considered, these associations are

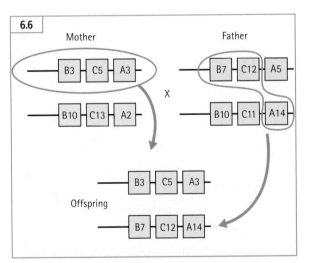

Fig. 6.6 Inheritance of MHC genes. In this example there is a simple recombination event before inheritance of the paternal haplotype, creating a subtly different MHC type in the offspring.

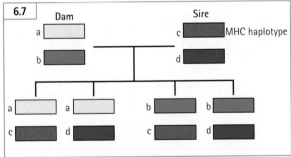

Fig. 6.7 Inheritance of MHC genes. Assuming *en-bloc* inheritance, MHC genes are inherited within a family by simple Mendelian genetics. This means that there is a theoretical one in four chance of any two siblings within a family sharing tissue type and being suitable donors for each other in case of the need for a transplant.

significantly stronger. The alleles within these disease-associated haplotypes frequently occur together in susceptible individuals and are said to be in '**linkage disequilibrium**'. The products of these susceptibility alleles may have a direct role in the pathogenesis of disease, or these haplotypes might simply serve as a marker for other genes that are more directly involved in the disease process. In contrast, other haplotypes may confer resistance, rather than susceptibility, to a particular disease state.

In such '**disease association**' studies, one would typically examine a population of affected individuals and a control group of clinically normal individuals. If a particular MHC allele or combination of alleles is found with higher frequency in the diseased population, then the statistical **odds ratio** can be calculated to indicate the relative risk of developing the disease if an individual inherited that particular MHC type.

As dogs develop a range of immune-mediated diseases very similar to those of humans, investigation of possible MHC–disease associations in this species has been ongoing since the 1970s. Recent molecular advances in the ability to rapidly 'tissue type' large numbers of dogs has led to dramatic developments in this area of science. Clear linkage has been shown between the inheritance of particular DLA haplotypes and the susceptibility or resistance to canine rheumatoid arthritis, immune-mediated haemolytic anaemia (IMHA), diabetes mellitus, lymphocytic thyroiditis, Addison's disease (hypoadrenocorticism), chronic hepatitis in Dobermanns, necrotizing meningoencephalitis, anal furunculosis, chronic superficial keratitis and leishmaniosis. To give a simple example, one study examined a population of 107 German shepherd dogs with anal furunculosis and 196 control German shepherd dogs without disease. Both groups had similar expression of the class II allele

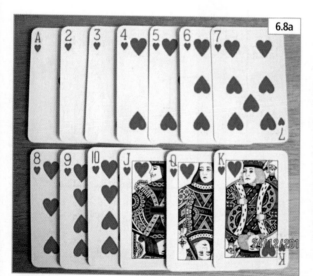
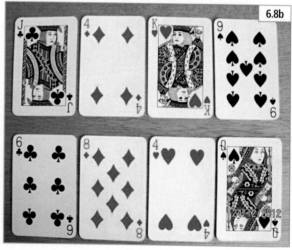

Figs. 6.8a, b Inheritance of MHC genes. A useful analogy for MHC inheritance is the pack of playing cards. (**a**) The four suits each represent a gene or locus at which there are 12 possible alleles. (**b**) The two hands of cards represent the MHC type of two individuals who have inherited different combinations of alleles from each locus. These individuals would be incompatible as a donor–recipient pair for transplantation.

DRB1*00102, but significantly more of the disease group expressed the allele *DRB1*00101*, with a very high odds ratio of 5.01 (**Figures 6.9, 6.10**).

OTHER APPLICATIONS OF TISSUE TYPING

As discussed above, the investigation of genetic susceptibility and resistance to disease has great relevance to veterinary medicine. Although most advanced for the dog, similar studies are being conducted for diseases in other species. For example, MHC links are proposed for susceptibility to bovine leukaemia virus and feline coronavirus infections, Marek's disease in chickens, muscular dystrophy in sheep and allergic disease and laminitis in the horse. In reality, MHC typing is unlikely to become commonplace for the purposes of refining transplantation medicine in veterinary species. The renal transplants that are currently performed are matched simply for blood group, although it would be entirely feasible to tissue type for MHC haplotype. A more important role for MHC typing in veterinary

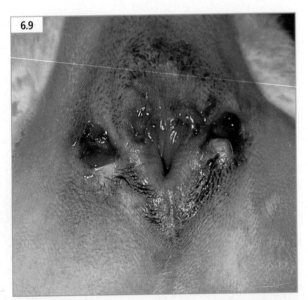

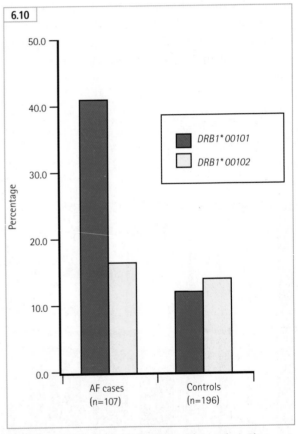

Figs. 6.9, 6.10 MHC disease association. (**6.9**) The perianal region of a German shepherd dog (GSD) with anal furunculosis. There is a region of ulceration and inflammation dorsal to the anus and bilaterally there are two ulcers that extend into the tissue as sinus tracts. GSDs have a particular predisposition for this disease (**6.10**) This graph displays the prevalence of two MHC *DRB1* class II alleles in populations of affected and unaffected dogs. The overrepresentation of allele *DRB1*00101* in the diseased population is highly significant. Inheritance of this allele by a GSD confers an odds ratio of 5.01 for development of the disease. (Data from Kennedy LJ *et al.* (2007) Risk of anal furunculosis in German shepherd dogs is associated with the major histocompatibility complex. *Tissue Antigens* **71**:51–56.)

medicine relates to the **identification** of individual animals. MHC type provides an unalterable means of identifying an animal for registration purposes and a means of determining the paternity of specific offspring. Indeed, MHC typing has already been used in legal cases where the blood line of pedigree dogs was at question. Of greater practical relevance is that MHC type is not simply linked to the development of disease but, for domestic livestock, may be associated with **production traits** such as meat or milk production or resistance to parasitism. Selection of stock on the basis of MHC type might be used to enhance economic output. Examples of such associations include linkage between MHC type and resistance of cattle to *Boophilus* ticks and infection by *Theileria*, resistance to intestinal endoparasitism in sheep, egg production in chickens and a range of parameters (piglet mortality, sow fertility, litter size, growth rate and carcase characteristics) in the pig. Recent intriguing studies have also shown that MHC type may be involved in the **selection of breeding partners** and be related to specific olfactory stimuli that indicate an optimal (different) MHC background in a potential mate. These studies were performed in mice and demonstrated that small peptides bound to MHC class I molecules are excreted in the urine. The peptides become detached from the MHC molecules and bind to receptors expressed by olfactory neurons within the vomeronasal organ. Several pheromone olfactory receptors are also encoded within the class I region of the MHC of some species, suggesting that MHC type may influence odour recognition and mate selection.

KEY POINTS

- Major histocompatibility antigens mediate graft rejection via the activation of alloreactive T and B lymphocytes in the recipient.
- GVHD may occur in highly immunosuppressed recipients of graft tissue containing viable donor leucocytes.
- Major histocompatibility class I antigens comprise an α chain and a β_2 microglobulin and are found on all nucleated cells of the body.
- Major histocompatibility class II antigens comprise an α and β chain and are mostly expressed by immune cells.
- Major histocompatibility molecules are part of the immunoglobulin superfamily.
- Major histocompatibility antigens are encoded by the MHC.
- The MHC comprises class I, II and III gene regions.
- MHC genes are the most highly polymorphic in the genome.
- MHC gene products are co-dominantly inherited.
- Due to polymorphism, MHC type is almost unique in individuals of an unrelated population.
- MHC haplotypes are inherited *en bloc*.
- MHC is inherited within a family by simple Mendelian genetics.
- There are associations between MHC type and the susceptibility or resistance of immune-mediated or infectious disease in man and other animals.
- In veterinary medicine MHC type may be used for identification purposes and can be associated with production traits in livestock.

Antigen Presentation and Cytokines

OBJECTIVES

At the end of this chapter you should be able to:
- Understand why antigen processing and presentation are required to initiate the adaptive immune response.
- Describe the different populations of dendritic cells in the body.
- Understand the differences between a dendritic cell and a macrophage.
- Define 'endogenous' and 'exogenous' antigen.
- Describe the antigen processing and presentation pathway for endogenous and exogenous antigens.
- Define 'pathogen-associated molecular pattern' and 'pattern recognition receptor'

and explain the role of these molecules in the immune response.
- Explain how events occurring within the innate immune system can determine the outcome of the ensuing adaptive immune response.
- Describe the role of the CD1 family of molecules in antigen presentation.
- Explain the circumstances under which antigen might be presented by B lymphocytes or non-professional antigen presenting cells.
- Define the role of cytokines as a means of intercellular communication in the immune system.

INTRODUCTION

This chapter addresses the transition stage between the innate and adaptive immune responses – that of antigen presentation. Previously we have considered how foreign antigen entering the body must be translocated from the site of entry to regional lymphoid tissue for initiation of the adaptive immune response, and how this process is largely mediated by **antigen presenting cells** (APCs) such as the **dendritic cell**. This action of APCs may be considered to occur in three stages:
- **Antigen uptake**.
- **Antigen processing**.
- **Antigen presentation**.

The end effect of this process is conversion of a large and complex antigenic structure into a 'user friendly' form for the adaptive immune system.

ANTIGEN PRESENTING CELLS

There are three types of APCs: **'professional'** and **'non-professional'** APCs and **'induced'** APCs. Professional APCs are purpose-designed for this role and include dendritic cells, macrophages and B lymphocytes. The most important of this group are the dendritic cells that mediate activation of a primary adaptive immune response in a naïve host who has not previously been exposed to the triggering antigen. Dendritic cells are considered much more potent than macrophages in this respect. Dendritic cells are named due to their octopus-like morphology. They are characterized by having multiple elongate cytoplasmic processes (dendrites), which may extend between cells in the surrounding matrix and provide a large surface area for contact with potential antigen.

Several subtypes of dendritic cells have now been defined. Dendritic cells are broadly divided into **conventional** and **non-conventional** groups. Conventional dendritic cells arise from a bone marrow dendritic cell progenitor (or pre-dendritic cell) and include two subcategories: **migratory** and **lymphoid** dendritic cells. Migratory dendritic cells are widely distributed in body tissues (e.g. in the intestine, liver, lung, kidney and dermis of the skin) where they capture antigen and migrate to regional lymphoid tissue in order to induce adaptive immune responses. In contrast, lymphoid dendritic cells remain within lymph nodes, but are also important in the induction of T-cell responses.

Non-conventional dendritic cells include two further subcategories: **plasmacytoid** and **monocyte-derived** dendritic cells. Plasmacytoid dendritic cells have a pre-dendritic cell origin and are found in both lymphoid and non-lymphoid organs (e.g. liver and lung). Plasmacytoid dendritic cells can migrate and are an important source of interferon production during viral infection. Monocyte-derived dendritic cells are widely distributed in tissues (e.g. intestine, liver, lung, kidney, dermis and epidermis of the skin) from where they take up antigen and migrate to regional lymphoid tissue. The **Langerhans cells** of the epidermis are monocyte-derived dendritic cells.

Dendritic cells are particularly prominent at body surfaces likely to come into contact with foreign antigen. The epidermal **Langerhans cell** is perfectly located to be able to interact with antigens that might penetrate into this barrier (**Figure 7.1**). Dendritic cells are also prominent in the airways (**Figure 7.2**) and intestinal tract (**Figure 7.3**) and in the latter

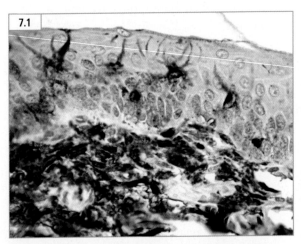

Fig. 7.1 Langerhans cells. Langerhans cells are the dendritic cells that reside in the epidermis of skin and are a first point of contact with antigen that penetrates this cutaneous barrier. Note the long cytoplasmic processes that arise from these cells and insinuate between keratinocytes. These cells are labelled to show that they express MHC class II antigens. (From Carter J, Crispin SM, Gould DJ *et al.* (2005) An immunohistochemical study of uveodermatologic syndrome in two Japanese Akita dogs. *Veterinary Ophthalmology* 8:17–24, with permission.)

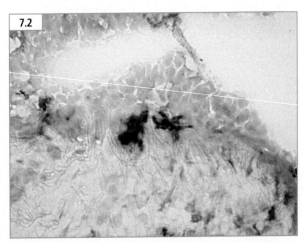

Fig. 7.2 Airway dendritic cells. These dendritic cells lie within the epithelial lining of the canine bronchus and are well positioned to be able to sample inhaled antigen that penetrates this epithelial barrier. These cells are labelled to show expression of the CD1 antigen presenting molecule.

location these cells are known to be able to extend their dendrites between enterocytes to 'sample' antigen passing through the intestinal lumen. Once dendritic cells have captured antigen, they must carry this to the regional lymphoid tissue via the afferent lymphatics. While in these lymphatic vessels, the cells undergo a morphological transformation whereby the cytoplasmic dendrites are replaced by broader and shorter cytoplasmic projections known as 'veils' (**'veiled dendritic cells'**). Once the cells have arrived in the lymph node they localize to the paracortex and revert to a dendritic morphology in order to optimize their contact with T lymphocytes (**Figure 7.4**).

Dendritic cells do not leave the lymph node in efferent lymph.

A specific population of **follicular dendritic cells** is located within the B-cell follicles of the lymph node. These cells are not bone-marrow derived and unlike the dendritic cells described above, they are non-phagocytic. Instead, these cells capture immune complexes of antigen and antibody on their surface and shed them in the form of bead-like structures (iccosomes), which are taken up by B cells that process and present the antigen to T cells. Follicular dendritic cells may act as a reservoir of antigen that may persist for many months on the cell surface in this form.

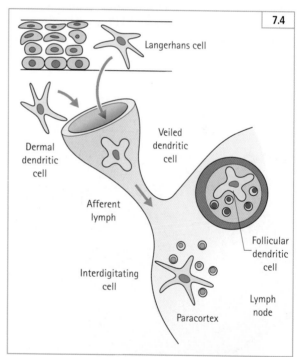

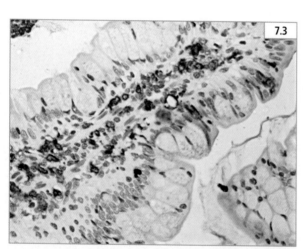

Fig. 7.3 Intestinal dendritic cells. The dendritic cells within the lamina propria of this intestinal villus are labelled to show expression of MHC class II. Some linear labelling is also present within the enterocyte layer and this likely represents the extension of dendritic processes through this barrier to sample luminal antigen. (From Waly N, Gruffydd Jones TJ, Stokes CR *et al.* (2001) The distribution of leucocyte subsets in the small intestine of normal cats. *Journal of Comparative Pathology* **124**:172–82, with permission.)

Fig. 7.4 Dendritic cell migration. Dendritic cells carry antigen from the site of entry into the body to the regional lymphoid tissue in order to activate the adaptive immune response. In the skin, both epidermal Langerhans cells and dermal dendritic cells may migrate in afferent lymph to the local lymph node. During migration the cell undergoes a morphological change to become a 'veiled' dendritic cell. In the lymph node, the cell transforms again to become an interdigitating dendritic cell within the paracortex. A separate population of follicular dendritic cells resides within the follicle.

Macrophages are also widespread throughout the tissues of the body and again are well-represented at mucocutaneous barriers. For example, within the alveoli of the lungs, a population of alveolar macrophages is responsible for phagocytosis of particulate debris that might evade filtration by the barriers of the upper respiratory tract. Within the liver, the sinusoidal **Kupffer cells** are also considered macrophage-like and have a similar role in collecting antigen from the circulating blood. Macrophages are large cells (15–30 µm) with an oval to kidney-shaped nucleus and plentiful cytoplasm that expands and becomes vacuolated when the cells are 'activated' (**Figures 7.5** and **7.6**). Activated macrophages may fuse together to form very large **multinucleated giant cells** that are characteristic in chronic inflammatory lesions. The role of B lymphocytes as APCs and the non-professional APCs will be discussed later in this chapter.

ANTIGEN UPTAKE

Antigens may generally be considered as one of two main types. The vast majority of antigens are '**exogenous**' foreign antigens that must be actively taken up into cytoplasmic endosomes of the APC. Exogenous antigens come from the wide array of infectious agents (e.g. bacteria, viruses, fungi, protozoa, helminths) or environmental substances (e.g. pollens, dust mites, foodstuff) to which the body is exposed. In contrast, an '**endogenous**' antigen is one that is already found within the cytoplasm of the APC (i.e. does not require active phagocytosis). Endogenous antigens include self-antigens (autoantigens), tumour antigens, alloantigens and viral antigens derived from the expression of viral proteins during virus replication in the cytoplasm of an infected cell.

There was once a belief that the uptake of exogenous antigens by the APC by **phagocytosis**,

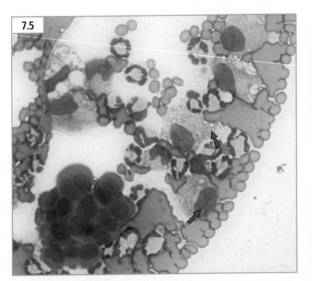

Fig. 7.5 Macrophages. The dominant cell type within this sample of abdominal fluid from a cat with feline infectious peritonitis (FIP) is an activated macrophage with abundant and finely vacuolated cytoplasm (examples arrowed). Some of these cells also have phagocytosed erythrocytes. Neutrophils and a cluster of mesothelial lining cells are also present.

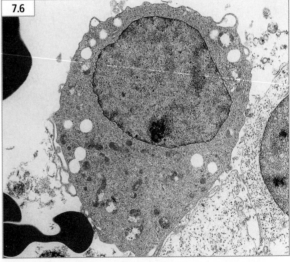

Fig. 7.6 Macrophage ultrastructure. This is a transmission electron microscope image of a canine macrophage showing the abundance of cytoplasm and the presence of a number of cytoplasmic compartments. Foreign antigen is incorporated into these compartments for degradation.

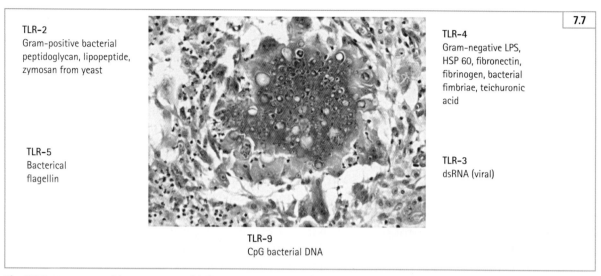

TLR-2
Gram-positive bacterial peptidoglycan, lipopeptide, zymosan from yeast

TLR-5
Bacterical flagellin

TLR-9
CpG bacterial DNA

TLR-4
Gram-negative LPS, HSP 60, fibronectin, fibrinogen, bacterial fimbriae, teichuronic acid

TLR-3
dsRNA (viral)

Fig. 7.7 Pattern recognition receptors. This figure gives examples of some of the key PRRs or TLRs and the PAMPs to which they bind. The central image shows a granulomatous inflammatory reaction, with multinucleate giant cells, surrounding a colony of fungal elements within the skin of a cat with mycotic dermatitis. The interaction of these fungi with APCs would involve PAMP–PRR binding.

pinocytosis or **macropinocytosis** was a relatively non-specific event that might be enhanced by the process of opsonization (see Chapter 3). It is now known that the interaction between antigen and APC has some specificity and involves molecular interactions between a family of receptors on the surface of the APC and ligands expressed by the antigen. The signalling events triggered by these molecular interactions are so significant that they determine how the APC will activate the adaptive immune response and which elements of adaptive immunity will be stimulated. This concept recognizes that the innate immune response, once considered relatively simplistic and primitive, actually directs the outcome of the adaptive response.

The APC, and in particular the dendritic cell, therefore carries a series of receptor molecules, which are collectively known as '**pattern recognition receptors**' (PRRs). Some of these receptors are also known as '**Toll-like receptors**' (TLRs), as the first recognized of these molecules was 'Toll', which is a receptor found in the fruit fly *Drosophila*. The PRRs interact with ligands associated with foreign antigens that are collectively known as '**pathogen-associated molecular patterns**' (PAMPs). More recently, alternative nomenclature has been proposed to encompass the fact that other antigens (in addition to pathogenic organisms) might interact with dendritic

cells in this fashion. Antigens from the commensal microbiota have similar interactions and so the term '**microorganism-associated molecular patterns**' (MAMPs) is more appropriate than PAMPs. Antigens associated with damaged or dying host cells (**damage-associated molecular patterns**; DAMPs) may also interact with the same range of PRRs, alerting the immune system to tissue damage (so called '**danger signals**').

The PRRs are molecules that are highly conserved throughout evolution such that similar receptors are found in plants, insects and mammals. Indeed, a number of such receptors are identified in domestic animals and their expression has now been studied in several disease states. The TLRs are best characterized, and there are at least ten of these molecules in those animal species examined (e.g. TLR-1 to TLR-10 in man and cattle, TLR-1 to TLR-9 and TLR-11 to TLR-13 in mice). The PAMPs with which these receptors interact are also relatively conserved molecules that are present in most organisms and are stable in structure and not readily altered antigenically by those organisms. PAMPs include a range of carbohydrate, protein, lipid and nucleic acid units. PAMPs and DAMPs also function as the activators of the lectin and alternative pathways of complement (see Chapter 3). Some examples of PRRs and their ligands are shown in **Figure 7.7**.

Some PRRs are located in the cell membrane of the APC and interact with PAMPs expressed on microbial membranes. These include TLRs 1, 2, 4, 5, 6 and 11. Other surface receptor molecules include dectin-1, dectin-2 and DEC205 (C-type lectin receptors), the mannose–fucose receptor, CD14, CD1, CD36 and CD48. Further PRRs are found within the endosomes and lysosomes of the cytoplasm of the APC and recognize internal PAMPs such as nucleic acids. These include TLRs 3, 7, 8, 9 and 10. Another group of PRRs is located within the cytoplasm of the APC, but they are similarly able to interact with microbial antigenic structures. The best characterized of these molecules are the nucleotide-binding oligomerization domain receptors (**NOD-like receptors; NLRs**) and retinoic acid inducible gene **(RIG)-like receptors**.

The PRRs on the surface of an APC have been likened to bar code readers that scan the surface of antigens to determine whether that antigen expresses molecules that might engage the receptors. Different antigens, depending on their PAMPs, will therefore engage different combinations of PRRs on the surface of the APC and one PRR may recognize several different PAMPs (**Figure 7.8**). Engagement of the PRR triggers activation of a cytoplasmic **signal transduction molecule**, which in turn stimulates a complex signalling pathway that results in the activation of specific genes mediated by the transcription factor **nuclear factor κB** (**Figure 7.9**). In this fashion, the interaction of different antigens with the dendritic cell will differentially activate particular combinations of genes and determine the influence that dendritic cell will have on the adaptive immune system. Different antigenic interactions with the APC lead to qualitatively distinct types of adaptive immune response, innate immunity directing the subsequent adaptive response. We shall return to this concept in Chapter 8.

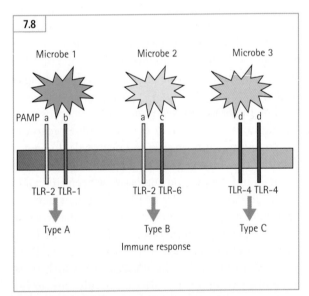

Fig. 7.8 PRR–PAMP interaction. This diagram shows three different microbial pathogens interacting with the surface of an APC. The three organisms express a different array of PAMPs and consequently engage different combinations of PRRs on the surface of the APC. Each organism therefore signals the cell in a different fashion, which will direct that APC to in turn stimulate a subtly different type of adaptive immune response.

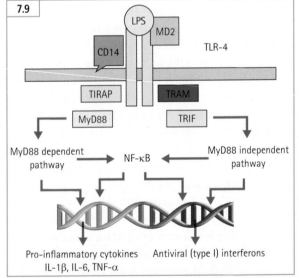

Fig. 7.9 PRR signalling. The engagement of PRRs by PAMPs leads to initiation of an intracellular signalling pathway via signal transduction molecules such as MyD88. The end effect of such pathways is to activate specific genes within the APC, an event which may be mediated by the transcription regulatory nuclear factor κB. In this diagram TLR-4 interacts with bacterial lipopolysaccharide acting as a PAMP, leading to activation of genes within the APC.

The molecular interactions between exogenous antigens and the membrane PRRs of the APC are therefore a precursor event to that APC internalizing the antigen into the cell cytoplasm by the process of phagocytosis, pinocytosis or macropinocytosis. The antigen is placed into a membrane-limited cytoplasmic compartment known as the **phagosome** or **endosome** where it may encounter further PRRs and then enter the second stage of the antigen presentation process.

The sensing of danger signals by cytoplasmic PAMPs and DAMPS (e.g. NLRs) leads to the assembly of a multiprotein complex called the **inflammasome**. Inflammasomes are key components of innate immunity and structurally different inflammasomes will form depending on the nature of the stimulating signal. The effect of inflammasome formation is to activate the molecule caspase 1, which stimulates the production and secretion of the pro-inflammatory cytokines IL-1β and IL-18. In addition, caspase 1 induces a form of cell death called **pyroptosis**, which combines features of apoptosis (DNA fragmentation) and necrosis (inflammation and cytokine release).

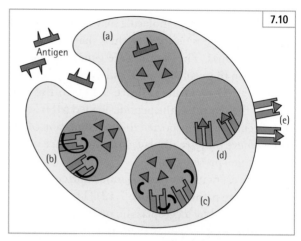

Fig. 7.10 Exogenous antigen presentation. (a) Exogenous antigen is taken up by phagocytosis and placed into the cytoplasmic early endosome. Enzymatic degradation reduces the antigen to constitutive peptide fragments. **(b)** The peptides are then transferred to a late endosome (the MHC class II compartment) where **(c)** enzymatic activity disrupts the invariant chain, detaching it from the MHC class II molecules that line the inner surface of this compartment. **(d)** The peptide fragments associate with the class II molecule. **(e)** The peptide-laden class II molecules are transported to the cell membrane where they are displayed on the surface of the APC.

ANTIGEN PROCESSING AND PRESENTATION

Once an exogenous antigen has been internalized (or at any time for a cytosolic endogenous antigen), the next stage in this sequence is antigen processing. This is the means by which a large, complex, conformational, multideterminant antigen is broken down into very small constituent segments that are of suitable size to be recognized by the receptor of the antigen-specific T lymphocyte. The processing pathways are often considered distinct for exogenous and endogenous antigens, but this is not necessarily always the case as sometimes exogenous antigen might enter the endogenous processing pathway and *vice versa* (this is known as '**cross-presentation**'). We shall, however, consider the two pathways separately here.

An exogenous antigen is placed into a cytoplasmic early endosome. Within this compartment there is a low pH, allowing acid proteases to degrade the protein antigen into small constituent components the size of **small peptides** in the order of **10–30 amino acids** in length. These peptides are then transferred from the early endosome to a late endosomal compartment termed the MHC class II compartment. The internal side of the limiting membrane forming the MHC class II compartment is lined by class II molecules with their variable ends oriented towards the centre of the compartment and the constant ends anchored within the limiting membrane. In an inactive compartment, these class II molecules are associated with another protein, the **invariant chain**, which wraps around the class II molecule and 'blocks' the variable region. Once an antigen enters the compartment, enzymes that break down the invariant chain become activated, leaving a small peptide (the class II-associated invariant chain peptide [CLIP]) in the space formed by the variable domains of the class II α and β chains. The peptide fragments of antigen generated within the early endosome displace CLIP and occupy the class II molecule by forming bonds between specific amino acids in the peptide sequence (the '**anchor residues**') and the class II structure (**Figure 7.10**).

A single MHC class II molecule may bind numerous different peptides as long as they share these key anchor residues. The peptides are generally slightly longer than the available space and overlap the edges of the class II molecule (**Figure 7.11**). In the next stage of the sequence, the peptide-loaded MHC class II molecules are transported to the membrane of the APC, where they are displayed on the surface of the cell ('antigen presentation').

The presentation of endogenous antigen occurs via a separate pathway (**Figure 7.12**). These antigens are first tagged by a cytoplasmic molecule known as **ubiquitin**, which enables them to enter a cytosolic compartment known as the **proteasome**, which resembles a hollow cylindrical structure. Degradation of the antigen to small peptide constituents occurs

within the proteasome and these peptides are then released back into the cytosol. The next stage of the sequence involves the peptides moving into the environment of the **endoplasmic reticulum** (ER), which they do by passing through a 'gateway' formed by '**transporter proteins**' (TAP1 and TAP2). The TAPs and some proteasome subunits are encoded within the class II region of the MHC. Within the ER the peptides encounter both MHC class I and class II molecules, but the latter are associated with an intact invariant chain. These peptide fragments therefore associate themselves with the variable domains of the class I α chain and form similar bonds between peptide contact residues and corresponding amino acids within the α chain. These peptides are generally smaller than those generated within the endosome and, therefore, are entirely contained within the class I structure (**Figure 7.13**). The next stages in the sequence involve the peptide-loaded MHC class I molecule transiting through the **Golgi apparatus** and then passing to the membrane of the APC to become displayed on the cell surface (antigen presentation). The finer mechanisms underlying these translocation events are not well understood, but the process probably involves transport in a membrane-limited compartment.

In this fashion, exogenous antigens are presented by MHC class II molecules and endogenous antigens are presented in the context of MHC class I molecules, although because of cross-presentation, peptides from exogenous antigens may be presented by MHC class I (when some peptides generated within the endosome escape to the cytoplasm and enter the proteasome) and endogenous peptides may be presented by MHC class II (when cytoplasmic material enters the endosome following the process of **autophagy**). Autophagy is a means by which a cell can remove unwanted or misformed proteins or organelles from its cytoplasm. The structure to be removed is first enclosed within a cytoplasmic double membrane (the autophagosome), which in turn fuses with a lysosome containing enzymes that digest the structure. The building blocks of the structure (e.g. amino acids, fatty acids and nucleotides) are released to the cytoplasm of the cell to be reused. The autophagy pathway may also be used to remove invading infectious agents (e.g. intracellular bacteria).

Fig. 7.11 Antigen presentation by MHC class II. This diagram shows the top surface of an MHC class II molecule presenting peptide antigen. The α and β chains of the molecule create a peptide-binding groove into which the peptide slots and forms specific points of contact with the MHC molecule through the anchor residues. The peptide is generally longer than the binding groove and slightly overlaps at either end.

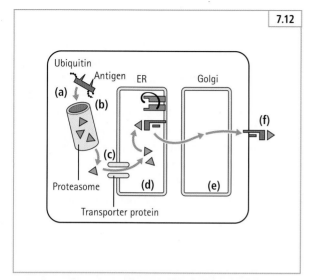

Fig. 7.12 Endogenous antigen presentation. Endogenous antigen is already located within the cell cytoplasm and is tagged by ubiquitin (**a**) before entering the proteasome, where it is degraded into peptide fragments (**b**). These fragments are released to the cytosol and migrate through the transporter protein (**c**) into the endoplasmic reticulum (ER). Although both MHC class I and II are found within the ER, only the class I molecule is able to bind peptide, as the class II invariant chain remains intact (**d**). The peptide-laden class I molecules move from the ER to the Golgi apparatus (**e**) and thence to the cell membrane for antigen presentation (**f**).

ANTIGEN PRESENTING BY CD1 MOLECULES

A distinct antigen presenting pathway is used for the presentation of **lipid antigen**, which is a major constituent of some pathogens such as *Mycobacterium* and therefore of great relevance to veterinary medicine (**Figure 7.14**). Such antigens are presented by one of a family of CD1 molecules that have an evolutionary relationship to MHC. CD1 is also a transmembrane glycoprotein with three extracellular domains that associates with the β_2 microglobulin. The CD1 molecules are encoded by a series of genes that lack the polymorphism that characterizes the MHC. The loading of CD1 with lipid antigen probably occurs within an endosome, with subsequent translocation of the antigen-laden CD1 molecule to the APC membrane.

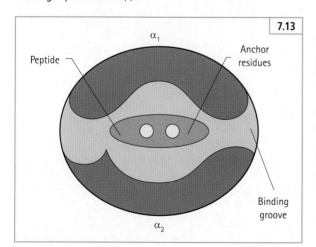

Fig. 7.13 Antigen presentation by MHC class I. This diagram shows the top surface of an MHC class I molecule presenting peptide antigen. The external α chain domains of the molecule form a peptide-binding groove into which the peptide slots and forms specific points of contact with the MHC molecule through the anchor residues. The short peptide fits entirely within this binding groove.

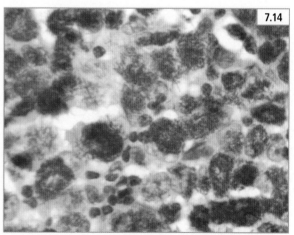

Fig. 7.14 CD1 antigen presentation. This section of spleen comes from a dog with disseminated mycobacterial infection and has been stained by the Ziehl–Neelsen method. The macrophages are distended by the large number of acid-fast bacilli within their cytoplasm. Lipid mycobacterial antigen would be expressed on the surface of these cells by members of the CD1 family of antigen presenting molecules.

ANTIGEN PRESENTATION BY B CELLS AND NON-PROFESSIONAL ANTIGEN PRESENTING CELLS

B lymphocytes are also capable of presenting antigen in the context of MHC class II. Antigen is bound by the BCR (immunoglobulin) and internalized into a cytoplasmic endosome; the same pathway described above for exogenous antigen is followed (**Figure 7.15**). B cells do not undertake antigen processing in order to compete with dendritic cells, as they are far less effective in this regard. However, as we shall see in Chapter 9, B-cell antigen presentation is integral to the activation of the B cell itself.

In certain circumstances a range of cells that do not normally present antigen can be induced to do so. **Epithelial**, **endothelial** and other **stromal** cells (e.g. fibroblasts) can all be made to express MHC class II and can presumptively present peptide within those molecules. The key signal required to induce such non-professional APCs to express class II is provided by the cytokine **interferon-γ** (IFN-γ). For example, the enterocytes lining the intestinal wall may express MHC class II and may act as functional APCs. Canine enterocytes normally express MHC class II on their basolateral surfaces, while such expression is induced on feline enterocytes in the presence of intestinal inflammation or neoplasia (**Figure 7.16**).

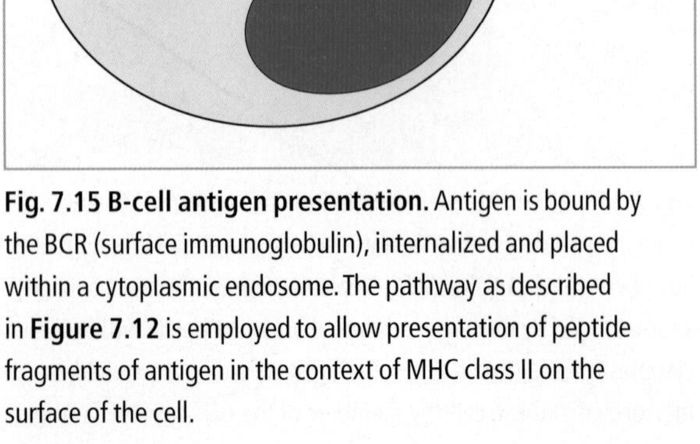

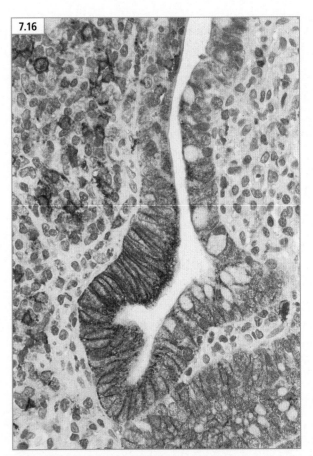

Fig. 7.15 B-cell antigen presentation. Antigen is bound by the BCR (surface immunoglobulin), internalized and placed within a cytoplasmic endosome. The pathway as described in **Figure 7.12** is employed to allow presentation of peptide fragments of antigen in the context of MHC class II on the surface of the cell.

Fig. 7.16 Non-professional APCs. Section of dog small intestine showing the basal region of a crypt. The enterocytes lining this structure express MHC class II molecules on their lateral and basal surfaces. It is suggested that these cells are able to present antigen to underlying lymphoid cells. Professional APCs expressing membrane MHC class II are also present within the adjacent lamina propria.

CYTOKINES

At this stage it is appropriate to consider another component of the immune system – the cytokines. **Cytokines** are soluble, low molecular weight (<80 kD), protein mediators released by one cell to bind to a specific **cytokine receptor** expressed by the same cell (autocrine action) or another cell nearby (paracrine action) (**Figure 7.17**). Cytokines are highly **potent** molecules that may have significant effect at picomolar concentration. The interaction of cytokine and receptor establishes signals that induce that target cell to perform a specific action. Some cytokines may circulate systemically and have distant (endocrine) actions. Cytokines are therefore one of the key means of **communication between cells** of the immune system (APCs, T and B lymphocytes, NK cells) and between immune cells and other cells of the body. The descriptor 'cytokine' is a generic term that encompasses a range of such molecules. These molecules are also referred to as lymphokines, monokines, interleukins, interferons and colony-stimulating factors.

Any one cell may produce multiple cytokines and multiple cytokines may act on any one target cell providing it expresses appropriate receptors. Any one cytokine may have multiple actions depending on the immunological circumstances and the nature of the target cell to which it binds. Cytokines often work in a **network**, whereby a series of cytokines has a concerted effect with a common end aim or, alternatively, where some cytokines antagonize the effects of others.

Several **families of cytokine** are recognized and many of these molecules will be considered further as we progress through the rest of this book. Some cytokines are important in bone marrow haemopoiesis and in the development of T and B lymphocytes, others are involved in the activation or suppression of immune cells and some are considered pro-inflammatory in their effects. Another large group of molecules, also grouped in families, are the chemoattractant cytokines or **chemokines**. As the name suggests, chemokines are important in the recruitment of leucocytes from blood into tissue and different chemokines are active in different types of immune or inflammatory response (**Figure 7.18**).

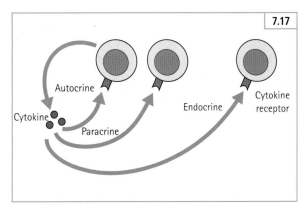

Fig. 7.17 Cytokines. A cytokine is a soluble messenger protein released by one cell to bind to a specific cytokine receptor expressed by the same cell (autocrine), a nearby cell (paracrine) or a distant cell (endocrine). Binding of cytokine to receptor activates intracellular signalling pathways and this results in some functional change to the target cell.

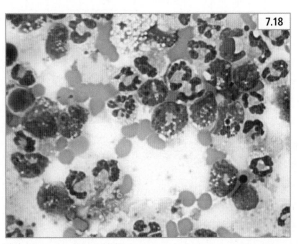

Fig. 7.18 Chemokines. Chemoattractant cytokines (chemokines) are important in the recruitment of leucocytes from blood into tissue. This cytological preparation shows eosinophils within the airway of a dog with parasitic respiratory disease. Eosinophils would have been recruited from blood into the bronchial lamina propria and then migrated through the epithelium into the bronchial lumen. This migration would be mediated by eosinophil chemotactic chemokines known as eotaxins.

The cytokines and chemokines of domestic animals are currently being characterized and ascribed a function in various disease states. It is now possible to detect both cytokine gene transcription in tissue by **quantitative real-time reverse transcriptase polymerase chain reaction** (RT-PCR) (**Figures 7.19–7.21**) and the presence of cytokine protein in tissue or fluid samples using capture ELISA or more complex bead-based multiplex assays.

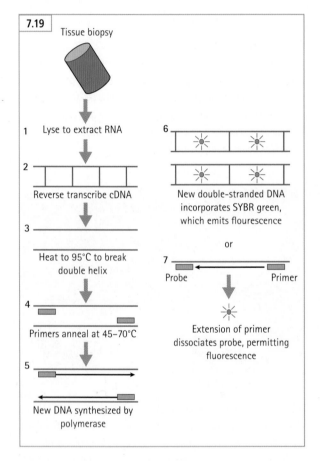

Figs. 7.19, 7.20 Real-time reverse transcriptase polymerase chain reaction (RT-PCR). (7.19) Real-time RT-PCR provides a means by which gene transcription within a tissue can be quantified. In this way the activity of genes encoding many inflammatory mediators can be assessed when reagents able to detect the proteins encoded by the genes are not available. In this process, RNA is first extracted from a tissue sample and then reverse transcribed to cDNA. The double-stranded DNA is heated to 94°C in a thermal cycler to denature the double helix. When the reaction is cooled to 45–70°C, small complementary sequences (primers) at each end of the gene sequence of interest are able to anneal to the appropriate nucleotides within the single-stranded DNA, following which a heat stable DNA polymerase adds bases complementary to those in the DNA strands to synthesize new double-stranded DNA. This cycle of heat and cooling is subsequently repeated up to 40 times, leading to an exponential increase in the amount of target gene. In the highly sensitive real-time method, the production of DNA is measured at each cycle (in 'real-time') using a fluorescence read out. Fluorescence is emitted (and measured) each time double-stranded DNA is produced in the reaction. This may be achieved via the use of an 'intercalating dye' (e.g. SYBR green), which only binds double-stranded DNA to emit fluorescence, or via the use of labelled reporter oligonucleotide 'probes' that emit fluorescence when they are dislodged from the template DNA by the process of extension mediated by the DNA polymerase. The point at which the fluorescence value crosses a threshold detection value (the Ct value) is related to the amount of target DNA in the sample. **(7.20)** In this graph from an experiment detecting mRNA within tissue samples, the samples on the left, which cross the threshold (the orange line parallel to the x axis) with lower cycle number, have more copies of the target DNA than the samples on the right, which require many more cycles of amplification to cross the threshold.

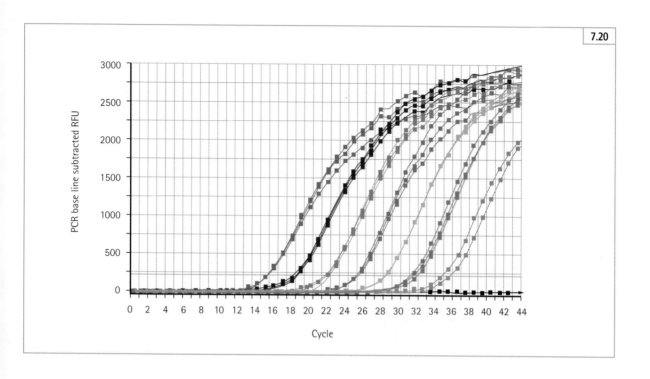

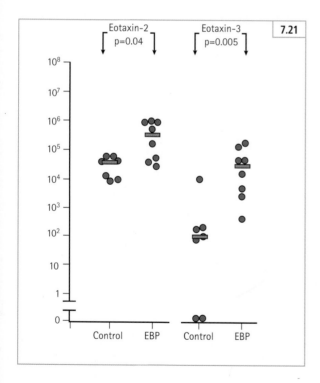

Fig. 7.21 Chemokine gene expression. This graph compares the level of transcription of genes encoding two eosinophil chemotactic proteins (eotaxin-2 and eotaxin-3) in bronchial mucosal biopsies taken from normal dogs and dogs with allergic respiratory disease (eosinophilic bronchopneumopathy). The affected dogs have significantly more gene expression as detected by real-time RT-PCR, which correlates with the presence of eosinophils within their airways. (Data from Peeters D, Peters IR, Clercx C *et al.* (2006) Real-time RT-PCR quantification of mRNA encoding cytokines, CC chemokines and CCR3 in bronchial biopsies from dogs with eosinophilic bronchopneumopathy. *Veterinary Immunology and Immunopathology* **110**:65–77.)

KEY POINTS

- APCs mediate the uptake, processing and presentation of antigen to the adaptive immune system.
- Professional APCs include dendritic cells, macrophages and B cells, of which the dendritic cell is most potent.
- Exogenous antigen derives from outside of the APC and includes most foreign antigens.
- Endogenous antigen is located within the host cell and includes autoantigen, tumour antigen, alloantigen and viral antigen.
- The initial interaction between APC and antigen is mediated by PRRs and PAMPs.
- PAMPs are relatively conserved microbial sequences (carbohydrate, protein, lipid, nucleic acid).
- PRRs are highly conserved throughout evolution.
- Signalling by PRRs leads to distinct pathways of APC induction of adaptive immunity; the innate immune response dictates the nature of the adaptive response.
- Exogenous antigen undergoes endosomal processing for presentation by MHC class II.
- Endogenous antigen is processed through the proteasome, endoplasmic reticulum and Golgi apparatus for presentation by MHC class I.
- The non-polymorphic CD1 family is important in presentation of lipid antigen.
- Non-professional APCs may be induced to express MHC class II and present antigen by IFN-γ signalling.
- Cytokines are one means of intercellular communication in the immune system.
- A cytokine binds to a specific cytokine receptor, leading to altered function of the target cell expressing the receptor.
- Chemokines recruit leucocytes from blood to tissue.

CHAPTER 8

The Biology of T Lymphocytes

OBJECTIVES

At the end of this chapter you should be able to:
- List the major molecules expressed on the surface of T lymphocytes and describe their function.
- Understand the concept of the 'immunoglobulin superfamily'.
- Describe the functional differences between CD4$^+$ and CD8$^+$ T cells.
- Understand how diversity in the T-cell receptor is achieved.
- Describe the intrathymic development of T cells and the processes of positive and negative selection.

- Describe the three signals required for activation of a T cell.
- Understand the concept of clonal proliferation and differentiation as it applies to T cells.
- Discuss the functional differences between naïve, Th1, Th2 and Th17 cells.
- Describe how target cells are recognized by CD8$^+$ cytotoxic T cells and NK cells.
- Define antibody-dependent cell-mediated cytotoxicity.
- Describe the stages in the cytotoxic response.
- Define what is meant by T-cell memory.
- Discuss the importance of $\gamma\delta$ T cells.

INTRODUCTION

Activation of antigen-specific T lymphocytes is pivotal to the generation of an adaptive immune response. In this chapter we consider further the nature of the T-cell receptor (TCR), T-cell development and maturation, T-cell activation and the roles of helper, cytotoxic and memory T lymphocytes. The suppressor function of T cells is discussed in Chapter 11.

THE T-CELL RECEPTOR

T lymphocytes are distinguished by the expression of a **TCR** and associated **CD3 complex**. The majority of T cells in the body fall into one of two non-overlapping subsets characterized by the expression of the CD4 molecule (the **helper T cells**; Th) or the CD8 molecule (the **cytotoxic T cells**; Tc).

The TCR of most T cells comprises an α and β chain, each of which has outermost variable domains and constant region domains closest to the cell membrane into which the chains anchor. This core receptor molecule is surrounded by a series of signal transduction molecules (δ, ε, γ and ζ chains) that collectively form the CD3 complex. The **CD4** molecule consists of a single elongate chain, while **CD8** may be composed of a shorter α and β chain or an alternative form consisting of two α chains (the CD8 homodimer). As for the TCR, CD4 and CD8 preserve the variable–constant region structure and all of these molecules are further members of the **immunoglobulin superfamily (Figure 8.1)**.

In accordance with Burnett's **clonal selection theory** (see Chapter 5), the vast number of T cells within the immune system must have almost unique antigen specificity in order to provide protection from the multitude of foreign antigens that may potentially enter the body. Each individual must therefore have an enormous 'repertoire' of different TCRs to make this possible. This extraordinary repertoire is created at the molecular level by rearranging the series of genes that encode different areas of the complete TCR α and β chains.

At the protein level the polypeptide **TCR α chain** consists of a variable domain (V_α) and a constant domain (C_α) linked together by a joining region (J_α). The **TCR β chain** is slightly more complex, as the V_β and C_β domains are linked by both a joining region (J_β) and a further diversity region (D_β) **(Figure 8.2)**. The series of genes that encodes each chain are found on distinct chromosomes. For the α chain there are numerous possible V_α genes ($V_{\alpha 1}$, $V_{\alpha 2}$...to $V_{\alpha n}$) and numerous possible J region genes ($J_{\alpha 1}$, $J_{\alpha 2}$... to $J_{\alpha n}$), but only a single constant region gene (C_α) **(Figure 8.3)**. Genes encoding elements of the TCR δ chain (see below) are integrated with the α chain genes. Immature T cells utilize the δ chain genes to form receptors, but as most T cells mature the series of δ chain genes is deleted and the α chain elements are utilized. The series of genes encoding the TCR β chain is more complex because at some point during evolution there was duplication of a portion of this area of the genome. So, although there is only one set of V_β genes ($V_{\beta 1}$, $V_{\beta 2}$...to $V_{\beta n}$), there are two sets of genes encoding the diversity, joining and constant regions. These are termed $D_{\beta 1}$, $J_{\beta 1}$ ($J_{\beta 1.1}$, $J_{\beta 1.2}$...to $J_{\beta 1n}$) and $C_{\beta 1}$, and $D_{\beta 2}$, $J_{\beta 2}$ ($J_{\beta 2.1}$, $J_{\beta 2.2}$...to $J_{\beta 2n}$) and $C_{\beta 2}$ **(Figure 8.4)**. In pigs, there are three such replicates of the D–J–C cluster. The number of genes encoding the various segments of the TCR chains is in the order of 100 V_α genes, 75 J_α genes, 75 V_β genes, 6 $J_{\beta 1}$ genes and 7 $J_{\beta 2}$ genes.

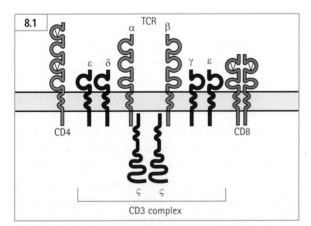

Fig. 8.1 T-cell surface molecules. This diagram depicts the structure of the $\alpha\beta$ TCR–CD3 complex and the T-cell molecules CD4 and CD8. Note that co-expression of CD4 and CD8 occurs only on immature T cells within the thymus. These are all members of the immunoglobulin superfamily with variable (V) and constant regions.

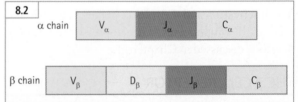

Fig. 8.2 Protein structure of the TCR. The α and β polypeptide chains of the TCR consist of a variable and a constant region separated by either a joining region (α chain) or diversity and joining region (β chain).

Therefore, for any individual T cell to create a TCR there must be selection and **rearrangement** of these various genetic elements. This is achieved by **looping out and deleting introns** from the V, D and J regions that are not required and bringing together those exons that will be transcribed. Following transcription of the VJ or VDJ segments, the constant region is attached by **RNA splicing** (**Figure 8.5**). The number of possible permutations and combinations of the V and J region genes for each of the two chains is the key to creating diversity in the TCR repertoire. The theoretical number of different TCRs that might be created (known as the '**germline repertoire**') is in the order of 10^{15}, but in reality this number is closer to 2×10^7 after the process of thymic selection (described below). Once a T cell has formed a specific TCR, the genes encoding this molecule tend not to undergo somatic mutation (single nucleotide deletions or substitutions), so the TCR repertoire remains relatively stable.

These numerical calculations expose a fundamental flaw in Burnett's clonal selection theory. A theoretical calculation of the number of possible peptide–antigenic epitopes to which the immune system could be exposed suggests that if each and every T cell in the body was absolutely monospecific for antigen, the volume of the T-cell compartment (for a mouse) would be 70 times greater than the body mass of the animal (**Figure 8.6**).

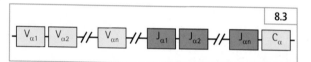

Fig. 8.3 TCR α chain genes. These comprise numerous variable and joining region genes, but only a single constant region gene.

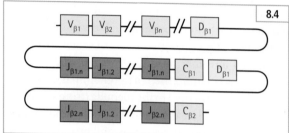

Fig. 8.4 TCR β chain genes. These comprise numerous variable region genes with a duplicated stretch of genome encoding the diversity, joining and constant regions. Each of these two sets of genes has a single diversity and constant region gene, with a limited number of joining region genes.

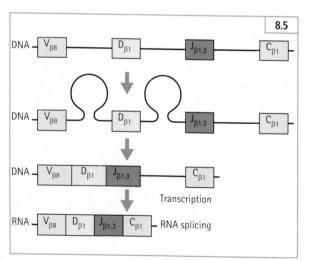

Fig. 8.5 Gene rearrangement for production of the TCR β chain. One variable, diversity and joining region gene is selected and the intervening intronic sequence is looped out and deleted. Following transcription the selected constant region is added by RNA splicing.

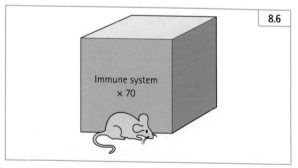

Fig. 8.6 The T-cell repertoire. According to Burnett's clonal selection theory, each individual T cell carries unique specificity for antigenic peptide. However, if this was the case, a mouse would require an immune system 70 times greater than its own body mass. T cells are therefore able to respond to multiple different peptides providing that they carry the appropriate contact residues.

As this is clearly not the case, the T cells within the immune system must have the ability to recognize multiple different antigenic peptides, a phenomenon known as '**TCR degeneracy**'. This becomes possible with the realization that within any one peptide only key '**contact residues**' are required to form a bond with any one TCR. Therefore, numerous peptides may potentially interact with a particular TCR as long as they carry the appropriate sequence of contact residues (**Figure 8.7**).

T-CELL DEVELOPMENT AND MATURATION

As discussed in Chapter 5, immature T cells are created within the bone marrow and exported via the blood to the thymus for their final development and maturation. This involves a series of stages that occur as the cell moves from the cortex (to where it first migrates as it enters the corticomedullary junction from the bone marrow) to the medulla (from where it is released to populate the secondary lymphoid tissues). Thymic maturation is a very wasteful process, as some 99% of immature T cells that enter the thymus do not leave. These cells **die by apoptosis** and the cellular debris is phagocytosed (**Figure 8.8**).

The first change to an early thymic immigrant is that the immature T cell forms and expresses a TCR. Additionally, this early cortical cell will co-express the CD4 and CD8 molecules, a phenomenon that generally is restricted to thymic T cells, as mature T cells express either one (but not both) of these markers.

The immature T cell must pass two 'examinations' before it is allowed to leave the thymus and enter the 'periphery' (to immunologists the thymus is '**central**' and the remainder of the immune system comprises the '**periphery**') (**Figure 8.9**). In the first examination,

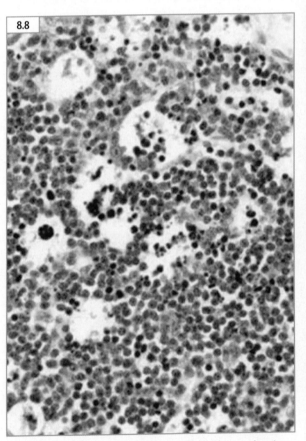

Fig. 8.8 Thymocyte apoptosis. Section of dog thymus showing numerous spaces within the sheet of small lymphocytes. These spaces contain apoptotic debris that will be phagocytosed by macrophages. Ninety-nine percent of immature T cells that enter the thymus die by apoptosis.

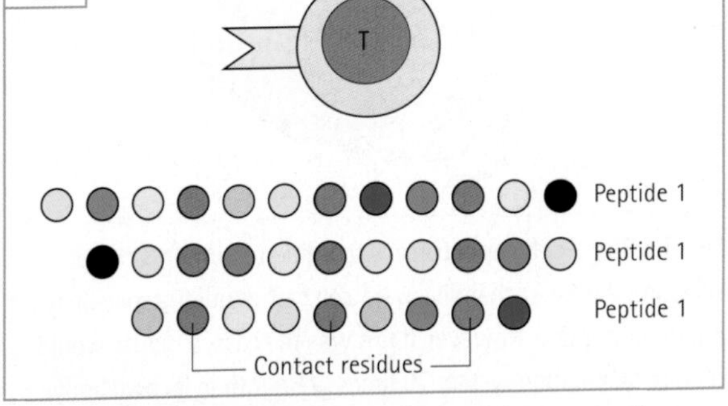

Fig. 8.7 TCR degeneracy. This T cell is able to recognize all three of these peptides when appropriately presented by MHC. Although the overall amino acid sequence of the peptides is different, each one carries the same 'contact residues' at the same position within the sequence.

called 'positive selection', the immature T cell must prove that it has created a TCR capable of interacting with peptide antigen presented to that T cell by an MHC molecule. Within the thymic cortex are numerous thymic epithelial cells. These display surface membrane MHC class I and II molecules that contain peptide fragments of self-antigens. Thymic epithelial cells have a high level of autophagy (see Chapter 7) enabling them to present a wide range of

normal tissue antigens. Each immature T cell must 'test out' its TCR to ensure that it can interact with the MHC–peptide complex, but only by having a moderate-affinity interaction. Cells that have such a functional TCR 'pass the test' of positive selection and are permitted to move on to the second examination. Cells that fail to mount such an interaction by having produced a TCR with no or low affinity for peptide-MHC, die by 'neglect'.

The positively selected T cells then move into the medulla of the thymic lobule where they undertake the second examination, called 'negative selection'. In this test the immature T cell meets a thymic dendritic cell displaying MHC class I or II molecules containing peptides derived from a wide array of self-proteins. For example, within the thymus it is known that there is expression of peptides derived from tissues such as the brain, endocrine pancreas and joint. Many thousands of such peptides from tissue antigens may be expressed by the phenomenon of 'promiscuous gene expression'. In this examination the T cell must prove that its TCR is incapable of responding to these self-antigens with high affinity. Cells that do not carry high-affinity autoreactive TCRs will pass this test and progress to the final stage of maturation. Cells that fail (i.e. are potentially autoreactive) will be instructed to undergo apoptosis. The high failure rate for these two examinations accounts for the marked loss of T cells during intrathymic development described earlier.

As part of positive selection, the developing 'double-positive' (CD4+CD8+) thymocyte loses either the CD4 or CD8 molecule. This decision is informed by whether the T cell encountered MHC class I or II molecules during its examination. Cells that interacted with MHC class I will become CD8+ T cells and those that were selected by MHC class II become CD4+ T cells. Only 'single-positive' T cells are exported from the thymus to enter the recirculating T-cell pool. There are, however, some unique species differences in the phenotype of circulating T cells. The majority (approximately 60%) of circulating T cells in the pig are double-positive, with most of the remainder being double-negative (CD4-CD8-). A significant proportion of circulating T cells in young cattle is also double-negative and expresses the γδ TCR (see below).

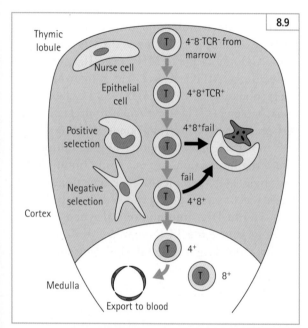

Fig. 8.9 Intrathymic T-cell maturation. Immature T cells enter the thymic cortex from the bone marrow and are induced to express a TCR together with both CD4 and CD8 molecules. The thymocyte then determines whether the TCR is functional by testing it against MHC class I or II (with peptide) expressed by a cortical epithelial cell. Thymocytes that do not carry functional receptors die by apoptosis in the process of 'positive selection'. The thymocyte subsequently determines whether the TCR has the potential for high-affinity interaction with self-peptide expressed by MHC on a thymic dendritic cell. Cells bearing such receptors die by apoptosis in the process of 'negative selection'. Within the medulla, the thymocyte expresses either CD4 or CD8 depending on whether it encountered MHC class II or class I molecules, respectively, during the selection process. Fully mature T cells leave the thymus to enter the recirculating T-cell pool.

T-CELL ACTIVATION

With that background we are now ready to consider the next stage in the adaptive immune response (the activation of T cells) and the reason for the complex mechanism of antigen presentation described in Chapter 7. Appropriately processed and presented antigen becomes accessible to T cells, which will respond through their TCRs to the combination of peptide and the MHC molecule in which the peptide sits. One key concept in antigen presentation is that peptides presented by **MHC class II** molecules stimulate only **CD4⁺ T cells**, whereas peptides presented by **MHC class I** are the signal for activation for **CD8⁺ T cells** (**Figure 8.10**). The TCR interacts both with contact residues on the peptide and also with residues on the surrounding MHC molecule, a phenomenon known as '**MHC-restriction**'.

The interaction between T cell and APC occurs within the paracortex of the lymph node. The APC (generally a dendritic cell) has carried antigen from tissue to that node and processed that antigen for presentation on MHC molecules. T cells within the recirculating pool continually enter the paracortex from blood. As the dendritic cell sits in the paracortex displaying antigen, large numbers of T cells will approach that APC and 'test out' whether their TCR is capable of responding to the antigen. Using real-time video microscopy it has been calculated that up to 500 different T cells may approach any one dendritic cell each hour.

Once an antigen-specific T cell has been selected from the T-cell repertoire, that T cell requires three specific signals to become fully activated and induce an adaptive immune response (**Figure 8.11**). The first of these signals (**signal 1**) is binding of **TCR** to the combination of antigenic **peptide and MHC** molecule. The second signal (**signal 2**) comprises a series of other **molecular interactions** between the APC and the T cell. One of these is the binding of the CD4 molecule to MHC class II, or the CD8 molecule to MHC class I, but numerous other interactions also occur (e.g. CD28 and CD80/86; see also Chapter 11). These intercellular interactions are very precise and form strong bonds, allowing the two cells to become closely apposed at the multiple foci where the interactions are occurring (multiple and not single TCR–peptide–MHC interactions occur). These foci of interaction between the two cells form what is termed the '**immunological synapse**', which has at its centre the TCR–peptide–MHC complex. Finally, a third signal (**signal 3**) is also required for

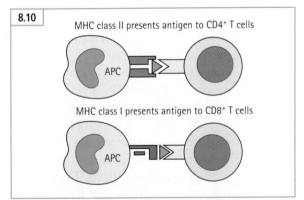

Fig. 8.10 MHC restriction. CD4⁺ T cells recognize peptide presented by MHC class II molecules, whereas CD8⁺ T cells recognize peptide in the context of MHC class I molecules.

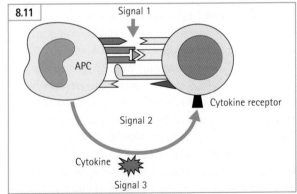

Fig. 8.11 T-cell activation. T-cell activation requires three signalling events: the recognition of peptide–MHC by the TCR (signal 1), the interaction of an array of APC and T-cell surface molecules that form the 'immunological synapse' (signal 2), and the binding of an APC-derived co-stimulatory cytokine to a T-cell cytokine receptor (signal 3).

full T-cell activation and this takes the form of a **co-stimulatory cytokine** that is released by the APC to bind to a cytokine receptor expressed by the T cell. A range of different cytokines can fulfil this role, and the selection of cytokine is determined by the nature of the stimulating antigen and the type of immune response required (see below). Only when all three signals have been received can that T cell become fully activated. The three signalling events trigger a series of intracellular pathways within the T cell that result in **gene transcription** events within the stimulated cell. For example, the interaction of cytokine and cytokine receptor leads to aggregation of the receptors and initiation of signalling via the activation of cytoplasmic tyrosine kinases ('Janus kinases', **JAKs**), which phosphorylate the cytosolic 'signal transducers and activators of transcription' (**STATs**) that subsequently migrate to the nucleus and initiate gene activation via the effects of specific transcription factors (**Figure 8.12**).

A number of actions follow T-cell activation. The first of these is the physical transformation of the activated T cell from a small lymphocyte to a **lymphoblast** (see Chapter 5). The activated T cell will start to secrete cytokines and express cytokine receptors, at least one of which (IL-2) acts in an autocrine fashion to maintain stimulation of the cell. Finally, the activated T cell will start to **divide** in a clonal fashion to generate a large number of identical T cells each bearing the same antigen-specific receptor (**Figure 8.13**). Most of these cells will become '**effector**' **T cells**, which participate in the immune response, and some will become a specialized population of '**memory**' **T cells**, which retain the immunological memory of this activation event.

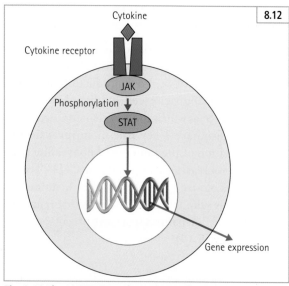

Fig. 8.12 The JAK/STAT pathway in T-cell activation. Key cytokines providing signal 3 for T-cell activation bind to cytokine receptors. Cytokine receptors consist of two identical or different transmembrane proteins. These proteins are dimerized by cytokine binding, which leads to activation of the associated Janus kinase (JAK) molecule. There are four different JAK molecules (JAK1–JAK4) used by receptors for different classes of cytokine. Activated JAK phosphorylates tyrosine residues on signal transducer and activator of transcription (STAT) molecules, which then dimerize, dissociate from JAK and move to the nucleus of the cell where they act as transcription factors in gene expression. STAT1 to STAT6 molecules are most important in T-cell activation pathways.

Fig. 8.13 T-cell clonal proliferation and differentiation. Activation of the T cell initiates clonal proliferation to produce large numbers of antigen-specific effector T cells and a smaller population of memory T cells.

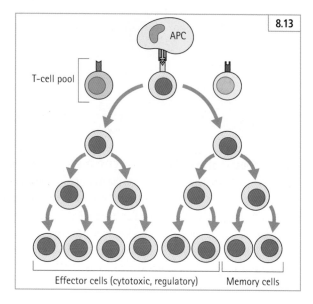

THE ROLE OF CD4⁺ T LYMPHOCYTES

CD4⁺ T cells are also termed 'helper' T cells (Th) and their major function is in providing such help for the generation of antibody production (**humoral immunity**) or cytotoxicity (**cell-mediated immunity**; CMI). However, as will become evident in Chapter 11, these cells also have a key role in **suppression** or down-regulation of the immune response. Since the mid 1980s increasing complexity in CD4⁺ T cells has been recognized and there are now numerous subsets of this subpopulation of T cells that represent different activation pathways of naïve precursor CD4⁺ T cells (**Figure 8.14**).

The first of these subsets to be recognized were the **T helper 1 (Th1)** and **T helper 2 (Th2)** cells (**Figure 8.15**). These are both CD4⁺ T cells that carry an αβ TCR that responds to antigenic peptide–MHC class II on the surface of an APC. These cells appear microscopically identical. In fact, it is very difficult to distinguish these cells on the basis of their surface molecular phenotype. The distinction is a functional one; the two subsets mediate (help) entirely different immunological events by virtue of the panel of cytokines that each subset produces. The **Th1** cells preferentially produce **IL-2** and **IFN-γ** and this latter cytokine stimulates cytotoxic effector

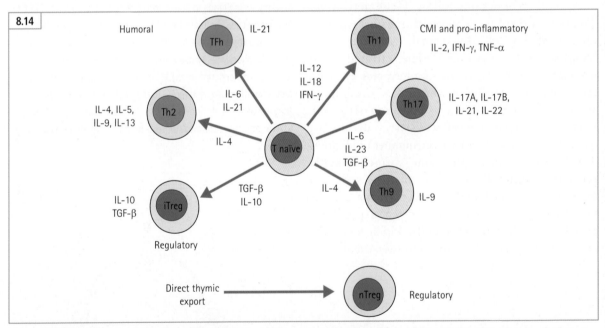

Fig. 8.14 Subsets of CD4⁺ T cells. Naïve CD4⁺ T cells may differentiate to become one of a number of effector T cells when activated by signals 1–3. The nature of signal 3 (i.e. the type of co-stimulatory cytokine indicated in the link between naïve and effector cell) is an important factor in this process. Effector T cell subsets are characterized by a specific cytokine signature (indicated adjacent to each cell type) and may function in cell-mediated/pro-inflammatory, humoral or regulatory roles. For example, Th17 cells are generated in the presence of IL-6, IL-23 and TGF-β signalling, and themselves produce the cytokines IL-17A, IL-17F, IL-21 and IL-22. Induced T regulatory (iTreg) cells are also generated from naïve CD4⁺ T cell precursors, while natural T regulatory (nTreg) cells are exported directly from the thymus. Regulatory T cells will be discussed in Chapter 11.

cells in a **cell-mediated immune response** (see below). Th1 cells are less able to provide help for B cells in the humoral immune response, although they can provide limited help for those B cells that will differentiate to produce the specific subclass of IgG antibody involved in cytotoxic responses (see below). In contrast, **Th2** cells preferentially produce **IL-4, IL-5, IL-9 and IL-13** and by virtue of this cytokine profile have a major role in providing help to B cells as they differentiate to become plasma cells, which secrete antibody (generally of the IgG, IgA or IgE classes) in the **humoral immune response**. Th1 and Th2 cells may follow selective recirculation pathways to different tissue sites, as they may express particular adhesion molecules and be chemotactically attracted by specific molecules (chemokines) for which they bear receptors.

In addition to these two cell subsets mediating distinctly different effector immune responses, they also tend to be **mutually antagonistic**, such that when one subset is activated the other is less so. This 'cross-regulation' again relates to the cytokines that each cell produces. IFN-γ produced by Th1 cells is inhibitory of the function of Th2 cells and the IL-4 and IL-13 produced by Th2 cells suppresses the action of Th1 cells. This effect means that many immune responses will have a relatively **polarized** outcome, with either CMI or humoral effects dominating in any one immune response. This phenomenon is referred to as '**immune deviation**' and there are several good examples of immune responses that are polarized in this fashion. However, in reality, for most immune responses elements of both types of immunity are important and polarization is not absolute.

The **Th17 cell** is characterized functionally by secretion of the cytokines IL-17A, IL-17F, IL-21 and IL-22. These cells mediate inflammation in various infectious, autoimmune and neoplastic diseases and are particularly effective in enhancing neutrophil recruitment. Th17 cells have an essential role in immune responses to fungi (see Chapter 13). The **Th9 cell** (characterized by dominant IL-9 production) has a role in the chronic phase of allergy. **T follicular helper cells** (TFh) reside in lymphoid follicles and are important in the formation and maintenance of germinal centres (see Chapters 5 and 9) and the

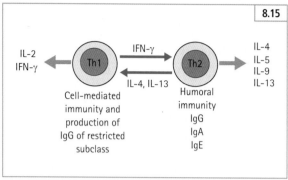

Fig. 8.15 Th1 and Th2 CD4+ T lymphocytes. These two subsets of CD4+ T cells are characterized functionally on the basis of the panel of cytokines that each produces. Th1 cells produce IL-2 and IFN-γ and stimulate cytotoxic cell-mediated immune responses. These cells provide limited help for those B cells that will eventually produce one IgG subclass involved in cytotoxic responses. Th2 cells produce IL-4, IL-5, IL-9 and IL-13 and preferentially provide help for B-cell differentiation and humoral immunity, leading to the production of IgG, IgA or IgE. The subsets are mutually antagonistic as IFN-γ is inhibitory of Th2 cells, and IL-4 and IL-13 are inhibitory of Th1 cell function.

regulation of B-cell differentiation to plasma cells and memory B cells (see Chapter 9). Induced and natural CD4+ T regulatory (Treg) cells will be considered further in Chapter 11.

These CD4+ T-cell subsets all arise from a common naïve CD4+ T-cell precursor and so the question arises as to what determines, in any one immune response, whether Th1, Th2, Th9 or Th17 immunity will dominate. The strongest influence would appear to be the **nature of the initiating antigen** and the way in which this antigen interacts (via PAMPs and PRRs) with the APC, which in turn determines how that APC will signal the naïve CD4+ T cell. The most important determining factors are the co-stimulatory cytokines released by the APC to provide signal 3 for activation of the T cell and the signalling from APC to T cell via one of a range of STATs (**Figure 8.16**). Other influences in this decision-making process may include the nature of the APC (e.g. dendritic cell, macrophage or B cell), the stage of the immune response and the tissue environment in which the immune response is being generated (as determined by regional environmental hormones or cytokines). A specific example of these effects is given in **Figure 8.17**. A dog with infection by the sand fly-transmitted obligate intracellular protozoan pathogen *Leishmania infantum* will require production of a strong cell-mediated immune response with production of IFN-γ to have any chance of containing the pathogen and recovering from infection. In this instance the protective immune response must be mediated by Th1 cells. In contrast, a dog with severe chronic diarrhoea and weight loss due to enteric infection with the bacterium *Escherichia coli* will require the production of IgA and IgG antibodies able to prevent receptor-mediated colonization of the intestine by these organisms. The protective immune response in this case must be mediated by Th2 cells. Both of these examples will be discussed in greater detail in Chapter 13.

These concepts have revolutionized the understanding of basic and clinical immunology in the past two decades and underpin current new developments in immunomodulatory medicine and vaccine development. Domestic animal species all have these CD4+ T cell subsets and this knowledge has enabled major steps forward in the understanding of diseases of our animals.

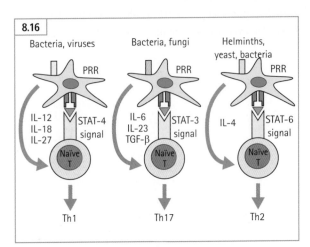

Fig. 8.16 Th0 decision making. The decision of the naïve CD4+ T-cell precursor to differentiate to become a Th1, Th2 or Th17 effector is determined by the signals that the cell receives from the APC. These in turn are determined by the nature of the antigen and the combination of PRRs that are engaged by PAMPs expressed by that antigen. Differentiation to a Th1 cell requires IL-12, IL-18 or IL-27 co-stimulation and signalling through STAT-4. Differentiation to a Th2 cell requires IL-4 co-stimulation and signalling through STAT-6. Differentiation to a Th17 cell requires IL-6, IL-23 and TGF-β co-stimulation and signalling through STAT-3.

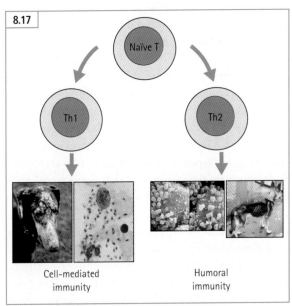

Fig. 8.17 Immune deviation. Some immune responses are polarized towards either a Th1 or Th2 effector response.
The dog with leishmaniosis (left) requires a strongly polarized Th1 response in order to control this protozoal pathogen. Failure to do so will lead to chronic multisystemic disease and death.
The dog with enteric *Escherichia coli* infection (right) must make a polarized Th2 response for the production of IgA antibody, which can block receptor-mediated colonization of the intestine.

CYTOTOXICITY

Cytotoxicity (destruction of a target cell) may arise in a number of different ways (**Figure 8.18**). In Chapter 3 we discussed how macrophages, antibody and complement can mediate such cellular destruction via opsonization, phagocytosis and formation of the MAC. It is also possible for mononuclear (lymphoid) cells to mediate cytotoxic destruction of a target, a role primarily performed by **CD8⁺ cytotoxic T cells** (Tc) and **natural killer** (NK) cells. These latter two cell types are characterized by the presence of cytoplasmic granulation and morphologically these cells are described as '**large granular lymphocytes**' (LGLs). Cytotoxicity proceeds through several stages: recognition, adhesion, cytolysis and detachment.

The **recognition** stage differs between Tc and NK cells, but the remaining steps in the sequence are similar. The targets of a cytotoxic immune response are abnormal cells within the body (e.g. virally infected cells, neoplastic cells or inappropriately transplanted cells). Cytotoxic responses also occur in some autoimmune diseases in which there is destruction of self-tissue via this mechanism.

NK cells are generally considered part of the **innate immune system** (see Chapter 1), are widely distributed at body surfaces and are able to act rapidly, when required, in a relatively non-specific fashion. NK cells may recognize a target cell in one of two ways (**Figure 8.19**). The first involves a series of **activating receptors** that are able to bind directly to surface molecules displayed on the surface of stressed

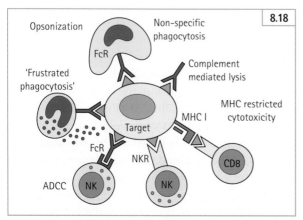

Fig. 8.18 Mechanisms of cytotoxicity. The cytotoxic destruction of a target cell may arise in a number of different ways. The target cell may be opsonized and phagocytosed by a macrophage, it may be damaged by extracellular degranulation of neutrophils or eosinophils, or antibody binding may activate the classical pathway of complement leading to formation of the MAC and osmotic lysis. The innate NK cells may recognize the target through an activating receptor (NKR) or, alternatively, by binding antibody through the FcR in the process of ADCC. NK cell activating receptors are members of the KIR, Ly49 or NKG2 receptor families. The adaptive CD8⁺ T cell recognizes the target in MHC-restricted fashion when that target expresses peptide in the context of MHC class I.

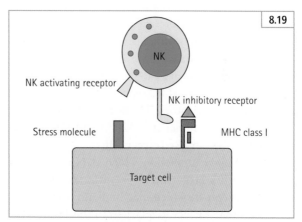

Fig. 8.19 NK cell recognition of target cells. The NK receptor families (KIR, Ly49 or NKG2) recognize cell surface molecules expressed by stressed cells directly, but the NK cell can only be cytotoxic if that target cell fails to express MHC class I. Where class I is present (i.e. on a normal cell) this is bound by an inhibitory member of one of the receptor families, which prevents activation of the NK cell.

target cells (stress-induced proteins). Note that there is no requirement for antigen processing for NK cell recognition. In addition to activating receptors, NK cells have **inhibitory receptors**, which bind to **MHC class I** molecules. This binding inhibits the NK cell and is a mechanism designed to protect normal cells of the body from cytolytic attack. Any NK cell that binds to a target expressing MHC class I will not be able to kill it, even if the activating receptor has recognized a suitable ligand. Therefore, only cells that have downregulated class I expression (e.g. virally infected or tumour cells) can become targets for an NK cell. The NK cell activating and inhibitory receptors are distributed within three families of NK cell receptors. **Killer cell immunoglobulin-like receptors** (KIRs) are the dominant form of human and primate NK receptor. Some KIRs bind MHC class I to inhibit NK function, while others play a role in activating NK cells. In mice and horses, the family of **Ly49 receptors** serve the same roles as KIRs, but these species lack KIRs (while primates and humans lack Ly49 receptors). In contrast, domestic animals other than horses may have both KIR and Ly49 receptors, but KIRs are the predominant and more important form. The third type of NK cell receptors are the **NKG2 receptors**. These molecules recognize MHC class I-like molecules (MICA and MICB) that are expressed on stressed target cells.

An alternative method by which an NK cell might interact with a target involves antibody. NK cells carry Fc receptors, which may bind antibody that is attached to the surface of a target. In this fashion the antibody is a bridge between the target and the NK cell, and the ensuing cytotoxic destruction is known as '**antibody-dependent cell-mediated cytotoxicity**' (ADCC). It should be recalled that antibody coating of a target cell may also permit interactions with other cells bearing Fc receptors. For example, a macrophage might phagocytose and destroy the target cell or a neutrophil or eosinophil may release cytoplasmic granule contents, leading to local damage to the target cell membrane. This latter process is referred to as '**frustrated phagocytosis**' and has a particular role in the immune response to parasites (see Chapter 13).

In contrast, the cytotoxicity mediated by **CD8+ T cells** is an **MHC-restricted** phenomenon that is part of an adaptive immune response. CD8+ T cells are activated by professional APCs in similar fashion to Th cells. The TCR of the cell recognizes antigenic peptide expressed by MHC class I, the CD8 molecule binds to MHC class I and further molecular interactions, including co-stimulatory cytokine production, occur between the two cells. While direct interaction between a CD8+ T cell and an APC is sufficient to activate the cell, a much more effective activation occurs when the APC has previously encountered a CD4+ Th1 cell specific for the same antigen. The interaction with the Th1 cell leads to prior activation of the APC, with up-regulation of peptide-loaded MHC class I and IL-12 expression. This allows more effective stimulation of the cytotoxic T cells. Further signalling of the CD8+ cell by Th1 derived cytokines (IL-2, IFN-γ) also contributes to activation. Activated CD8+ T cells then recognize target cells in an MHC-restricted fashion through the peptide–MHC class I–TCR complex, with additional interactions between other surface membrane molecules expressed by the target cell and cytotoxic cell.

Following recognition the next stage in the cytotoxic sequence is **adhesion (Figure 8.20)**. At this point the target and cytotoxic cells form membrane interdigitations and intercellular '**tight junctions**', which form a **contained microenvironment** in the narrow space between the two cells. The cytoplasmic granules within the cytotoxic cell move through the cytoplasm to polarize against the surface of the cell in apposition to the target.

Adhesion is followed by **cytolysis** and this may be mediated by one or more of several different mechanisms (**Figure 8.21**). The first of these involves release of the contents of **cytotoxic cell granules** into the confined space between the two cells. The presence of tight junctions prevents these toxic molecules from diffusing away and causing damage to nearby normal cells. The granule contents include the molecule **perforin**, which polymerizes and inserts into the membrane of the target cell to form a channel similar to the MAC of the complement pathway.

In fact, there is sequence homology between these molecules. Although perforin may establish an osmotic imbalance (akin to the MAC), the more important effect is that this channel provides a route by which other granule contents (enzymes known as **granzymes** and **fragmentins**) enter the cytoplasm of the target. These enzymes may cause direct damage but also, importantly, they activate intracellular pathways that lead to **apoptosis** of the target cell. Apoptosis ('programmed cell death' or 'cell suicide') is a carefully regulated process by which an aged, damaged or abnormal cell may kill itself. The process is characterized by blebbing of the cell membrane, loss of cytoplasmic organelles and clumping of the nuclear chromatin leading to nuclear fragmentation. The final stages of apoptosis are the generation of 'apoptotic bodies' (cellular remnants), which are phagocytosed. Granzymes activate the **intrinsic pathway of apoptosis** in which damaged cells produce pro-apoptotic bcl-2 proteins that cause mitochondria to release cytochrome C, leading to formation of the 'apoptosome' (a multiprotein complex). The apoptosome activates the 'initiator caspase' (caspase-9), which in turn activates the 'effector caspases' (caspase-3, -6 and -7) that are responsible for the physical effects of apoptosis described above.

Secondly, the cytotoxic T cell may secrete the cytokine tumour necrosis factor-α (TNF-α), which binds to receptors on the target cell and provides further signalling events leading to apoptosis via the **extrinsic pathway**. The extrinsic pathway of apoptosis involves activation of initiator caspases-8 and -10, leading to effector caspase induction. The same pathway is triggered following interaction between the molecules **Fas** (expressed by the target cell) and the **Fas ligand** (expressed by the Tc), which also activates apoptosis. Co-stimulatory cytokines such as IFN-γ may amplify these effects.

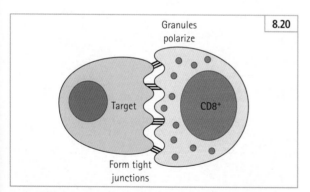

Fig. 8.20 Adhesion. After recognition, the cytotoxic cell forms close adhesion to the target cell. This involves interdigitation of the cell surface and the formation of tight junctions between the cells in order to create a contained microenvironment. The cytotoxic cell cytoplasmic granules polarize to the surface of the cell in apposition to the target.

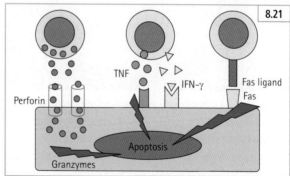

Fig. 8.21 Cytolysis. Several mechanisms are used by the cytotoxic cell to destroy the target. The cytoplasmic granule contents are released into the space between the two cells. One of these molecules (perforin) polymerizes and inserts into the target cell membrane to form a channel that has homology to the MAC of complement. Enzymes (granzymes) enter the target cell through this channel and cause direct damage in addition to activating the apoptotic pathway in the target. Apoptosis is also induced in the target following signalling through the TNF-γ receptor and the molecule Fas. The effects are amplified by cytokines such as IFN-γ.

Once the target cell is destroyed, the cytotoxic cell may detach and move on to locate and kill another target. In this fashion, cytotoxic cells are '**multi-hit**' cells that may destroy a number of targets. A good clinical example of the value of the cytotoxic response is provided by the benign canine skin tumour known as histiocytoma (**Figures 8.22–8.24**). These are the most common skin tumours of the dog and generally occur in younger animals. The small nodular lesions grow very rapidly, but in a matter of weeks undergo spontaneous regression. The regression of the tumour is a direct consequence of active infiltration of CD8+ cytotoxic T cells into the lesion. This is one of the rare examples of an immune response to a tumour being able to resolve the neoplastic lesion.

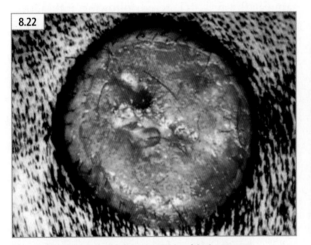

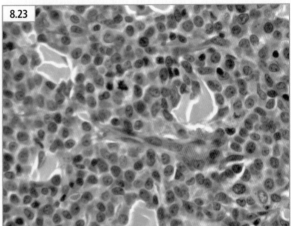

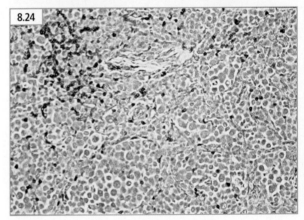

Figs. 8.22–8.24 Cytotoxicity in canine histiocytoma.
(**8.22**) This small, raised, nodular mass is an example of the most common canine cutaneous tumour, the histiocytoma. (**8.23**) This is a tumour of Langerhans dendritic cells that most often occurs in young dogs and undergoes spontaneous regression over a period of weeks. (**8.24**) This section of a histiocytoma is labelled to show an infiltrate of T cells expressing the CD3 complex. These are CD8+ cytotoxic T cells and are responsible for destruction of the tumour. This lesion provides one of the few examples of the immune system successfully destroying a neoplastic growth.

MEMORY CELLS

As discussed in Chapter 1, a key feature of the adaptive immune response is that it carries the memory of past antigen exposure so that on re-encounter with that same antigen a more potent 'secondary' immune response is generated. Both T and B **memory lymphocytes** exist, but they are poorly characterized. Immunological memory can be **long-lived** (for the lifetime of humans), as epitomized by observations made many years ago of native populations living on remote islands. When such islands were first visited by European explorers, new infectious agents (e.g. measles virus) were introduced to these populations and caused outbreaks of disease. After departure of the Europeans the virus failed to become endemic. Many decades later, when virus was reintroduced by further visitors, natives that had been alive at the time of the first exposure were resistant to infection, whereas those who had been born since became ill. The principle of immunological memory underlies the process of vaccination, which we shall consider in Chapter 20.

Despite firm evidence for the existence of T-cell memory, it has proven very difficult to isolate and characterize memory T cells. In some species, different isoforms of the leucocyte common antigen (CD45) are expressed by naïve and memory T cells, with the truncated CD45R0 form associated with the memory population. As discussed in Chapter 5, it is also possible that memory cells have selective recirculation pathways and homing receptor expression. Such cells may also display greater sensitivity to antigen and have functional differences (e.g. in terms of cytokine production) relative to naïve T cells.

A contentious aspect of memory cell biology is the longevity of such cells. Although individual memory cells are probably relatively long-lived, throughout a lifetime they likely require some form of periodical restimulation to maintain their presence. Antigen is required to effect such restimulation and several models are proposed to account for the availability of such antigen. One theory is that in every immune response, small **reservoirs of antigen** may be stored (perhaps associated with dendritic cells in lymphoid tissue) and periodically presented to the memory population. An alternative theory is that ubiquitous environmental antigens provide **cross-reactive epitopes** that permit restimulation of memory lymphocytes. The required antigen may also be provided by **re-exposure** to an infectious agent (or field virus) or via deliberate booster vaccination.

γδ LYMPHOCYTES

As discussed above, the majority of T cells in the immune system express an αβ TCR. An alternative form of TCR is composed of γ and δ chains with the CD3 complex. **γδ TCR-bearing cells** (γδT cells) are not as well characterized as the αβ TCR-bearing population. These T cells also undergo **intrathymic development** and it is suggested that the γδ TCR may be an evolutionarily older form of T-cell antigen-recognition molecule. Diversity in γδ TCRs is achieved as described earlier. The δ chain genes are clustered together with those that encode the TCR α chain, whereas there is a distinct cluster of genes encoding elements of the γ chain. There is a **single δ chain constant region gene**, but there are **species differences in the number of γ chain constant region genes** ranging from two in humans to five or six in ruminants. In most species there are **few variable region genes** in both gene clusters, meaning that γδ TCRs have **limited antigenic specificity**. However, in ruminants and pigs these receptors have greater diversity, as there are more variable, diversity and joining region genes.

γδ T cells are highly enriched at the **mucocutaneous surfaces** of the body and often live within epithelial barriers (**Figure 8.25**) where they are well-located to provide one of the first points of contact with the immune system. γδ T cells are in fact readily activated by exposure to bacteria that colonize such surfaces (e.g. *Listeria*, *Escherichia coli*, *Salmonella*, *Mycobacterium*). These cells generally do not express CD4 or CD8 and it is thought that they are not MHC restricted. They are generally considered to be part of the **innate immune system**. There may be functional subsets of γδ T cells determined by polarized cytokine production akin to that of Th1 and Th2 cells.

There are particular species differences in the distribution of γδ T cells, which are enriched in the circulation of cattle, sheep and pigs and are the dominant T-cell population at the mucocutaneous surfaces of these species. Porcine γδ T cells have broad antigen specificity at birth, but develop more restricted specificity with age. Bovine γδ T cells comprise two separate subsets. The WC1+ subset is considered part of innate immunity, but it shows a Th1-like function by producing IL-12 and IFN-γ, whereas cells that do not express WC1 have a regulatory function. In dogs, γδ T cells comprise up to one third of the T cells in the spleen.

NATURAL KILLER T CELLS

Natural killer T (NKT) cells are a T-cell subset distinct from CD4+ and CD8+ T cells. Two NKT subsets are reported. **Type I NKT cells** express a TCR that comprises an **invariant α chain** combined with a limited number of β chains. **Type II NKT** cells have **greater variability in α chain usage**. Both cell types are also defined by recognition of **antigen expressed by the CD1d** molecule, and therefore predominantly respond to glycolipid molecules. Type I NKT cells have been described in the dog.

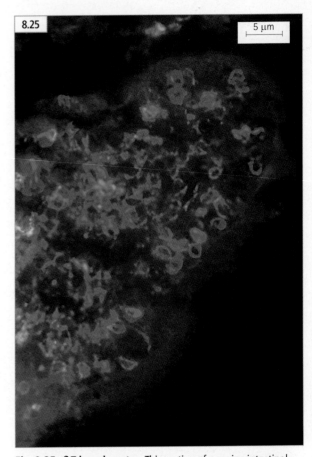

Fig. 8.25 γδ T lymphocytes. This section of a canine intestinal villus is labelled with two fluorescent antibody markers that show the location of T cells expressing the αβ TCR (green) within the lamina propria, and T cells expressing the γδ TCR (red) within the epithelial barrier. The latter population is well situated to be able to provide first-line defence of the intestine from pathogens that attempt to colonize the surface or invade. (From German AJ, Hall EJ, Moore PF *et al.* (1999) Analysis of the distribution of lymphocytes expressing the αβ and γδ T cell receptors and expression of mucosal addressin cell adhesion molecule-1 in the canine intestine. *Journal of Comparative Pathology* **201**:249–263, with permission.)

KEY POINTS

- Most T cells carry an αβ TCR and CD3 complex with either CD4 or CD8.
- Generation of diversity in the T-cell repertoire is achieved by rearrangement of genes encoding segments of the α and β chains of the TCR.
- One TCR may recognize numerous antigenic peptides as long as these have the same contact residues.
- Most T cells that enter the thymus die by apoptosis.
- T cells with a functional TCR are positively selected during thymic development.
- T cells with a high-affinity autoreactive TCR are negatively selected during thymic development.
- Antigen presentation by MHC class II activates CD4$^+$ T cells; presentation by MHC class I activates CD8$^+$ T cells.
- T-cell activation requires signal 1 (TCR–peptide–MHC interaction), signal 2 (co-stimulatory molecular interaction) and signal 3 (APC-derived co-stimulatory cytokine).
- Activated T cells undergo clonal proliferation and differentiation to effector and memory T cells.
- CD4$^+$ T cell subsets include Th1, Th2, Th9 and Th17 cells.
- Th1 cells produce IL-2 and IFN-γ and generate CMI.
- Th2 cells produce IL-4, IL-5, IL-9 and IL-13 and mediate humoral immunity.
- Naïve CD4$^+$ T cells give rise to Th1, Th2, Th9 or Th17 cells depending on the nature of the simulating antigen and signalling by the APC that presents it.
- Th1 and Th2 cells are mutually antagonistic, allowing polarized immune responses (immune deviation).
- Cytotoxicity is mediated by NK cells and CD8$^+$ T cells.
- NK cells are part of the innate immune system.
- NK cells recognize a target via an activating receptor.
- NK cells can only destroy a target cell if the target does not express MHC class I, which would be recognized by the NK cell inhibitory receptor.
- NK cells may bind an antibody-coated target cell via the FcR in ADCC.
- CD8$^+$ T cells recognize target cells in an MHC class I-restricted fashion.
- Cytotoxicity involves adhesion, cytolysis and detachment.
- Cytolysis involves granule release, perforin insertion and entry of granzymes into the target cell.
- Target cell apoptosis is induced by intracellular granule contents, cytokine–cytokine receptor interaction and Fas–Fas ligand interaction.
- Memory T cells are poorly characterized, but are likely to require periodical restimulation with antigen.
- γδ T cells are concentrated at mucocutaneous barriers and provide first-line defence from bacterial pathogens.

CHAPTER 9

The Biology of B Lymphocytes

OBJECTIVES

At the end of this chapter you should be able to:
- Describe the difference in how T and B lymphocytes recognize antigen.
- Distinguish between a T-independent and a T-dependent antigen.
- Summarize the development of B cells in man, other animals and birds.
- Describe the three signals required for B-cell activation.
- Summarize the events that occur within the secondary lymphoid follicle during B-cell activation.

- Understand how BCR diversity develops in man, other animals and birds.
- Understand the mechanism of the immunoglobulin class switch.
- Describe the differences between the primary and secondary humoral immune response.
- Relate the secondary immune response to B-cell memory.
- Describe how monoclonal antibodies are produced.

INTRODUCTION

One of the main roles of Th cells is to provide help to B lymphocytes in order that they may become fully activated to transform into plasma cells for the production of antibody. This chapter considers the development and maturation of B cells, diversity in the BCR and the effector and memory functions of this lymphoid subset.

ANTIGEN RECOGNITION BY B CELLS

T and B lymphocytes are both able to respond to the same antigenic stimulus, but in an entirely distinct fashion. The TCR recognizes a small peptide fragment from the antigen presented in association with an MHC molecule. In contrast, the **BCR** (surface membrane immunoglobulin) interacts with a much **larger** area of an **intact antigenic epitope** that generally has **conformational or planar structure**. Consequently, the B cell has no requirement for antigen processing and may directly recognize antigen. Although antigen may sometimes be associated with the surface of an APC, the epitopes remain intact and are bound by the BCR without prior processing.

B-cell antigen recognition may be **thymus independent** or **thymus dependent**. Thymus-independent (T-independent) recognition is a relatively uncommon event and is restricted to antigens composed of polymers of simple repeating structural units. Such antigens are able to cross-link BCRs and trigger stimulatory signals for B-cell activation in the absence of T-cell help (**Figure 9.1**). The end effect of T-independent stimulation is generally production of IgM antibody.

In contrast, the majority of antigens recognized by the BCR are not able to fully activate these cells, which require assistance from Th cells (T-dependent). This process will be examined in detail below.

DEVELOPMENT AND MATURATION OF B LYMPHOCYTES

As for all haemopoietic and immune cells, B lymphocytes derive from bone marrow stem cells. B-cell maturation is not as well characterized as the intrathymic development of T cells. Some stages of maturation likely occur within the bone marrow, but in most domestic animal species the final stages of B-cell maturation are thought to occur in extramedullary locations such as the ileal Peyer's patch (e.g. in ruminants) or, in avians, the bursa of Fabricius (see Chapter 5).

The earliest form of B cell recognized (the **pre-B cell**) is a precursor that produces the μ heavy chain within the cytoplasm. In the next stage of development, complete IgM monomers are synthesized and the **immature B cell** displays these on its surface membrane. The final step in development is the co-expression of surface membrane **IgM and IgD**

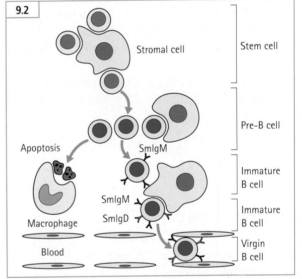

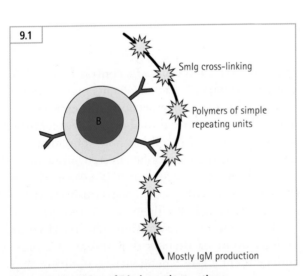

Fig. 9.1 Recognition of T-independent antigen.
A T-independent antigen consists of a polymer of repeating subunits that are able to cross-link BCRs and activate the B cell in the absence of T-cell help. SmIg, surface membrane immunoglobulin.

Fig. 9.2 Development of B lymphocytes. B cells originate from the bone marrow stem cell and undergo a series of maturation events involving interactions with stromal cells that supply stimulatory cytokines such as IL-7. The pre-B cell expresses cytoplasmic μ heavy chain, while immature B cells express first surface membrane IgM and then a combination of IgM and IgD. Some apoptosis of developing B cells that fail to produce appropriate receptors is likely to occur. In man, these developmental stages occur within the bone marrow, but in other animals the latter stages may occur in extramedullary tissues such as the ileal Peyer's patch or, in avians, the bursa of Fabricius. The naïve or virgin B cell-bearing surface membrane IgM and IgD enters the recirculating and secondary lymphoid tissue B-cell pool.

molecules by **naïve or 'virgin' B lymphocytes**. At this stage, the naïve B cells are released from their place of development to become part of the recirculating and secondary lymphoid tissue B-cell pool (**Figure 9.2**).

Immature bone marrow B cells undergo a process similar to the **negative selection** of developing intrathymic T cells. Contact of the BCR with self-antigen may lead to deletion (by apoptosis) of that cell. Alternatively, the B cell may undergo further gene rearrangements within the light chain (see below) and express a new BCR. If this new receptor is still self-reactive, the cell will be deleted but if not, the cell will be exported for further maturation in the periphery. This process is known as **receptor editing**. Some **autoreactive B cells** do escape this process and enter the peripheral immune system where they remain **anergic** (with lack of T-cell help) or **ignorant** of their cognate antigen that may be sequestered within the body.

ACTIVATION OF THE B LYMPHOCYTE

The activation of a naïve B cell is not dissimilar to the process of T-cell activation described in Chapter 8. The B cell requires three specific signals in order to become fully activated (**Figure 9.3**):
- **Signal 1** for B-cell activation is the **recognition of antigenic epitope** by the surface membrane BCR. Signal transduction for the BCR is undertaken by a complex of CD79a and CD79b molecules (similar to the function of CD3 for the TCR).
- **Signal 2** comprises **intermolecular interactions** between surface molecules on that B cell and the appropriate antigen-specific Th cell. One such interaction results from the B cell internalizing antigen and presenting peptide fragments associated with MHC class II molecules. These are in turn bound by the TCR of the helper T cell with CD4 binding to the MHC molecule. A second key interaction between the two cells involves the B-cell surface molecule **CD40** binding to the **CD40 ligand** expressed by the Th cell.

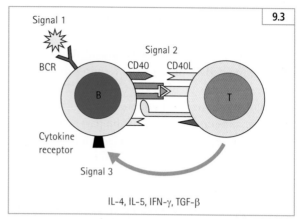

Fig. 9.3 Activation of the B lymphocyte. B-cell activation requires three signalling events. Signal 1 for the B cell is the recognition of antigenic epitope by the BCR. Signal 2 involves the interaction between molecules on the surface of the B cell and Th cell. The most important of these involves the B-cell presentation of peptide antigen by MHC class II for recognition by the TCR and CD4 molecules. Other intermolecular interactions, including that between CD40 and the CD40 ligand, also occur. Signal 3 is the delivery of co-stimulatory cytokine derived from the Th cell to cytokine receptor on the surface of the B cell.

- **Signal 3** for B-cell activation takes the form of a **co-stimulatory cytokine** released by the Th cell that binds to a cytokine receptor on the surface of the B cell. A range of cytokines act in this fashion (depending on the nature of the antigen, the subset of Th cell and the type of immune response required) including IL-4, IL-5, IL-13, TGF-β and IFN-γ.

The delivery of all three signals permits activation of the B cell. The activated cell transforms morphologically to become a **B lymphoblast**, upregulates expression of surface MHC class II and undergoes a unique phenomenon, the **'immunoglobulin class switch'**, whereby the cell replaces its surface membrane IgM and IgD with a receptor of a single immunoglobulin class (IgG, IgA or IgE). The means by which this class switch occurs will be discussed below. In addition, the activated B cell will undergo **clonal proliferation and differentiation**, generating large numbers of antigen-relevant B lymphocytes (**Figure 9.4**). The effector stage of B-cell activation involves transformation of these B cells into **plasma cells**, a process that requires the input of further cytokine signalling (e.g. IL-6, IL-11). Plasma cells will synthesize and secrete immunoglobulin of the same antigen specificity as the parent B cell and of the same immunoglobulin class determined by class switching. In addition to effector cells, some activated B cells differentiate to become **memory B lymphocytes**.

At this point it is possible to consider all the stages of the adaptive immune response that lead to antibody production (**Figure 9.5**) and involve the triad of APC, Th cell and B cell. The question arises as to where anatomically these cells interact with

each other. This has been defined by studies in which antigen-specific T and B lymphocytes were labelled and tracked within lymphoid tissue as the adaptive immune response was generated. The **interaction between APC and Th cell** occurs within the lymph node **paracortex**, as Th cells from the recirculating pool of naïve and memory T cells enter the node through HEVs. The activated T cell then migrates to the edge of the **primary follicle** where it encounters the antigen-specific B cell and provides co-stimulatory signals for activation of that cell.

Activation of the B cell and clonal proliferation take place within the follicle, which transforms to become a **secondary follicle** with a germinal centre and surrounding mantle zone. The **germinal centre** comprises a **dark zone** and a **light zone**, the former

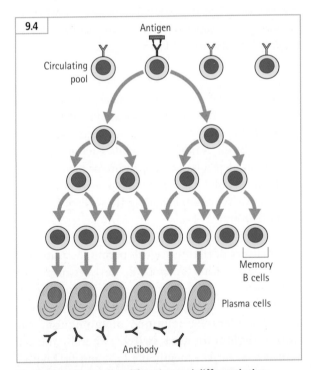

Fig. 9.4 B-cell clonal proliferation and differentiation. Activation of the B cell leads to clonal division, which is further assisted by Th cell-derived cytokines. The terminal stage of differentiation for a B cell is the effector B cell or plasma cell that is the source of antibody. These plasma cells may be short or long lived. A population of long-lived B memory cells is also produced.

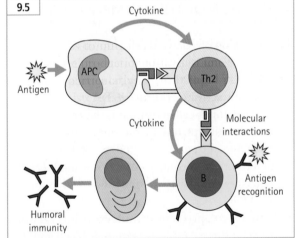

Fig. 9.5 Generation of the adaptive immune response. This diagram summarizes the key stages in the generation of the adaptive immune response as discussed in preceding chapters. Antigen is taken up by APCs, processed and presented by MHC class II. The naïve CD4+ T cell is activated by the APC following the delivery of signals 1–3. The nature of these signals and the type of initiating antigen determines whether a Th1, Th2, Th17 or T-regulatory phenotype is induced. In this model, Th2 differentiation provides appropriate help for the subsequent activation of B cells via provision of signals 1–3. B-cell activation leads to terminal differentiation to an antibody-producing plasma cell.

being the site of the most active proliferation and containing 'centroblasts'. The B cells that form by clonal proliferation migrate from the dark to the light zone, where they are known as 'centrocytes' and are able to re-encounter antigen associated with **follicular dendritic cells** and also re-encounter antigen-specific Th cells. This provides an opportunity for the B cell to 'test out' its BCR. B cells with **low-affinity receptors** (see Chapter 1) will undergo **apoptosis** within the germinal centre, while those cells carrying **high-affinity receptors** are allowed to leave the follicle to eventually become **effector B cells** (plasma cells) or **memory B cells** (**Figure 9.6**). Mature plasma cells are distributed throughout the lymph node medullary cords, splenic red pulp, bone marrow and mucosal lamina propria. The elimination of B cells carrying low-affinity receptors (**negative selection**) occurs on a large scale, with almost one in every two developing B cells being eliminated. Similar to the thymus, evidence of this may be seen on microscopic examination of a germinal centre in which there is significant macrophage phagocytosis of apoptotic cell debris.

B-CELL RECEPTOR DIVERSITY

The fundamental principles underlying the generation of BCR diversity are very similar to those discussed for formation of the TCR in Chapter 8. In accordance with Burnett's **clonal selection theory**, the adaptive immune system must carry a large **repertoire of antigen-specific B cells** to account for the possible interactions with antigen that might occur throughout life. This diversity appears to be achieved in a different fashion in man and domestic animals.

In humans and mice, any one B cell selects from a series of genes encoding different regions of the immunoglobulin heavy and light chains, and diversity in the variable region of these chains is achieved in a number of ways. For example, the **heavy chain variable region** is encoded by three segments: **variable** (V), **diversity** (D) and **joining** (J) regions. There are in the order of 40 V region genes, 25 D region genes and 6 J region genes for the heavy chain. One each of these gene segments is selected and the intervening **intronic sequence is looped out and deleted**. This

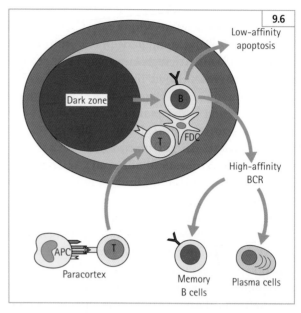

Fig. 9.6 Anatomical location of T- and B-cell activation. Antigen-laden dendritic cells enter the lymph node paracortex where they activate antigen-specific T cells from the recirculating pool that enter the paracortex via HEVs. Antigen-specific T cells migrate to the edge of a primary follicle where they encounter antigen-specific B cells from the recirculating B-cell pool. Activation of the B cell leads to formation of the germinal centre. Active B-cell proliferation occurs within the dark zone of the germinal centre. B cells thus formed migrate into the light zone where they re-encounter the Th cell and antigen present on the surface of a follicular dendritic cell (FDC). B cells that have formed low-affinity BCRs fail to recognize antigen and receive T-cell help and so die by apoptosis. B cells with high-affinity receptors are allowed to undergo terminal differentiation to plasma cells or memory B cells.

process involves a complex of enzymes that cleave and ligate the DNA. The complex is collectively known as the **V(D)J recombinase** and includes two important enzymes encoded by the **recombination activating genes RAG-1** and **RAG-2**. Similar to the TCR (Chapter 8), the selected **constant region gene** is added by **RNA splicing** after transcription. There are species differences in the arrangement of heavy chain constant region genes, but most have a single C_μ, C_δ and C_ε gene, with separate gene segments encoding constant regions for those immunoglobulins with subclasses (IgG and IgA).

These are arranged in the order C_μ, C_δ, C_γ, C_ε and C_α (**Figure 9.7**). The immunoglobulin **light chain genes** include **V** and **J segments** (with no D region) and either C_κ or C_λ must be selected for addition by RNA splicing after transcription. In man there is a single C_κ gene, but a series of several C_λ gene segments.

The theoretical calculation of the possible **germline repertoire** for BCRs produces a figure of approximately 2×10^8 permutations and combinations of these gene segments. However, unlike for the TCR, B cells can further increase diversity in their receptors by the processes of **alternative junctional recombination** and **somatic mutation**. Junctional alternatives are simply variable boundary recombinations between V–J or V–D–J segments (for light and heavy chains, respectively), which join at different points in their sequences. Somatic mutation refers to **single nucleotide substitutions** (point mutations) in a gene sequence that again would result in an immunoglobulin polypeptide of different sequence. These two additional processes expand the theoretical germline repertoire to a factor of approximately 10^{30}, but in reality it has been calculated

that the **recirculating B-cell pool** probably includes around 10^9 BCR specificities at any one time.

In domestic animals the process of generation of BCR diversity is largely achieved in a different fashion. In sheep, cattle, pigs, horses, rabbits and birds there are limited V, D and J heavy chain gene segments, and these are rearranged to achieve a **restricted range of VDJ regions** in immature bone marrow B cells. These precursor B cells, either within bone marrow or after migration to lymphoid tissue such as the spleen, express surface membrane immunoglobulin and start to proliferate. During proliferation a process of '**gene conversion**' allows the introduction of multiple

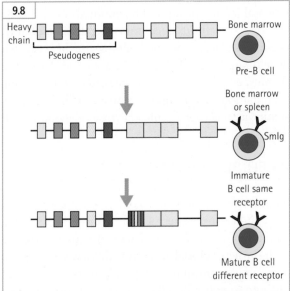

Fig. 9.8 Generation of diversity in animal and bird BCRs. Formation of the BCR differs in birds and domestic animals, in which there are restricted V, D and J heavy chain gene segments. Within the bone marrow or spleen, these segments are combined within immature B cells to form limited primordial variable regions. These immature B cells express the BCR formed of those limited variable regions and start to proliferate. During proliferation there is incorporation of small segments from up-stream V region pseudogenes into the V region by the process of 'gene conversion'. If these modified BCRs are expressed on the cell membrane, the cell will survive. Cells that fail to express the modified receptor die by apoptosis. Finally, the immature B cells migrate to the specialized sites of the ileal Peyer's patch, appendix or bursa of Fabricius (depending on species), where further diversity is achieved through somatic mutation.

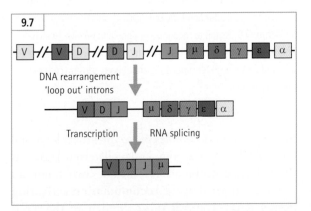

Fig. 9.7 Generation of diversity in the human BCR. The human BCR heavy chain is formed by initial recombination of V, D and J gene segments by looping out and deleting intronic sequence via the action of the V(D)J recombinase enzyme complex. Following transcription, the heavy chain region is added by differential RNA splicing. Shown is the formation of an IgM heavy chain protein. Similar rearrangement occurs for the formation of the immunoglobulin light chain.

short areas of sequence from a series of **up-stream V region pseudogenes** into the expressed V region gene segment (**Figure 9.8**). This process generates diversity in the V region sequence of the heavy chain. In contrast, **light chain** formation (at least in ruminants) is known to occur through **gene recombination**, as defined above for humans and mice. If gene conversion produces an immunoglobulin protein that can be expressed on the surface of the B cell, that cell will be maintained within the B-cell pool; if not, the cell will undergo apoptosis. The immature B cells then migrate to the specialized environments of the ileal Peyer's patch (most animals), the appendix (the rabbit) or the bursa of Fabricius (birds). In these locations, BCR diversity is further expanded by somatic mutation. In many animal species the C_λ gene is preferentially used, so that most immunoglobulins comprise a λ light chain.

THE IMMUNOGLOBULIN CLASS SWITCH

As stated above, one feature of B-cell activation is the replacement of surface membrane IgM and IgD by a single immunoglobulin class (IgG, IgA or IgE) of the same antigen-binding specificity. The decision as to which immunoglobulin class the naïve B cell 'switches' to is probably **cytokine driven** and determined by the nature of the **Th cell** and, accordingly, by the **nature of the initiating antigen**. An exception to this lies in the case of IgA production, where class switching may be T dependent or T independent in nature. T-dependent IgA class switching involves classical T-cell help with TCR–MHC–peptide and CD40–CD40 ligand interactions, as described above. T-independent IgA class switching is induced by binding of the cytokines BAFF (B-cell activating factor), APRIL (a proliferation-inducing ligand) and transforming growth factor (TGF)-γ to receptors on the surface of a mucosal B cell. These stimulatory cytokines are produced by mucosal dendritic cells and epithelial cells.

The class switch is achieved by the ability of the B cell to undertake **multiple DNA rearrangements**. In the immature B cell the variable region genes (e.g. VDJ) are initially selected and then, following transcription, there is alternative RNA splicing to allow the formation of both IgM and IgD. During

class switching, a **second DNA rearrangement** permits the RNA splicing of an alternative constant region gene, leading to the formation of the final species of immunoglobulin (**Figure 9.9**). This comes about through recombination between 'switch regions', which are sequences of intronic DNA that lie up-stream of each constant region gene (except for C_δ). The μ chain switch region (Sμ) recombines with the switch region of the selected immunoglobulin class (e.g. Sα) with looping out and deletion of intervening sequences in a process that probably involves enzymes similar to those of the V(D)J recombinase complex.

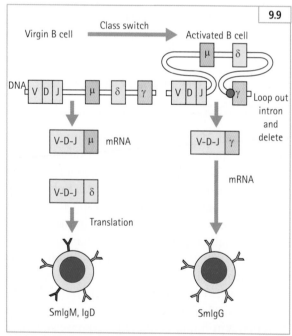

Fig. 9.9 The immunoglobulin class switch. All naïve B cells co-express surface membrane (Sm) IgM and IgD. This is permitted by differential RNA splicing of the C_μ or C_δ region after VDJ recombination. Following antigen-specific activation of the B cell there is a second DNA rearrangement. The C_μ and C_δ gene segments are looped out and deleted and the switch region intronic sequence preceding the C_μ is brought into apposition with the switch region for the chosen immunoglobulin class (IgG in this example). Following transcription, the C_λ chain mRNA would now be added by RNA splicing, and the B cell would express surface membrane IgG.

AFFINITY MATURATION

Affinity maturation of the B-cell response is based on the **somatic mutations** in BCR sequences that occur during B-cell activation within the **germinal centre**. During **clonal proliferation**, each generation of dividing B cells may acquire further somatic mutations, leading to slight modifications in the expressed BCR. If these mutations create a receptor with **lower affinity** for antigen, the B cell will fail to effectively capture antigen and present it to Th cells within the germinal centre light zone, resulting in **apoptosis** of that B cell. In contrast, those B cells with **high-affinity receptors** will effectively capture antigen and receive T-cell help, thus progressing to become effector or memory B cells. Early in an immune response, when antigen is abundant, a greater number of B cells may be positively selected in this fashion; however, in the late stages of the adaptive response only those B cells with the highest-affinity receptors will be selected.

KINETICS OF THE HUMORAL IMMUNE RESPONSE

In a naïve individual who has never before encountered a particular antigen, there is a pre-existing capacity for immunoglobulin to bind that antigen as it first enters the body. Mucosal surfaces are bathed in **low-affinity polyreactive antibodies** that bear receptors capable of interacting with numerous epitopes. Such antibodies may be considered part of the innate immune defence of these surfaces. If the antigen is **T independent**, the activation of antigen-specific B cells may be relatively rapid and specific antibody may be detected within the serum within **2–7 days**. In contrast, generation of a **T dependent** humoral immune response generally takes somewhere between **4 and 10 days** because it involves the sequential stages of antigen presentation, T-cell activation, B-cell activation and the generation of an effector population of plasma cells.

B1 AND B2 LYMPHOCYTES

The B cells described in this chapter are 'conventional' B cells that arise from bone marrow stem cell precursors and play a major role in the adaptive immune response by producing antigen-specific antibody, primarily of the IgG class. These classical B lymphocytes (known as B2 cells) are in fact just one of two B-cell subsets. B1 lymphocytes are thought to arise from stem cell precursors in the fetal liver or abdominal omentum, and are produced only in early life. There is, however, debate as to whether B1 and B2 cells derive from unique precursors or have a common precursor from which particular selection processes give rise to the two lineages. They produce polyreactive immunoglobulins (IgM and IgA) with a broader antigenic reactivity in a T-independent fashion, as they have more restricted receptor diversity with limited V region repertoire. B1 cells are recognized in a number of species including pigs and ruminants. In rodents they are found in the abdominal and thoracic cavities and are self-renewing (as opposed to being replaced from the bone marrow). A large proportion of IgA plasma cells in the intestinal tract are of B1 origin.

MEMORY B LYMPHOCYTES

The phenomenon of B-cell memory is readily demonstrated in a classical immunological experiment that describes the kinetics of a **primary and secondary humoral immune response** (**Figure 9.10**). In this experiment a naïve animal is injected with foreign antigen on day 1 in order to induce the primary response. The development of this response is monitored by daily blood sampling and testing for the titre of antigen-specific antibody within the serum. For the first few days of the experiment, no serum antibody will be detectable, but after 5–7 days, low-titred IgM antibody will appear. Over the following few days, as the immunoglobulin class switch proceeds, this will be joined by detectable IgG antibody that gradually becomes the dominant class of immunoglobulin. This humoral response will peak at around 2–3 weeks after primary exposure and the concentration of serum antibody will gradually decline, as most immunoglobulins have a half-life of around 10–14 days.

Once the primary immune response has subsided, the presence of a population of **memory B cells** is readily demonstrated by reimmunizing that animal with the same antigen. This will induce a serum antibody response with strikingly different kinetics:

- There will be a **minimal lag phase** before antibody becomes evident within the serum.
- The antibody **titre will be significantly greater** than in the primary response and this higher titre will be **achieved relatively rapidly.**
- The antibody will **primarily be IgG** (or whichever class of immunoglobulin was selected during the primary response).
- The antibody will persist within the serum with a **plateau of high titre** before **gradual decline.**

The secondary immune response is therefore considerably more potent than that following primary exposure. The antibodies produced will also be of much **higher affinity** than in the primary response and the proliferating B cells within germinal centres will continue to undergo **affinity maturation.** The secondary response is, of course, mediated by the memory B cells that were generated within the primary activation event. These cells, as memory T cells, are poorly understood, but are thought to be a relatively **long-lived population** that might undergo periodical low-level division on restimulation by antigen held by follicular dendritic cells. In man these memory B cells are likely to survive for the life of the individual. Additionally, there are populations of **long-lived plasma cells** that survive for years (decades in man)

and continue to produce specific antibody. These cells may preferentially reside in the bone marrow. The induction of memory B cells and long-lived plasma cells and the persistence of serum antibody derived from the latter population are fundamental to the process of vaccination, which will be further discussed in Chapter 20.

MONOCLONAL ANTIBODIES

Discussion of B-cell biology would not be complete without considering the production and use of **monoclonal antibodies,** an immunological advance that has revolutionized the practice of medicine and led to the award of the 1984 Nobel Prize to Jerne, Kohler and Milstein, who first described this technique.

As described previously, immunization of an animal with a complex antigen bearing many epitopes will lead to generation of a **polyclonal immune response** as numerous clones of T and B lymphocytes respond to the different antigenic epitopes. Serum from such an animal will contain antibodies of many different specificities and affinity for antigen. Such serum may be used as a **polyclonal antiserum** in immunological testing. In contrast, a monoclonal antibody derives from a single clone of activated B cells and therefore represents a single species of high-affinity antibody

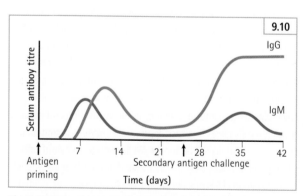

Fig. 9.10 The primary and secondary humoral immune response. The kinetics of serum antibody production following primary and secondary immunization with a non-replicating antigen are shown. The secondary response has a shorter lag phase, is of greater magnitude, mostly comprises class-switched immunoglobulin (IgG) of greater affinity and persists for a longer period of time. Memory B cells mediate this secondary response.

of a single immunoglobulin class. Monoclonal antibodies therefore provide a much more refined means of serological testing and these reagents have found wide application in diagnostic medicine and research. As will be discussed further in Chapter 21, monoclonal antibody therapy has had a major impact in human medicine. Because of the exquisite specificity of such antibodies, if injected intravenously they will target and bind only the antigen with which they are designed to interact. Such antibodies may be used to block receptors for infectious agents, to target toxins or drugs to tumours, and to block immunological pathways by neutralizing specific cell surface molecules or cytokines.

Although monoclonal antibodies are produced *in vivo*, their generation does initially require the use of an experimental animal (**Figure 9.11**). Mice are most widely used for this stage, but it is possible to use animals of any species (including man). A **mouse is first injected with the target antigen**, which is generally a relatively complex molecule that bears numerous epitopes. The mouse will make a polyclonal immune response to the antigen. Some time after immunization (multiple exposures may be given and the mouse may be tested for seroconversion) the mouse is sacrificed and the spleen is removed. The spleen is carefully teased apart and the lymphocytes (**splenocytes**) within it are placed into liquid suspension. This complex lymphoid population will contain some B cells that are specific for the antigen and others that are not.

The second component required to produce a monoclonal antibody is a **myeloma cell line**. A myeloma is a malignant **tumour of plasma cells** (see Chapter 14) and a myeloma cell line is one that initially derived from such a tumour but has been propagated *in vitro* by maintaining the tumour in **cell culture** (with appropriate media and growth factors), which is periodically replenished as subcultures of cells are established. As with all neoplastic cells, providing the myeloma cell line is appropriately maintained it will survive indefinitely (i.e. is **immortal**). The myeloma cell lines chosen do not secrete their own immunoglobulins.

In producing a monoclonal antibody, the key stage is the process of cellular '**fusion**'. In this procedure the suspension of immunized mouse splenocytes is mixed with a suspension of myeloma cells in the presence of a

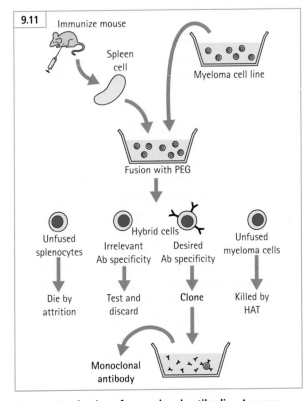

Fig. 9.11 Production of monoclonal antibodies. A mouse is immunized with multideterminant antigen so that multiple clones of B cells are activated in that animal. The spleen is taken and a suspension of splenic lymphocytes (splenocytes) is fused with a myeloma cell line by addition of polyethylene glycol (PEG). This results in four populations of unfused splenocytes, unfused myeloma cells and fused hybrid cells of required or irrelevant antibody specificity. Aliquots of this mixed population are plated out in a medium containing hypoxanthine, aminopterin and thymidine (HAT). Unfused splenocytes die by attrition and unfused myeloma cells die as they lack appropriate enzymes to metabolize HAT, while hybrid cells will survive. Wells containing hybrid cells of required antibody (Ab) specificity are diluted to a point where a single hybrid cell is present within a well. That cell is expanded and, if it produces an antibody of required specificity, the clone is bulk cultured for the harvesting of monoclonal antibody.

sticky polymer known as **polyethylene glycol** (PEG). Some of the splenocytes will fuse together with some of the myeloma cells to produce a genetically **hybrid cell** that has the properties of both parent cells. These hybrid cells are morphologically plasma cells, which will now produce antibody of the specificity of the immunized mouse splenocyte, but retain their *in-vitro* immortality. Following fusion, there will be four populations of cells within the test tube:

- Fused hybrid plasma cells of desired antibody specificity.
- Fused hybrid plasma cells of irrelevant antibody specificity.
- Unfused myeloma cells.
- Unfused mouse splenocytes.

In order to separate these populations, the cells are transferred to a medium containing a combination of **hypoxanthine, aminopterin and thymidine** (HAT) and the cells are aliquotted over the wells of a plastic microtitration plate. Unfused myeloma cells are sensitive to these substances, as they lack the enzyme **hypoxanthine–guanine phosphoribosyl transferase** (HGPRT) and will die in the presence of HAT. Unfused mouse splenocytes will die simply because they are not immortal. Fused hybrid cells, however, will survive in HAT because the myeloma cell obtained the HGPRT gene from the splenocyte during the fusion process.

At this stage, therefore, some wells of the microtitration plate will contain mixtures of hybrid cells, some of which will have the desired antibody specificity. In order to identify these wells, a small sample of medium is collected and utilized in a **serological test** (most commonly an ELISA). The cells from wells that are positive in this test will be harvested and subjected to the process of '**cloning**', whereby the cells are diluted to the point where a newly seeded well contains only a single hybrid cell. These single hybrid cells are then cultured so that they divide to produce a **hybridoma**, which represents a single cell type producing a single immunoglobulin that is the monoclonal antibody. After further serological testing, the desired hybridomas are **bulk cultured** to produce large quantities of monoclonal antibody, which is harvested from the cultures and concentrated for application in research, diagnosis or therapy.

KEY POINTS

- The BCR directly recognizes a large conformational determinant of antigen.
- T-independent antigens are polymers of repeating units that cross-link BCRs and directly activate B cells.
- T-dependent antigens require T-cell help for B-cell activation.
- B cells evolve in the bone marrow, but may undergo final maturation in extramedullary tissues in some species.
- Naïve or virgin B cells co-express surface membrane IgD and IgM.
- B-cell activation requires signal 1 (BCR antigen recognition), signal 2 (interaction with T-cell co-stimulatory molecules) and signal 3 (Th cell-derived cytokine signalling).
- Activated B cells undergo clonal proliferation and differentiation to form effector B cells (plasma cells) and memory B cells.
- B-cell clonal proliferation occurs within the germinal centre of a secondary follicle.
- Affinity maturation of the BCR during clonal proliferation leads to selection of those B cells bearing high-affinity receptors.
- BCR diversity is achieved by different means in man, domestic animals and birds.
- In man, recombination of V, D and J region genes with RNA splicing of the C region occurs for the heavy and light chains of immunoglobulin.
- The V(D)J recombinase complex mediates V(D)J recombination.
- The germline repertoire of BCRs is further increased by alternative junctional recombination and somatic mutation.
- Animals have restricted heavy chain V, D, J genes and must generate diversity by gene conversion and somatic mutation.
- B-cell activation leads to a second DNA rearrangement that underlies the immunoglobulin class switch from IgD/IgM to IgG, IgA or IgE.
- The secondary humoral immune response has a short lag phase and a more rapid and higher-titred production of class-switched antibody, which persists for a longer period.
- The secondary humoral immune response is mediated by long-lived memory B cells.
- Monoclonal antibodies are a single specificity high-affinity antibody generated *in vitro* by fusing immunized splenocytes with a myeloma cell line.
- Monoclonal antibodies have wide application in research, diagnosis and teaching.

CHAPTER 10

Testing of Cellular Immune Function

OBJECTIVES

At the end of this chapter you should be able to:
- Understand why it would be useful to test the function of lymphoid or phagocytic cells in a clinical situation.
- Describe the principle of the lymphocyte stimulation test.

- Describe the principle of evaluation of lymphocyte or NK cell cytotoxic function.
- Describe how the ability of phagocytic cells to move along a chemotactic gradient, to phagocytose particulate antigen and to kill phagocytosed microbes may be evaluated *in vitro*.

INTRODUCTION

The major components of the immune system are humoral immunity and cell-mediated immunity (CMI). In Chapter 4 we considered how the interaction between antigen and antibody might be evaluated *in vitro* by the use of a range of different serological tests. Other serological tests are used to quantify the amount of immunoglobulin (see Chapter 19), complement factors (see Chapter 3) and cytokines (see Chapter 7) produced in various body fluids. CMI may also be studied *in vitro* by the application of an array of techniques. We have already discussed how elements of the **cellular immune response** may be evaluated and enumerated within tissue by **immunofluorescence microscopy** or **immunohistochemistry**, or within fluid suspensions by the use of **flow cytometry** (see Chapter 5). In this short chapter we consider how the function of lymphoid and phagocytic cells might be evaluated *in vitro*. Such diagnostic procedures have widespread potential application in determining whether an individual patient has a fully competent immune system; unfortunately, the complexity of these tests means that they are rarely available to practising veterinarians.

LYMPHOCYTE STIMULATION TESTS

The lymphocyte stimulation test (or lymphocyte blastogenesis test) aims to determine whether the lymphocytes in a sample (generally blood, although teased apart lymphoid tissue can also provide a suitable suspension) are able to respond to stimulation *in vitro* (**Figure 10.1**). The simplest means of stimulating these cells is via the use of substances called '**mitogens**', which bind in a non-antigen-specific fashion directly to glycoslyated proteins expressed on the lymphocyte cell membrane, and so activate the cells. The most commonly used mitogens are derived from plants or other natural sources. Some mitogens more effectively activate T lymphocytes or subsets of T lymphocytes (concanavalin A [ConA]; phytohaemagglutinin [PHA]), while others are preferential B-cell stimulants (lipopolysaccharide [LPS]) and some stimulate both populations (pokeweed mitogen [PWM]). An alternative means of stimulating T cells is to incubate them with **antibody specific for CD3**, which binds to this signal transduction complex and directly activates the cells, again in a non-antigen-specific fashion. The most satisfying (but technically complex) procedure is to attempt to stimulate the lymphocytes in an antigen-specific fashion. This generally entails using an antigen to which the animal has been previously exposed and thus carries immunological memory (typically a vaccinal antigen), although it is also possible to demonstrate a primary immune response in such a culture system to a previously unseen antigen (which will have slower kinetics). This latter methodology requires that the lymphocyte culture is supplemented with a source of autologous APCs or that the mononuclear cell suspension incorporates blood monocytes. These are required to process and present the antigen for recognition via the antigen-specific TCR.

In practical terms, heparinized blood is collected from the test animal and from one or two control animals that are closely age and breed matched for comparative purposes. Although the test can be performed with whole unfractionated blood, it is best to separate the mononuclear cell fraction from the erythrocytes, platelets, granulocytes and serum. This is readily achieved by **density gradient centrifugation** in which a diluted sample of whole blood is carefully layered onto the top of a dense clear medium and, following centrifugation of the tube, the more dense cell types (erythrocytes and granulocytes) separate to the bottom of the tube (i.e. spin through the density gradient), whereas the less dense **mononuclear cells** and platelets form a distinct layer at the top of the density gradient from where they can be carefully aspirated, washed and resuspended at a known cell concentration following counting of the cell yield. Different density gradient media are required for isolation of lymphocytes from different animal species. The '**viability**' of the population can also be assessed by taking a small aliquot of the cells and staining them with '**vital dye**' (e.g. trypan blue), which is taken up by dead cells. The percentage viability in a good sample should be >98%.

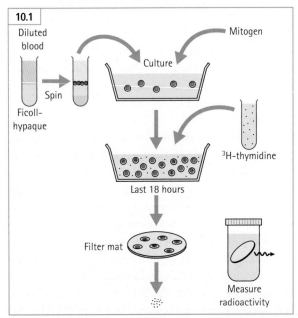

Fig. 10.1 The lymphocyte stimulation test. Mononuclear cells may be separated from whole blood by density gradient centrifugation and cultured *in vitro* in the presence or absence of mitogen or antigen. Stimulated cells will start to divide and, during the final stages of culture, radiolabelled thymidine added to the cultures will be incorporated into the DNA of newly dividing cells. At the end of the culture period the cells within the wells are trapped within a filter mat and the amount of radioactivity within stimulated versus unstimulated cells provides an index of the stimulation that has occurred.

The purified mononuclear cells (generally a mixture of lymphocytes and monocytes) are seeded into the wells of microtitre plates in tissue culture medium supported with nutrients, antibiotics and a buffering serum (ideally autologous serum, but fetal calf serum is often used). The mitogen or antigen is added (often by titration with appropriate unstimulated controls to indicate 'background' reactivity) and the trays are incubated at 37°C in a specific atmosphere containing optimum concentration of CO_2. Most such cultures are incubated for a **72-hour period**, although longer periods (with replenishment of medium) may be required in primary response experiments.

There are different approaches to determining whether lymphocyte stimulation has occurred. The most commonly used method involves the addition of **radiolabelled (^{3}H) thymidine** into the culture for the last 18 hours of incubation. The thymidine is incorporated into the DNA of newly dividing cells, such that at the end of the culture period, when the cells are washed free of unbound thymidine, the amount of radioactive label within the cell pellet (as determined by a beta irradiation counter) is proportional to the amount of cell division. The most accurate means of expressing this cell division is as counts per minute (cpm), with background counts (in unstimulated control wells) subtracted. Many investigators chose to calculate the ratio of signal in stimulated versus unstimulated cultures (the **stimulation index** [SI]), but this method should be discouraged as it does not report the true level of stimulation obtained. There are also non-radioactive, colourimetric alternatives for read-out of cell division, although these are not as widely utilized. In larger cell cultures it is also possible to harvest the cells after culture for flow cytometric analysis to determine whether (for example) there has been expansion of the CD4+ or CD8+ T cells. Finally, yet another alternative means of determining outcome is to **assay the culture supernatant** for proteins that may have been elaborated by the stimulated cells. Classically, the production of antigen-specific **immunoglobulin** can be detected by ELISA. It is also possible to measure the production of **cytokine** by activated cells, also by **capture ELISA**. The measurement of cytokine is often best achieved by sampling earlier in the culture period. Recently, commercial assays for the detection of animal cytokines, such as IL-4, IL-10, IFN-γ and TNF-α, have become available. A newer **bead-based technology for multiplex detection** of canine cytokine protein is used increasingly. An alternative means of evaluating cytokine protein production within a fluid sample is the **bioassay**. This test measures the ability of cytokine within the sample to support the growth and division of an **indicator cell line** that has an absolute requirement for that cytokine for maintained growth.

The enzyme-linked immunospot (**ELISPOT**) assay may also be used to detect cytokine production by mononuclear cells (**Figure 10.2**). The principle of this test is similar to that of the capture ELISA described in Chapter 4; however, ELISPOT is up to 200 times more sensitive than ELISA and can detect cytokine production by individual cells. In this test, capture antibodies (specific for cytokine) are coated to a membrane made of nitrocellulose or polyvinylidene fluoride (PVDF), which sits at the base of a well in an ELISPOT plate. Mononuclear cells are then added to the well together with stimulating antigen or mitogen. Alternatively, mononuclear cells may be pre-activated (as above) before being added down to the wells. As these cells produce cytokine, it is captured by the antibody adjacent to the position of the cell. After a culture period, the mononuclear cells are washed from the well. Cytokine is detected using a secondary enzyme-linked antibody. The addition of substrate leads to formation of a spot of colour on the base of the well that corresponds to the position of a single cytokine-producing cell. The membranes with 'developed' spots may be examined microscopically or removed and analysed by an ELISPOT reader. The production of two separate cytokines by individual cells may be determined using the related FLUOROSPOT system, in which two capture antibodies are coated to the membrane and two fluorochrome-linked detecting antibodies are employed. A fluorescence reader is used to evaluate the outcome.

In the absence of appropriate reagents for detection of cytokine protein, the expression of cytokine genes within harvested cell pellets may be evaluated by real-time RT-PCR (see Chapter 7).

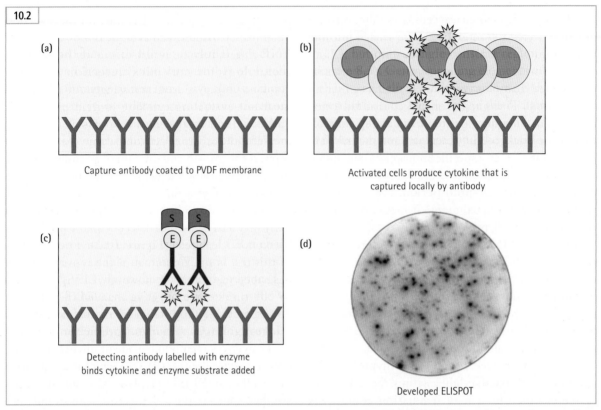

10.2

(a) Capture antibody coated to PVDF membrane

(b) Activated cells produce cytokine that is captured locally by antibody

(c) Detecting antibody labelled with enzyme binds cytokine and enzyme substrate added

(d) Developed ELISPOT

Figs. 10.2 The ELISPOT assay. The enzyme-linked immunospot test is a highly sensitive means of detecting production of a protein (e.g. cytokine) by single cells in a culture. (**a**) A capture antibody specific for the molecule of interest is coated to a polyvinylidene fluoride (PVDF) membrane in the base of a microtitration well. (**b**) Cells of interest are added and activated (e.g. by antigen or mitogen) so that some cells in the population produce the molecule of interest. Cells are washed from the plate and the bound molecule is identified by a second detecting antibody conjugated to an enzyme. (**c**) Addition of substrate produces a colour change with each spot correlating to local cellular production of the target molecule. (**d**) Spots can be evaluated microscopically or with purpose-designed ELISPOT readers. **E**; enzyme, **S**; substrate.

TESTS OF CYTOTOXIC FUNCTION

Much less commonly performed in veterinary medicine have been tests for determining the function of **cytotoxic lymphocytes** *in vitro*. These generally involve the use of a 'target cell' that will readily be killed by a cytotoxic lymphocyte or NK cell (e.g. an MHC-matched tumour cell line), which is radiolabelled, often with ^{51}Cr. These labelled target cells are incubated with the '**effector cells**' derived from the patient (generally at a range of different target to effector cell ratios) and after a period of culture, the free radioactive label within the culture supernatant is measured as an index of destruction of the targets.

TESTS OF PHAGOCYTIC CELL FUNCTION

A range of tests of the *in-vitro* function of **neutrophils** and **macrophages** has been applied to animal samples. Neutrophils are readily fractionated from blood by the use of density gradient media, as described above, and monocytes may be separated from lymphocytes by short-term incubation on glass coverslips (monocytes will adhere to the coverslip, whereas lymphocytes will not and will be subsequently washed away). The most important functions of phagocytic cells are their ability to **migrate towards a chemotactic stimulus**, to **phagocytose particles** and to **destroy** the particles that have been phagocytosed.

The chemotaxis of phagocytes can be detected in a variety of ways. The cells can be placed into one half of a '**Boyden chamber**', which is divided by a filter membrane permeable only to protein molecules. The chemotactic stimulus (e.g. molecules derived from bacteria or serum complement components) is placed into the second half of the chamber and diffuses to establish a chemotactic gradient. Phagocytic cells that are attracted towards the gradient will become caught in the dividing membrane and may be identified by removing and staining the membrane after culture (**Figure 10.3**). In the '**under agarose' assay**, phagocytic cells placed into one well in an agarose gel will migrate towards a chemotactic substance placed into a distant well, by moving under the agarose layer towards the stimulus.

The phagocytic ability of these cells can also be readily assessed by incubating the purified cells with a target particle of optimum size for phagocytosis. Classically, **staphylococci** or **latex spheres** have been used for this purpose and the phagocytosis is generally enhanced when these particles are appropriately **opsonized** by pre-incubation with fresh autologous serum as a source of antibody and complement (see Chapter 3). The relative phagocytic ability of cells from test and control animals can be determined by stopping the reaction and staining cytospin preparations of the culture in order to count the numbers of intracytoplasmic versus unphagocytosed particles. Alternatively, the process can be automated by the use of fluorescein-labelled particles that can be detected by subsequent flow cytometric analysis (**Figure 10.4**).

The efficiency of phagocyte **killing of particles** and the activation of the intracellular enzymatic pathways involved can also be measured. Viable bacteria (e.g. staphylococci) are used as targets and pre-incubated with the phagocytic cells such that an optimum number of these are taken into the cytoplasm of the phagocytes. After a period of incubation (or a series of time points throughout an incubation period), phagocytic cells can be removed from the culture well and lysed by exposure to water. The lysates may then be cultured in order to determine the number of viable organisms remaining at that time point relative to the

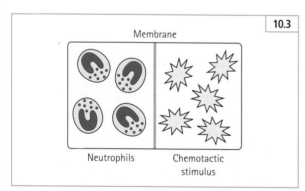

Fig. 10.3 Tests of chemotactic migration. The Boyden chamber has two halves separated by a semi-permeable membrane. A chemotactic stimulus is added to one half of the chamber and purified phagocytic cells (e.g. neutrophils) to the other. The neutrophils migrate towards the source of the chemotactic stimulus and adhere to the membrane. At the end of the culture period the membrane is removed, fixed and stained and the number of adherent neutrophils provides an index of the chemotactic ability of the cells.

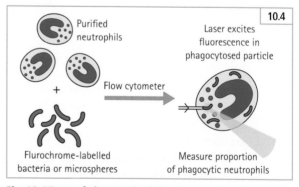

Fig. 10.4 Tests of phagocytic ability. A suspension of phagocytic cells is incubated with microparticles labelled with a fluorochrome. The particles may previously be opsonized by serum antibody and complement. After incubation and uptake of particles, the neutrophil suspension is run through the flow cytometer. The interrogating laser beam indicates the proportion of neutrophils that have phagocytosed fluorescent particles.

total number of starting organisms (**Figure 10.5**). Alternatively, the **respiratory burst** of the neutrophil can be measured after phagocytosis of particulate material by an enzymatic reaction producing a colour change (the nitroblue tetrazolium test) or by emission of light in a **chemiluminescence** reaction.

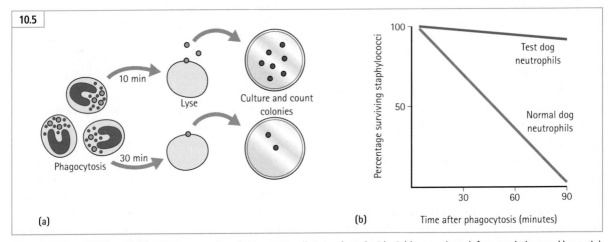

(a)   (b)

Fig. 10.5 Tests of killing ability. (a) A suspension of phagocytic cells is incubated with viable organisms (often staphylococcal bacteria) that may previously have been opsonized by serum antibody and complement. Over the period of incubation, increasing numbers of the phagocytosed bacteria will be killed. The progression of this killing can be monitored in replicate cultures that are halted at different times after phagocytosis. These cultures are washed to remove bacteria that have not been phagocytosed and then the neutrophils are lysed by the addition of water. Viable bacteria released from the cytoplasm may be cultured on agar plates and the number of colonies enumerated. Neutrophils from a normal animal will progressively kill increasing numbers of organisms so that there are fewer colonies at each time point of the experiment (generally 30 minute intervals over a 2-hour period). (b) A 'killing curve' can be generated and used to compare this function between neutrophils taken from different animals.

KEY POINTS

- Tests of lymphocyte or phagocytic cell function are clinically useful, but rarely available in veterinary medicine.
- Lymphocytes may be stimulated to divide *in vitro* by incubating them with mitogens, anti-CD3 antibody or specific antigens.
- Mononuclear cells can be separated from blood by density gradient centrifugation.
- Cellular division may be measured by quantifying the incorporation of radiolabelled thymidine into the nucleic acid of newly generated lymphocytes.

- Release of immunoglobulin or cytokine into culture medium can also be evaluated by techniques such as ELISPOT.
- The ability of cytotoxic T cells or NK cells to kill a radiolabelled target cell can be measured *in vitro*.
- Phagocytic cells will migrate along a chemotactic gradient *in vitro*.
- The ability of phagocytic cells to take up particulate antigen and kill microbes can be assessed *in vitro*.

Immune Suppression

OBJECTIVES

At the end of this chapter you should be able to:
- Understand why suppression of an immune response is necessary.
- Outline how antibody plays a role in downregulation of an immune response.
- Explain the concept of the neuroendocrine–immunological loop.
- Discuss how Th1 and Th2 cells are counter-regulatory.
- Describe the phenotype and mode of action of natural and induced Treg cells.

INTRODUCTION

Until this point, our discussion of the adaptive immune response has centred on the activation and amplification of effector T and B lymphocytes and the various positive signals that must be delivered to induce such reactions (positive regulation or up-regulation). This chapter examines the opposite immunological phenomenon, that of switching off (**suppressing** or **down-regulating**) an adaptive immune response when it is no longer required. Once the immune system has eliminated foreign antigen, it has no need to maintain the large population of effector cells and molecules. In fact, if such cells persisted in the absence of antigen, there would be a risk that they might turn upon normal tissue and induce **secondary immunopathology**. Therefore, the immune system must have evolved strategies to detect the elimination of antigen and to suppress effector cell function. At the same time, it is crucial that the memory lymphocyte populations are retained in case of secondary antigenic exposure.

Suppression is one of the least well understood areas of immunology and receives a great deal of attention from researchers. Understanding of suppression holds the key to developing new strategies to controlling unwanted immune responses such as those that occur in autoimmune (see Chapter 16) or allergic (see Chapter 17) diseases. In reality, suppression is probably a complex event that involves combinations of the various strategies that will be outlined in this chapter. Different combinations of these mechanisms might be applied to any one immune response.

ANTIGEN USAGE

The simplest means of switching off an immune response is to eliminate the source of antigen. If antigen is required to initiate and expand an adaptive immune response, then **removal of antigen** and slowing of antigen presentation will remove the source of stimulation for the immune system. We have already encountered this concept in discussing **affinity maturation** of the B-cell response where, as antigen becomes less available, only those B cells with high-affinity receptors are able to successfully capture and present antigen to obtain T-cell help in order to maintain their activity. It should also be recalled that a small reservoir of antigen may be sequestered away in lymphoid tissue (associated with follicular dendritic cells) to aid in the maintenance of memory.

ANTIBODY-MEDIATED SUPPRESSION

Antibody can have a down-regulatory function at several different levels. At the simplest level, antibody may be involved in the elimination of antigen, thereby reducing antigen concentration, as discussed above (**Figure 11.1**). Alternatively, **immune complexes** of antigen and antibody are generally removed, once formed, by phagocytic cells such as **macrophages**. There is evidence that the uptake of immune complexes may induce macrophages to release **immunosuppressive substances** (e.g. prostaglandin E_2, IL-10 or TGF-β) that in turn inhibit the function of lymphoid cells (see below). Another means of antibody-mediated suppression acts at the level of the antigen-specific B cell. As B cells carry surface Fc receptors, it is possible for antibody derived from a different B cell with distinct epitope-binding specificity to occupy receptors on the surface of a B cell (**Figure 11.1**). The presence of intact antigen may **cross-link** the B cell's own **surface membrane immunoglobulin with the Fc receptor-bound antibody**. This induces a negative signalling event that prevents that B cell from becoming activated. An example of this phenomenon with relevance to human medicine is the management of **haemolytic**

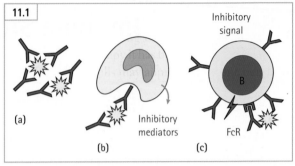

Fig. 11.1 Antibody-mediated suppression. (**a**) Antibody may bind to and eliminate antigen, making it unavailable for perpetuation of the immune response. (**b**) Alternatively, immune complexes of antigen and antibody that are phagocytosed by macrophages may induce those cells to release immunosuppressive mediators. (**c**) Finally, antibody may occupy B-cell surface Fc receptors such that antigen may cross-link the BCR with the FcR-bound antibody and inhibit that B cell.

disease of the newborn. This arises when a mother who is Rhesus blood group antigen negative (Rh⁻) carries a child who has inherited the Rhesus blood group antigen from the father (**Figure 11.2**). At the time of parturition at the end of the first pregnancy there is an opportunity for Rh⁺ fetal red cells to enter the maternal circulation and for the mother to mount an immune response to Rh. During second and subsequent pregnancies, these maternal anti-Rh antibodies may cross the placenta and cause haemolytic destruction of fetal red cells, with severe consequences for the developing child. The anti-Rh

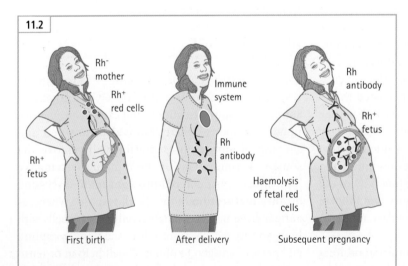

Fig. 11.2 Haemolytic disease of the newborn. A mother negative for the Rhesus blood group antigen (Rh⁻) carrying a Rh⁺ fetus may be exposed to fetal red blood cells at the time of parturition. If that mother generates anti-Rh antibody, during second and subsequent pregnancies this antibody may cross the placenta and cause haemolysis of fetal red cells. Formation of antibody may be avoided by administration of pre-formed anti-Rh antibody at the time of first parturition.

immune response can be effectively prevented at the time of first parturition by injecting pre-formed anti-Rh antibody into the maternal system. These antibodies in part bind and destroy Rh⁺ red cells, but they may also work through occupying Fc receptors on those B cells in the maternal repertoire able to recognize the Rh antigen and, through cross-linking, prevent activation of those cells. Similar mechanisms may be involved in the suppression of the endogenous immune response in neonatal animals by maternally derived immunoglobulin (see Chapter 18).

IMMUNOREGULATORY MACROPHAGES

In Chapter 1 we briefly discussed the functional differences between 'classically activated' M1 macrophages and 'alternatively activated' M2 macrophages. Subsets of M2 macrophages have been proposed including: (1) M2a macrophages generated in the presence of IL-4 and IL-13 that promote Th2 responses; (2) M2b macrophages generated in the presence of immune complexes, IL-1β and ligands for particular TLRs that also promote Th2 responses; and (3) M2c macrophages generated in the presence of IL-10, TGF-β and glucocorticoids that have immunosuppressive function. Suppressive tumour-associated macrophages will be discussed further in Chapter 14.

THE NEUROENDOCRINE–IMMUNOLOGICAL LOOP

This is the name given to describe the concept that these three key body systems are linked, in that soluble mediators from one system are able to **cross-regulate** aspects of function of the other systems (**Figure 11.3**). There are numerous examples of such cross-regulation and some involve suppression of immune responses:

- The range of macrophage-derived pro-inflammatory cytokines (IL-1, IL-6 and TNF-α) is responsible for the induction of pyrexia by influencing the hypothalamic body temperature regulatory centre (see Chapter 1).
- Chronic neurological stress leads to elevated release of endogenous glucocorticoid from the adrenal cortex, which has an immunosuppressive function. This explains the common occurrence

of coughs and colds in students around the time of examinations!

- Similarly, in the endocrine disease hyperadrenocorticism, inappropriate elevation of endogenous glucocorticoid or excessive iatrogenic administration of medical immunosuppression leads to atrophy of lymphoid tissue, blood leucopenia and susceptibility to secondary infectious disease (**Figure 11.4**).

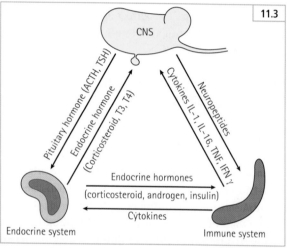

Fig. 11.3 The neuroendocrine–immunological loop. Soluble mediators produced within each of these three body systems may cross-regulate elements of the other systems. Examples of such effects are given within the text.

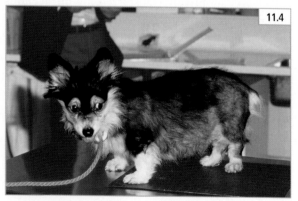

Fig. 11.4 Hyperadrenocorticism. This dog displays the classical cutaneous, muscular and hepatic changes of hyperadrenocorticism. Elevated endogenous glucocorticoid in this disease causes atrophy of lymphoid tissue and circulating lymphopenia.

- The hormonal changes during pregnancy imbalance the immune system. During pregnancy the maternal immune system becomes dominated by Treg cell immunity in an attempt to suppress Th1 responses, which could potentially mediate cytotoxic placental damage and cause abortion (see Chapter 15). A striking example of this effect occurs in pregnant females who have the Th1-mediated autoimmune disease rheumatoid arthritis. During pregnancy, this disease will often go into remission, only to recur after parturition. This effect also has a role in the development of an allergic phenotype (see Chapter 17).

REGULATORY (SUPPRESSOR) T LYMPHOCYTES

Although each of the mechanisms described above may have a role in immunoregulation, the single most important means of controlling the adaptive immune response is through the action of specific populations of T lymphocytes that are suppressive rather than effector in function. The phenomenon of **T-cell-mediated suppression** was first identified in the important experiment conducted by Richard Gershon and published in 1974 (**Figure 11.5**). In this study, mice were injected with sheep red blood cells (SRBCs) and several days later the spleen was removed and a suspension of splenocytes prepared. These cells were 'adoptively transferred' by intravenous injection into naïve mice of the same strain. When the recipient mice were subsequently injected with an immunogenic dose of SRBCs, they failed to mount an appropriate serum antibody response. As only splenic lymphocytes were transferred to these recipients, these cells must have been responsible for suppressing the primary immune response in those animals. Since that experiment, numerous studies have unequivocally shown that **T lymphocytes** are the cell type required to mediate this effect. Experimental animals depleted of T cells by various strategies, or genetically modified so that T cells are insufficiently activated, will generally develop various manifestations of autoimmunity, and replenishment of T cells may counteract this effect.

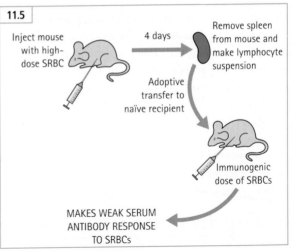

Fig. 11.5 Recognition of suppressor lymphocytes. This experiment provided the first evidence for the presence of a regulatory lymphocyte population. A mouse is immunized with SRBCs and, shortly after, the spleen is taken and a suspension of splenic lymphocytes produced that is adoptively transferred into a naïve recipient. The recipient mouse is immunized with an immunogenic dose of SRBCs, but fails to mount a significant serum antibody response to the antigen. The activated splenic lymphocytes have suppressed the primary immune response in the recipient.

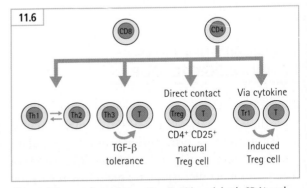

Fig. 11.6 Types of regulatory T cell. Although both CD4+ and CD8+ T cells may be suppressive, the former is the more significant population in this respect. CD4+ T cell suppression may reflect cross-regulation between Th1 and Th2 cells or the action of natural or induced Treg cells.

It is now recognized that although both CD4+ and CD4+ T cells may have an immunosuppressive function, it is the CD4+ subset that is responsible for most of this effect. Indeed, there are several distinct **subsets of CD4+ T cell that are immunoregulatory** and these are described (**Figure 11.6**).

Th1 versus Th2 immune deviation

In Chapter 8 we discussed the generation of **Th1 and Th2 CD4+ T lymphocytes**, which stimulate, respectively, cell-mediated or humoral immunity. These cells may be **cross-regulatory** by virtue of the cytokine profile that each elaborates. Th1-derived IFN-γ is inhibitory of Th2 function and Th2-derived IL-4 and IL-13 may inhibit Th1 function. This effect may sometimes (but not always) lead to polarization of the immune response, with a dominant cellular or humoral effector phase, and this effect is known as 'immune deviation'. This counter-regulatory effect was first demonstrated using the murine model of *Leishmania* infection. The C57BL/6 strain of mouse responds to experimental infection by mounting a strongly polarized Th1 immune response that allows these animals to control the parasite and remain clinically healthy. This effect is mediated by IFN-γ,

which signals infected macrophages and allows them to eliminate the intracellular protozoan organisms. In contrast, infection of mice of the BALB/c strain results in the induction of a Th2 immune response with high levels of serum antibody, which fails to protect from infection. These mice develop severe multisystemic disease and die.

To further support the observation that disease outcome depends on genetically determined immune responsiveness, these mice may be experimentally manipulated to alter their disease phenotype. For example, a resistant C57BL/6 mouse injected with monoclonal antibody specific for IFN-γ at the time of infection will develop severe terminal infection and high concentration of serum antibody. The monoclonal antibody neutralizes the cytokine, preventing macrophage activation and parasite destruction and allowing expansion of the Th2 immune response that would normally be inhibited by IFN-γ. Similarly, injection of a susceptible BALB/c mouse with monoclonal antibody specific for IL-4 at the time of infection leads to neutralization of that cytokine, inhibition of the Th2 response, activation of the Th1 response and killing of the organism, (**Figure 11.7**).

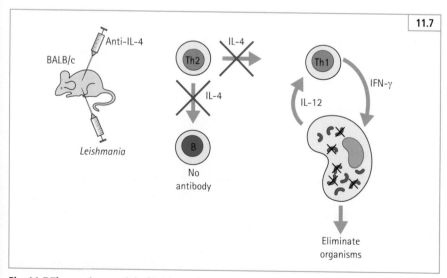

Fig. 11.7 The murine model of leishmaniosis. The natural resistance of C57BL/6 mice and susceptibility of BALB/c mice to infection by *Leishmania* can be manipulated by injection of anti-cytokine monoclonal antibody at the time of infection. In this experiment, BALB/c mice co-injected with organism and anti-IL-4 make a protective Th1 immune response, leading to elimination of the organisms. The Th2 response is inhibited following neutralization of IL-4.

The most recent studies in the same model system suggest that there may be further **lineage development** in these T-cell subsets. Once a robust Th1 response has contained and controlled the *Leishmania* infection, there appears to be a phenotypic change whereby the IFN-γ-producing Th1 cell alters its cytokine expression profile and begins to secrete immunosuppressive IL-10. This form of '**self-regulation**' may be important in preventing the Th1 cells from mediating secondary immunopathology (tissue damage), but has the downside that it also prevents total elimination of the infectious agent and allows a low-grade chronic infection to occur.

Regulatory cells

There are several key populations of T regulatory (Treg) cells. They are defined by the expression of various cell surface molecules, by the use of particular transcription factors or by their production of particular cytokines.

The first of these are the **natural Treg** (nTreg) cells, which are always active in the body (therefore 'natural') and are thought to have a major role in controlling lymphocytes that might potentially trigger **autoimmune disease**. In fact, it is now well recognized that reduced function of nTreg cells does occur in individuals with such disorders. These cells are derived directly from the thymus and are characterized phenotypically by the expression of CD4 and **CD25** (the α chain of the IL-2 receptor) and use of the transcription factor **Foxp3** (forkhead box p3). Expression of Foxp3 has enabled the characterization of nTreg cells in cats and dogs. nTreg cells also express **GITR** (glucocorticoid-induced TNF-receptor-regulated [gene]), **CTLA-4** (cytotoxic T lymphocyte antigen-4) and some PRRs. Although these cells also produce the immunosuppressive cytokine **IL-10**, they appear to require direct contact (**cognate interaction**) with the cell that they intend to suppress.

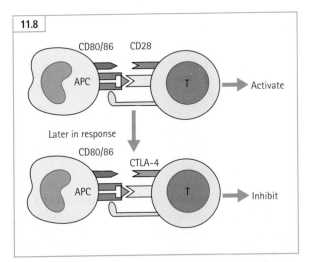

Fig. 11.8 The role of CTLA-4 in suppression. During activation of an immune response, CD28 on the surface of the T cell interacts with CD80/86 expressed by the APC. In the latter stages of the immune response, the T cell down regulates CD28 expression and begins to express CTLA-4. Interaction of CTLA-4 with CD80/86 generates inhibition of the T cell.

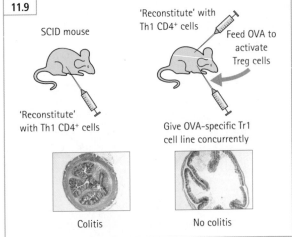

Fig. 11.9 Recognition of Tr1 cells. When SCID mice are reconstituted with Th1 cells the cells home to the intestinal tract and induce severe colitis. If SCID mice are reconstituted with both Th1 cells and a Tr1 cell line specific for ovalbumin (OVA), both populations home to the colonic mucosa. Feeding OVA to the reconstituted mice activates the Tr1 cells and reduces the severity of colitis.

The expression of CTLA-4 warrants further discussion (**Figure 11.8**). During induction of the adaptive immune response, one of the intermolecular interactions that occurs within the immunological synapse between the APC and the Th cell is pairing between the T-cell molecule **CD28** and the APC ligand **CD80/86**. Later in the immune response, at the stage of suppression, T cells appear to lose expression of CD28 and replace this with CTLA-4. CTLA-4 is also able to engage CD80/86 expressed by the APC, but this interaction leads to **inhibition** of the T cell rather than activation.

The second population of regulatory cells are the **induced Treg** (iTreg) cells, which develop in the periphery (i.e. not in the thymus) following antigen-specific activation of naïve CD4+ T cells in the presence of cytokines such as IL-10 and TFG-β. At least three subsets of iTreg cells are characterized. These cells do not require cognate interaction with their target, but work via the production of immunoregulatory cytokines that signal the target cell.

The first of these subsets are the **Tr1 cells**, which are CD4+CD25+Foxp3- and produce IL-10. Tr1 cells were first identified in an elaborate murine experimental system. A strain of mice known as 'severe combined immunodeficient' (SCID) mice essentially lack an immune system and must be housed in sterile isolators to survive. These mice are a valuable immunological resource, as they can be repopulated ('reconstituted') with different combinations of lymphocytes (including lymphocytes from other species such as man and dog) and used to monitor the interaction of those cell types *in vivo*. When SCID mice are reconstituted with a pure population of Th1 cells, these cells preferentially migrate to the intestinal tract and establish a severe colonic inflammation. When the same mice are concurrently given a population of IL-10-producing Tr1 cells carrying a TCR specific for the antigen OVA, these cells also establish in the host colon. When the dually reconstituted mice are fed OVA, the Tr1 cells are activated and produce IL-10, which inhibits the pathogenic Th1 cells and prevents colitis (**Figure 11.9**). The pathogenic Th1 cells are not OVA specific, so Tr1 cells must be able to non-selectively inhibit T cells of any specificity in the vicinity, a phenomenon known as '**bystander suppression**'. Tr1 cells have recently been defined in the horse.

The second subset comprises iTreg cells that are CD4+Foxp3+ and produce IL-10 and TGF-β and the third group of iTreg cells are the **Th3 cells**, which are CD4+CD25+Foxp3+ and also produce IL-10 and TGF-β. Th3 cells are thought to be crucial to the development of '**oral tolerance**', which will be discussed in Chapter 15.

It is thought that such regulatory cells are induced in similar fashion to Th cells. iTreg cells carry antigen-specific TCRs and must recognize epitopes from the stimulating antigen, although it is possible that these are distinct from the epitopes that drive the effector immune response. Moreover, the dendritic cells that present antigen to regulatory cells may be of a particular type known as '**semi-mature' dendritic cells** and may preferentially stimulate the developing regulatory cell through cytokines such as **IL-10** or **TGF-β** (**Figure 11.10**).

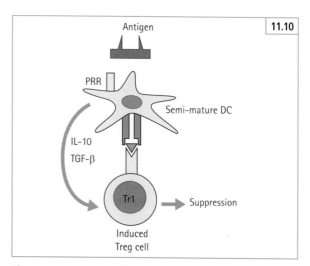

Fig. 11.10 Activation of induced regulatory T cells. Induced Treg cells are activated in a similar fashion to effector T cells. However, antigen may be presented by a specific population of 'semi-mature' dendritic cells that signal the precursor T cell through IL-10 or TGF-β.

KEY POINTS

- Regulation or suppression is required to avoid secondary immunopathology once antigen is eliminated by effector cells.
- Elimination of antigen removes the stimulus for maintaining the effector immune response.
- Antibody may be regulatory by eliminating antigen, by forming immune complexes that cause macrophages to release immunosuppressive substances on phagocytosis, or by binding B-cell FcRs to cross-link with that cell's normal BCR.
- The concept of the neuroendocrine–immunological loop indicates that these three body systems may cross-regulate each other.

- Regulatory or suppressor T cells deliver the most important means of suppression and CD4$^+$ T cells are the most significant regulatory subset.
- Th1 and Th2 cells cross-regulate each other, leading to immune deviation.
- CD4$^+$CD25$^+$Foxp3$^+$ nTreg cells are important in the control of autoreactive T cells.
- nTreg cells secrete IL-10, but require cognate interaction with their targets.
- iTreg cells develop from naïve CD4$^+$ T cells during a specific immune response and mediate their effect via IL-10 and/or TGF-β production and non-cognate bystander suppression.

Hypersensitivity Mechanisms

OBJECTIVES

At the end of this chapter you should be able to:
- Define hypersensitivity.
- Discuss the Gell and Coombs classification of hypersensitivity and the mechanisms underlying types I–IV hypersensitivity.
- Give examples of where hypersensitivity mechanisms are used in a protective immune response.

- Give examples of where hypersensitivity mechanisms are used in a pathological immune response.
- Understand that hypersensitivity mechanisms may occur sequentially or concurrently in some instances.

INTRODUCTION

This chapter explores how the components of the adaptive immune system described previously can interact to produce a series of distinct and standard immune responses. These standard immune responses are generally termed '**hypersensitivity mechanisms**'. A hypersensitivity response involves **sensitization** to an antigen by prior exposure (often repeated and over time). Once an individual is sensitized, subsequent **re-exposure** to that antigen may lead to an **inappropriately excessive immune response** termed a **hypersensitivity reaction**. Hypersensitivity is often equated to **allergy**, where repeated exposure to antigen (termed '**allergen**') leads to immunological sensitization and an inappropriate **allergic response** on re-exposure. In this context, the hypersensitivity or allergic response has led to unwanted tissue pathology

and clinical signs of allergic disease. Many allergens are ubiquitous environmental substances (e.g. grass pollens, house dust mite particles) to which only genetically susceptible individuals will mount an inappropriate allergic response.

The equating of hypersensitivity mechanisms to allergic disease is somewhat unfortunate because the same fundamental mechanisms are often used in other forms of disease (e.g. autoimmune disease, see Chapter 16), but, more importantly, in productive and protective immune responses. In fact, these standard immune responses initially evolved to deal with particular types of pathogen, but have become subverted into the occasional generation of pathological immune responses. For this reason it may be simpler to consider these standard responses as '**immunopathological mechanisms**' rather than 'hypersensitivity mechanisms'.

THE GELL AND COOMBS CLASSIFICATION OF HYPERSENSITIVITY

In 1963, P.G.H. Gell and R.A.A. Coombs published the influential text *Clinical Aspects of Immunology*, which laid the foundation for the development of the discipline of clinical immunology. It is worth noting that Robin Coombs (who also gave his name to the Coombs test, see Chapter 16) was in fact a veterinarian by primary training. Within this book, Gell and Coombs proposed the classification of hypersensitivity reactions that forms a cornerstone to immunology to this day. The **classification scheme** groups these immunopathological mechanisms into four categories:

- Type I or immediate (or IgE-mediated) hypersensitivity.
- Type II or antibody-mediated cytotoxic hypersensitivity.
- Type III or immune complex hypersensitivity.
- Type IV or delayed-type hypersensitivity (DTH).

TYPE I HYPERSENSITIVITY

As for all four types of hypersensitivity, the type I reaction has two phases. The first phase is the period of sensitization of the immune system to the antigen (**Figure 12.1**) or allergen and the second phase is re-exposure of the sensitized individual to antigen with clinical expression of the hypersensitivity response.

The antigens that induce type I hypersensitivity are generally encountered at the **mucosal and cutaneous surfaces** of the body. So, for example, a dendritic cell within the bronchial epithelium may encounter an inhaled antigen or a Langerhans cell within the epidermis may capture a percutaneously absorbed antigen (see Chapter 7). The nature of PRR signalling to this APC will mean that once the dendritic cell has migrated to regional lymphoid tissue it will preferentially signal the antigen-specific naïve CD4[+] T cell to differentiate to a **Th2 cell**. In turn, the Th2 cell will promote a humoral immune response, with expansion of antigen-specific B cells that class switch towards **IgE production**. The net effect of this form of sensitization is the generation of high concentrations

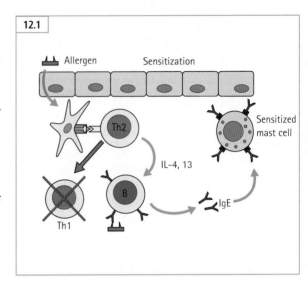

Fig. 12.1 Sensitization phase of type I hypersensitivity. Repeated exposure to allergen absorbed across an epithelial barrier leads to Th2-regulated production of allergen-specific IgE antibodies that occupy Fcε receptors on tissue mast cells or circulating basophils.

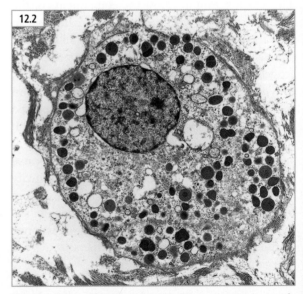

Fig. 12.2 Mast cells. Transmission electron microscope image of a feline mast cell showing numerous cytoplasmic granules.

of **antigen-specific IgE**, which may be detected in the bloodstream and, more importantly, which bind to **Fcε receptors** on the surface of circulating **basophils** and tissue **mast cells (Figure 12.2)**. Many of these IgE-coated mast cells will reside beneath the epithelium of the body surface at which the antigen was originally encountered. Additionally, there is likely to be some class switching towards production of a restricted subclass of IgG that is able to bind to Fcγ receptors on the same cells (termed '**homocytotropic IgG**'). The individual with allergen-specific IgE-coated mast cells is now sensitized, but at this stage displays no tissue pathology or clinical signs.

The second phase of the type I hypersensitivity reaction therefore occurs when a sensitized individual re-encounters the antigen or allergen (**Figure 12.3**). On this occasion, the absorbed antigen meets the IgE-coated mast cells as it penetrates the particular mucosal or cutaneous barrier. The antigen is bound by two or more IgE molecules, thus **cross-linking** these antibodies and initiating a signalling pathway within that mast cell. The consequences of mast cell activation are the rapid release (within seconds) of cytoplasmic granules (**degranulation**) containing numerous potent, pre-formed, biologically active mediators including histamine, heparin, serotonin, kininogenase, tryptase, chymase and exoglycosidases. In addition, the synthesis of a range of other mediators is initiated within minutes (e.g. platelet activating factor). The most important of these derive from arachidonic acid, which forms by cleavage of membrane phospholipids. Arachidonic acid modified by the cyclooxygenase pathway gives rise to thromboxanes and prostaglandins and, if modified by the lipoxygenase pathway, to leukotrienes. Mast cells may also produce a range of pro-inflammatory and immunoregulatory cytokines (e.g. IL-4, IL-5, IL-6, IL-13, TNF-α), which are synthesized over several hours following initial degranulation.

Mast cell degranulation and release of pre-formed mediators occurs very rapidly after antigen exposure and the speed of this response (with clinical effects seen within **15 – 20 minutes**) is why the reaction is termed '**immediate hypersensitivity**'. The consequences of mast cell degranulation include:

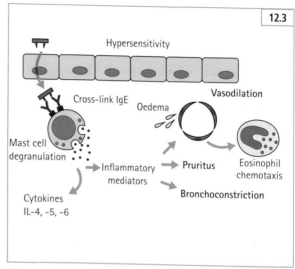

Fig. 12.3 Type I hypersensitivity. When a sensitized individual re-encounters allergen, this cross-links mast cell-bound IgE, leading to degranulation of that cell and release of potent bioactive molecules that mediate the local tissue changes of vasodilation, oedema, inflammation, bronchoconstriction and pruritus.

- **Vasodilation** with resulting tissue **oedema**, leakage of serum proteins and extravasation of **inflammatory cells**.
- Contraction of smooth muscle, which has greatest relevance in the airways and leads to **bronchoconstriction**.
- Interaction of mediators with local nerve endings (pruiceptors) that are linked to specific centres in the brain mediating itch (**pruritus**). This has greatest relevance in the skin and pruritus is a major part of cutaneous allergic disease. The mediators responsible for this effect include histamine, some prostaglandins and leukotrienes, and neuropeptides. A key mediator of pruritus is IL-31, which is derived from Th2 cells and mast cells

It is now also appreciated that there is a second stage of this reaction, known as the 'late-phase response', that occurs **4–24 hours** after antigen exposure. During the late-phase response there is active **recruitment of eosinophils and macrophages** into the tissue, and the presence of eosinophils in particular is regarded as a hallmark of the type I hypersensitivity reaction (**Figures 12.4, 12.5**). Type I hypersensitivity reactions may also become chronic in nature following recurrent episodes of allergen exposure or the effects of secondary infections or self-trauma (in the skin). Chronicity may alter the nature of the tissue immune response, which may become dominated by Th1 immunity stimulated by infectious agents (e.g. staphylococcal bacteria or *Malassezia* yeasts in the skin) or involve tissue remodelling mediated by cytokines (e.g. fibroblast or epithelial growth factors) and enzymes (e.g. matrix metalloproteinases).

The majority of type I hypersensitivity reactions are **localized** and affect the tissue that comes into contact with the inciting antigen. The multitude of allergic diseases that afflict man and domestic animals (see Chapter 17) are excellent examples of localized allergic responses affecting the **skin** (e.g. atopic dermatitis, flea allergy dermatitis [**Figure 12.6**], equine 'sweet itch' or 'insect bite hypersensitivity'),

respiratory tract (allergic rhinitis, asthma) or **intestinal tract** (food allergy). In contrast, some type I hypersensitivity reactions are **systemic** and involve degranulation of circulating basophils or tissue mast cells in multiple locations. These may be severe and life-threatening events and are known as **anaphylactic reactions** (the process is **anaphylaxis**). The sensitizing allergens in this instance are often drugs (e.g. penicillin sensitivity) or insect stings (e.g. bee sting). The mechanisms of the anaphylactic reaction differ between species, but in man, for example, the onset of severe bronchoconstriction and laryngeal oedema often underlies the rapid demise that typifies such responses. In ruminants the so-called '**shock organ**' is also the respiratory tract, whereas in horses, pigs and cats both the respiratory and intestinal tracts may be affected. In contrast, the canine shock organ is the liver, where there is massive pooling of blood leading to reduced venous return to the heart, which in turn results in reduced cardiac output and blood pressure.

Although type I hypersensitivity is generally equated with this range of allergic diseases, the same mechanism likely evolved to form a protective immune response to **parasitic infestation**. This will be discussed further in Chapter 13.

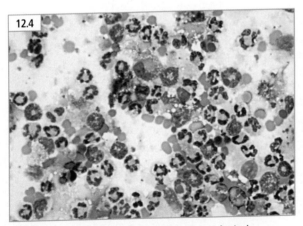

Fig. 12.4 Eosinophil recruitment. This is a cytological preparation of bronchoalveolar lavage fluid from a dog with pulmonary disease (eosinophilic bronchopneumopathy) presumptively caused by a type I hypersensitivity reaction. Numerous eosinophils are recruited into the airways of affected dogs.

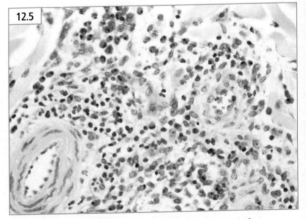

Fig. 12.5 Eosinophil recruitment. This skin biopsy is from a horse with sweet itch (*Culicoides* sensitivity) and shows a perivascular infiltration of mononuclear cells and eosinophils typical of the more chronic stages of disease.

TYPE II HYPERSENSITIVITY

Type II hypersensitivity (or **antibody-mediated cytotoxicity**) makes use of the range of immunopathological mechanisms discussed in Chapters 3, 7 and 8. This form of hypersensitivity involves destruction of a **target cell** and sensitization is to an antigen displayed on the surface of that target. Sensitization leads to production of **IgG** (mostly) or **IgM** antibodies that may bind to target cells and cause their destruction. The cytotoxic reaction may be relatively rapid where it involves activation of the classical pathway of complement and formation of the terminal pathway MAC, or may take days to weeks where the target cell destruction involves macrophage phagocytosis or even NK cell destruction via ADCC (**Figure 12.7**).

The classic example of a type II hypersensitivity reaction is that of an **incompatible blood transfusion** where a recipient animal carries **alloantibodies** specific for **blood group antigens** expressed on the donor red blood cells (RBCs). Such an incompatible transfusion might lead to an **acute haemolytic reaction** or a **chronic haemolytic reaction** involving destruction of transfused erythrocytes within days of transfusion (whereas such cells would normally be expected to survive for several weeks). In the case of whole blood transfusions, acute **anaphylactic reactions** may also occur, but these generally involve type I hypersensitivity with sensitization to serum proteins within the donor blood.

Blood transfusion reactions are relatively uncommon in the dog and are mostly related to expression of the blood group antigen termed **dog erythrocyte antigen 1** (DEA1). Most dogs do not carry this blood group antigen (i.e. are DEA1⁻) and DEA1⁻ dogs do not have spontaneously arising alloantibodies to the DEA1 antigen. However, a DEA1⁻ dog that has been previously transfused with DEA1⁺ blood will generally develop IgG antibody to that blood group antigen (i.e. become sensitized) so that second and subsequent incompatible transfusions may result in hypersensitivity. Other canine blood group antigens may rarely cause transfusion reactions.

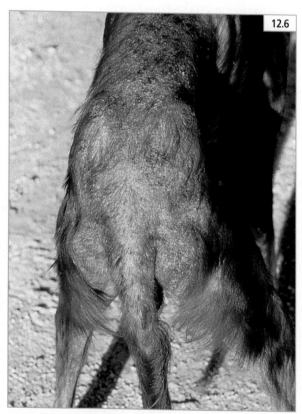

Fig. 12.6 Flea allergy dermatitis. This dog has severe flea allergy dermatitis. Much of the skin damage relates to intense pruritus and self-trauma by the dog and there is a classical distribution centred over the base of the tail.

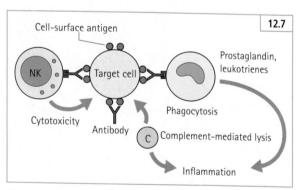

Fig. 12.7 Type II hypersensitivity. In this form of hypersensitivity reaction, a target cell is destroyed following binding of IgG or IgM antibody to the cell-surface antigen. Cytolysis may be due to the effects of complement or mediated by NK cells, or the entire target may be phagocytosed by a macrophage.

Although it is often said that the first transfusion is relatively safe in the dog, best clinical practice would dictate that **blood typing and cross-matching** (see Chapter 22) must be performed before any blood transfusion (**Figure 12.8**).

A much greater risk of incompatible blood transfusion occurs in the cat. Cats may phenotypically be of blood groups A, B or AB. **Type A cats** may sometimes have **low-titred anti-B** alloantibodies, but **type B cats** invariably have **high-titred anti-A** alloantibodies (and type AB cats have no alloantibodies). As the prevalence of blood group B is relatively high in some pure breeds, there is a much greater risk of transfusion reaction occurring when a type B cat receives type A blood. Therefore, blood typing and cross-matching is of great importance in feline transfusion medicine (see Chapter 22).

Although not a classical hypersensitivity reaction, the type II mechanism also forms the basis for a range of **autoimmune diseases** mediated by autoantibodies, and alloantibody formation has a role in graft rejection (see Chapter 6). Autoimmune diseases such as **autoimmune haemolytic anaemia, thrombocytopenia or neutropenia** utilize this immunopathological mechanism, as do those autoimmune diseases in which autoantibody binds to specific **receptor molecules**. Two such antireceptor autoimmune disorders are often considered when discussing type II hypersensitivity. The first is human **Grave's disease** (for which there is no animal equivalent) in which an autoantibody specific for the thyroid-stimulating hormone (TSH) receptor leads to uncontrolled activation of thyroid follicular epithelial cells, with excessive production of thyroid hormones (T3, T4) and enhanced systemic metabolism (hyperthyroidism) (**Figure 12.9**). The second is **myasthenia gravis** (recognized in dogs and cats) in which autoantibody specific for the acetylcholine receptor of the neuromuscular junction causes blockade or destruction of these receptors, leading to episodic skeletal muscle weakness (**Figure 12.10**). Again, it should be recalled that antibody-mediated cytotoxicity has an important role in many protective immune responses such as in the **clearance of virus-infected cells** (see Chapter 13) and that this immunopathological mechanism evolved for that primary purpose.

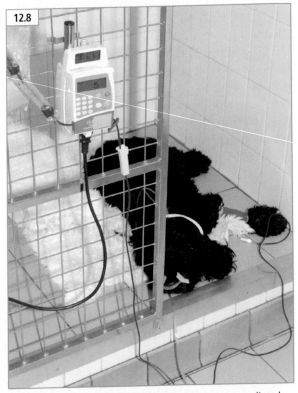

Fig. 12.8 Blood transfusion. This dog with immune-mediated haemolytic anaemia is receiving a whole blood transfusion after blood typing and cross-matching to ensure that the donor blood is compatible and that the recipient does not have pre-formed alloantibodies to blood group antigens on the surface of the donor cells. (Photo courtesy S. Warman)

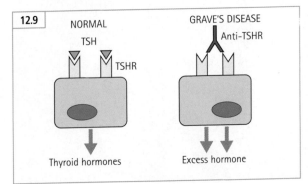

Fig. 12.9 Grave's disease. In this autoimmune disease of man, autoantibodies specific for the thyroid-stimulating hormone receptor inappropriately stimulate the receptor, leading to excessive production of thyroid hormone (hyperthyroidism).

TYPE III HYPERSENSITIVITY

Type III hypersensitivity (or **immune-complex hypersensitivity**) involves the formation and tissue deposition of immune complexes with activation of complement as described in Chapter 3. An immune complex may form with a variable ratio of antigen to antibody, and there are two subtypes of type III reaction recognized: antibody excess or antigen excess.

Antibody excess type III hypersensitivity involves repeated sensitization to antigen such that a **high concentration of antigen-specific IgG** antibody forms in the body. When antigenic re-exposure of a sensitized individual occurs (generally via inhalation), the relatively small quantity of antigen is bound by antibody almost immediately after it penetrates through the epithelial barrier. This antibody excess immune complex tends to be **localized to the site of antigen penetration** and **complement activation** at that site leads to a **localized tissue inflammatory reaction (Figure 12.11)**. The components of this inflammatory response have been discussed in Chapter 3. This localized inflammatory reaction is known as an **Arthus reaction** and generally occurs in the lung. Pulmonary Arthus reactions (hypersensitivity pneumonitis) are recognized in man and generally relate to occupational exposure to allergen. The most classic such reaction occurs in 'Farmer's lung' in which repeated sensitization to the spores of

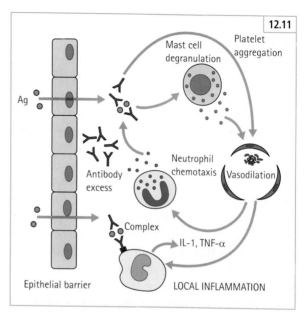

Fig. 12.11 Antibody excess type III hypersensitivity. In this form of hypersensitivity, repeated exposure to antigen leads to high concentrations of IgG antibody. Re-exposure to antigen results in the formation of immune complexes with an excess of antibody at the site of antigen penetration. Activation of the classical pathway of complement triggers a local tissue inflammatory reaction involving vasodilation, recruitment of granulocytes and monocytes, mast cell degranulation and platelet aggregation within local capillaries. Activated macrophages phagocytose immune complexes and release pro-inflammatory cytokines.

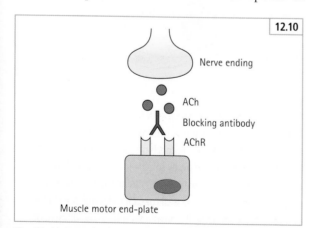

Fig. 12.10 Myasthenia gravis. In this autoimmune disease of man, dogs and cats, autoantibodies specific for the acetylcholine receptor of the neuromuscular junction block the receptor for binding by acetylcholine. The antibodies may also cause damage to the receptors and the postsynaptic membrane.

the thermophilic actinomycete *Saccharopolyspora rectivirgula* in bales of mouldy hay (stored indoors in warm temperatures while still damp) leads to IgG production and the potential for a hypersensitivity response on re-exposure to the allergen. Clinical signs of pulmonary disease usually become manifest **within 24 hours** of exposure. The same disease may occur in **cattle housed over winter** and fed hay containing these spores, which are small enough (1 μm) to pass through the upper respiratory tract defences and into the lungs. A similar pathogenesis is involved in **equine recurrent airway obstruction** (RAO), which is believed to result from sensitization to moulds and other allergens in dusty stable air and to involve elements of type I and III hypersensitivity (see Chapter 17). **Canine 'blue eye'** is a further example of localized type III hypersensitivity. This occurs in some dogs that are infected by or vaccinated with canine adenovirus-1. Immune complexes form within the uveal tract and lead to localized inflammation, corneal endothelial damage and corneal oedema (**Figure 12.12**).

Antigen excess type III hypersensitivity is characterized by a relatively low-level sensitization with only **moderate amounts of circulating IgG** antibody. The hypersensitivity reaction is triggered by subsequent exposure to a **high concentration of circulating antigen**, leading to the formation of immune complexes in antigen excess within the circulation. These complexes are generally relatively **small and soluble** and circulate in the bloodstream until they deposit within the wall of small capillaries in the predilection sites of the **renal glomerulus, uveal tract, synovium** and **cutaneous epidermal basement membrane**. Once lodged within the capillary wall there is complement fixation and triggering of the same inflammatory pathways described above, but now the inflammatory reaction occurs within the vascular wall (**vasculitis**) rather than the surrounding tissue (**Figure 12.13**). The consequences of small vessel vasculitis may be the formation of a **thrombus** that occludes the capillary lumen, leading to **ischaemic necrosis** of the tissue supplied by that vessel (**Fgure 12.14**). Vasculitis is best observed within the skin, where discrete round foci of necrosis may develop (**Figure 12.15**) or there may be necrosis and loss of the tips of the ears or tail tip (**Figure 12.16**).

Whether circulating immune complexes will induce such a reaction is determined by a number of factors:

- The **biochemical nature** of the antigen and antibody.
- Whether the normal immune complex **clearance mechanisms** (e.g. macrophage phagocytosis in spleen or liver) are impaired.
- Whether there are pre-existing **lesions in the vascular wall** resulting in contraction of endothelial cells and exposure of subendothelial collagen.

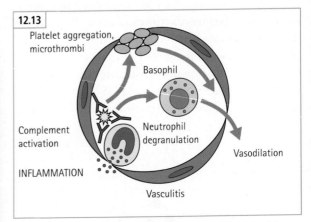

Fig. 12.13 Antigen excess type III hypersensitivity. In this form of hypersensitivity the sensitized individual has low levels of IgG antibody. Re-exposure to a high concentration of antigen leads to the formation of small, soluble immune complexes in antigen excess. In areas of high-pressure turbulent blood flow these are forced against the walls of capillaries and may lodge at these sites. Complement activation results in recruitment of neutrophils and inflammation within the vessel wall (vasculitis). Local platelet aggregation may result in the formation of microthrombi and ischaemic necrosis of tissue supplied by the vessel. Platelets and basophils release vasoactive amines to cause vasodilation and increased vessel permeability.

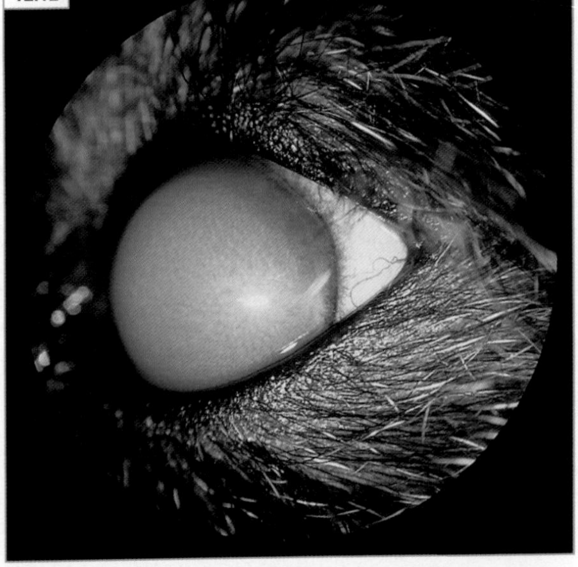

Fig. 12.12 Antibody excess type III hypersensitivity. This dog has 'blue eye', which is corneal oedema that occurs secondary to local uveal tract inflammation triggered by the formation of immune complexes of canine adenovirus-1 antigen with antibodies formed in infected or vaccinated dogs.

- The **nature of blood flow** in the capillary bed. As the renal glomerulus has a turbulent and high pressure flow, more likely to force complexes against the vascular walls, this is a clear predilection site for deposition and induction of immune complex glomerulonephritis (**Figure 12.17**).

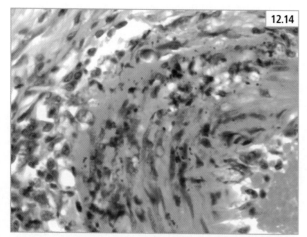

Fig. 12.14 Vasculitis. This image shows part of the wall of an arterial blood vessel in the kidney of a dog with multisystemic immune complex disease secondary to *Leishmania* infection. There is neutrophilic inflammation, necrosis and fibrin deposition within the smooth muscle wall of the vessel.

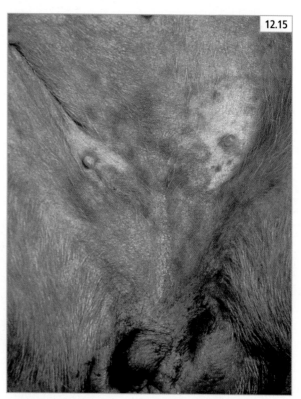

Fig. 12.15 Vasculitis. The ventral abdomen of this dog has numerous discrete round 'target' lesions consistent with vasculitis. This dog had septicaemia and it is likely that immune complexes of bacterial antigen and antibody had formed and deposited within the walls of cutaneous capillaries.

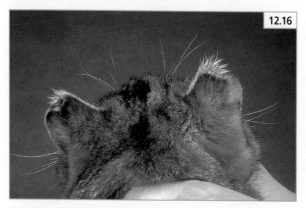

Fig. 12.16 Vasculitis. The tips of the ears of this cat have become necrotic and detached. The underlying cause was vasculitis with thrombosis of small capillaries and ischaemic necrosis of the skin.

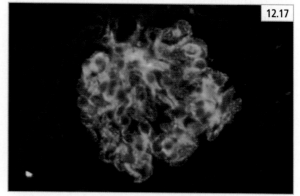

Fig. 12.17 Immune complex glomerulonephritis. This section of kidney from a cat with protein-losing nephropathy has been probed with antibody specific for feline IgG and detected by immunofluorescence microscopy. The fine granular deposits around the capillary loops of the glomeruli are immune complexes that have deposited in the walls of these vessels. The causative antigen is unknown.

Antigen excess immune complex disease may therefore be **multisystemic** and include clinical signs such as lameness, joint pain or swelling, visual impairment and ocular pain, cutaneous lesions and protein-losing nephropathy. This form of immune complex disease is certainly recognized in animals, but often the antigenic cause is not determined. In these instances the disease is often described as '**idiopathic**' or '**immune-mediated**', but that simply reflects an inability to identify the causative antigen. In some truly autoimmune immune complex diseases the antigen may be derived from self-tissue.

As for the other hypersensitivity reactions, immune complex formation evolved as a means of clearing infectious agents. In fact, this mechanism is a classical means of producing an immune-mediated reaction secondary to an infectious disease, where the infectious agent might be eliminated or be persistent, but complexes of residual antigen and antibody now perpetuate clinical disease by causing **secondary immunopathology**. There are many excellent examples of this phenomenon in veterinary medicine, and canine leishmaniosis provides one such instance. Although this disease involves granulomatous inflammatory lesions in skin and other organs, some of the clinical changes arise via secondary immune complex formation, with deposition of complexes within the synovium, glomerulus and uveal tract (**Figure 12.18**).

TYPE IV HYPERSENSITIVITY

Type IV hypersensitivity has two features that distinguish it from type I, II and III reactions. Whereas types I–III hypersensitivity are all mediated by antibody, the type IV reaction is **cell mediated**. Additionally, and because of this cellular nature, the type IV reaction has a prolonged onset (**24–72 hours**) and is therefore known as '**delayed-type hypersensitivity**' (**DTH**).

The sensitization phase of a type IV response leads to the generation of antigen-specific T lymphocytes, in particular **Th1 cells**. Subsequent exposure to the sensitizing antigen leads to antigen presentation and reactivation of those sensitized T cells. These cells home to the tissue site of antigen exposure and release

IFN-γ and chemokines, which in turn results in the formation of HEVs and up-regulation of vascular addressins, and **recruitment of mononuclear inflammatory cells** including macrophages, CD4+ and CD8+ T cells and some granulocytes. Further pro-inflammatory cytokines are elaborated by the infiltrating cells (**Figures 12.19, 12.20 a, b**).

The most significant pathological manifestation of the type IV hypersensitivity reaction is **contact allergy** in man and other animals. In this disease there is topical sensitization to an allergen and re-exposure

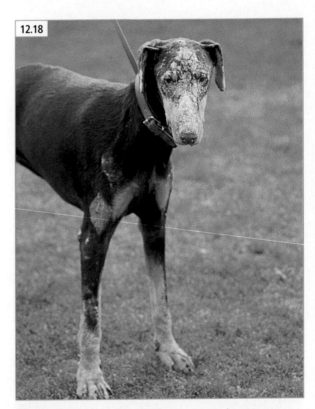

12.18

Fig. 12.18 Canine leishmaniosis. This dog is infected by *Leishmania infantum*. A sandfly has transmitted the infection to the skin establishing a granulomatous dermatitis apparent as areas of alopecia and scaling over the face of the dog. This dog is also lame and has protein-losing nephropathy. These two clinical signs relate to the development of circulating immune complexes and their deposition in capillaries of the synovium and renal glomerulus. This secondary immunopathology is a sequela to the primary infection.

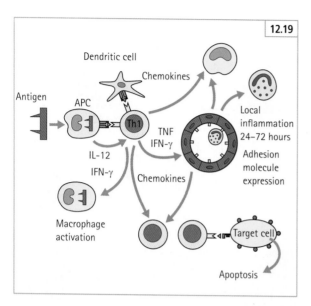

Figs. 12.19 Type IV hypersensitivity. In this form of hypersensitivity the sensitized individual develops populations of memory Th1 cells that become activated on re-exposure to antigen and home to the site of antigen exposure. At the site of antigen exposure these cells produce cytokines (particularly IFN-γ) and chemokines that enhance the local tissue development of HEVs and the recruitment of a range of mononuclear inflammatory cells. The recruited cells amplify local inflammation.

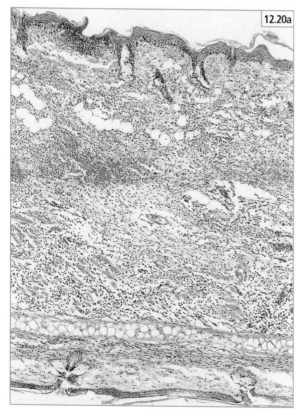

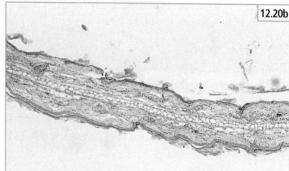

Figs. 12.20a, b Type IV hypersensitivity. In this experimental demonstration of type IV hypersensitivity, a rat is sensitized by injection of a synthetic peptide in adjuvant. Following sensitization the rat is re-exposed to peptide injected into the dermis of the hair covering the ear. Within 24 hours the site of injection had become raised, reddened and firm. Biopsy reveals that this is attributed to an influx of mononuclear inflammatory cells into the dermis. This inflammatory response is shown (**a**) together with a control section from the contralateral ear injected with another peptide to which the rat had not been sensitized (**b**).

leads to an inappropriate inflammatory response at the cutaneous site of challenge (**Figures 12.21, 12.22**). Consistent with the other immunopathological mechanisms, the type IV reaction evolved to counteract infectious diseases, particularly those caused by intracellular pathogens. A classical example of such an agent is *Mycobacterium* spp. (**Figure 12.23**) and the cutaneous DTH reaction is used in diagnosis and monitoring of vaccine efficacy in both man and other animals (**Figures 12.24-12.26**).

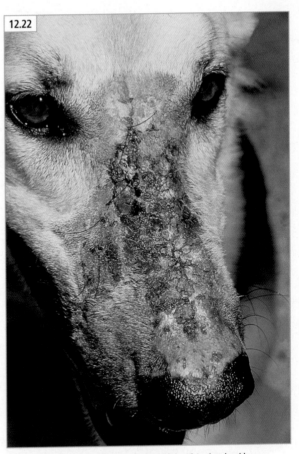

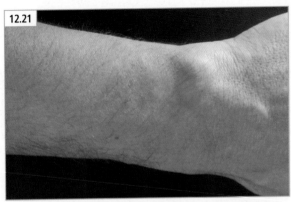

Fig. 12.21 Contact allergic dermatitis. In man, metal jewellery is a common contact sensitizer. The author has a stainless steel backed wrist watch that triggers a localized area of redness within 72 hours of wearing the watch. In this instance, metal (e.g. nickel) acts as the antigenic sensitizer.

Fig. 12.22 Contact allergic dermatitis. This dog had been treated with a topical aural medication containing neomycin. Subsequently, the dog developed a small lesion on the bridge of its nose to which the owner applied the same medication, leading to development of this extensive alopecic and crusting lesion. The lesion spontaneously regressed after the medication was halted.

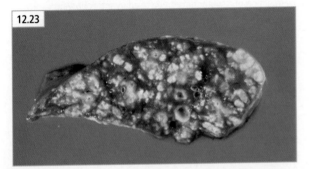

Fig. 12.23 Mycobacterial infection. This section of lung is from a captive sea lion. Within this colony of sea lions there is a background of mycobacterial infection. The lung displays the classical coalescing granulomas that form during myobacterial infection. The type IV immunopathological mechanism evolved to deal with obligate intracellular pathogens such as *Mycobacterium* spp.

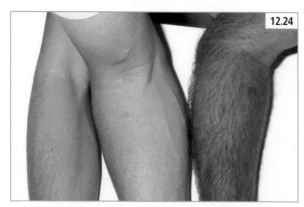

Fig. 12.24 Tuberculin testing. A classical example of a type IV hypersensitivity reaction involves the intradermal injection of tuberculin via the Heaf or Mantoux test. These tests are read 48–72 hours after injection of tuberculin, as this time is required to mount a DTH response. Alternative newer tests involve *in-vitro* stimulation of blood lymphocytes and measurement of the ability of those cells to produce IFN-γ, which may be detected by methods such as capture ELISA.

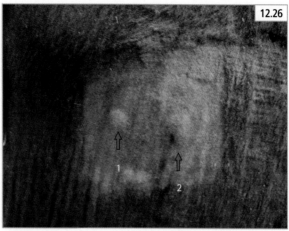

Fig. 12.26 Tuberculin testing. Tuberculin testing of cattle remains a major veterinary activity worldwide. Skin sites on the lateral neck are selected, clipped and the thickness of a skin fold measured with callipers. Two intradermal injections (of avian and bovine tuberculin) are given. The test is read 72 hours later by repeating the calliper measurement. If the thickness of the skin fold at the site of injection of the bovine tuberculin is more than 4 mm greater than the fold for the avian tuberculin, the animal is considered a 'reactor'. An alternative procedure, used in some countries, involves detection of IFN-γ after stimulating blood lymphocytes with mycobacterial antigen *in vitro*. 1, *M. avium*; 2, *M. bovis*.

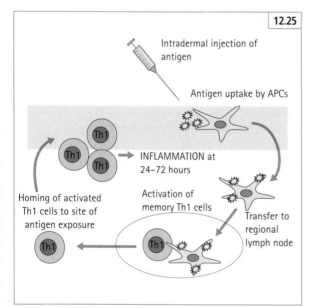

Fig. 12.25 Mechanism of tuberculin testing. Injected antigen is transported to regional lymph nodes where memory Th1 cells are activated and then home back to the site of injection to mediate an inflammatory response.

KEY POINTS

- Hypersensitivity involves an initial period of sensitization to antigen. On re-exposure of the sensitized individual there is an inappropriately excessive response to antigen.
- Allergy is the pathological manifestation of hypersensitivity.
- An allergen is an antigen that triggers an allergic response.
- Hypersensitivity responses evolved to protect from infectious disease, but they have been subverted to cause allergy.
- Gell and Coombs classified types I–IV hypersensitivity.
- In type I (immediate) hypersensitivity, sensitization leads to Th2-regulated production of IgE antibody that coats mast cells and basophils.
- Re-exposure to antigen in type I hypersensitivity leads to IgE cross-linking, mast cell degranulation and release of bioactive molecules.
- Mast cell degranulation leads to vasodilation, bronchoconstriction and pruritus within 15–20 minutes of exposure to allergen.
- The late-phase response (4–24 hours) of type I hypersensitivity involves tissue recruitment of eosinophils and macrophages.
- Type I hypersensitivity reactions may be localized (skin, respiratory and intestinal tracts) or generalized (anaphylaxis).
- In type II hypersensitivity (antibody-mediated cytotoxicity), sensitization leads to production of IgG or IgM antibody, which mediates destruction of a target cell on re-exposure.
- Blood transfusion reactions are an example of a type II hypersensitivity reaction.
- The type II hypersensitivity mechanism also underlies a range of autoimmune diseases including those in which antireceptor antibodies form (Grave's disease, myasthenia gravis).
- Type III hypersensitivity (immune complex hypersensitivity) may occur in antibody excess or antigen excess.
- In antibody excess type III hypersensitivity, immune complex forms at the site of tissue exposure to antigen, leading to localized tissue inflammation (the Arthus reaction).
- In antigen excess type III hypersensitivity, soluble circulating immune complexes lodge in capillary walls in the renal glomerulus, uveal tract, synovium or skin.
- The basic lesion of antigen excess type III hypersensitivity is vasculitis, which may progress to thrombosis and ischaemic necrosis.
- Antigen excess immune complex formation is an important cause of post-infectious secondary immunopathology.
- Type IV or DTH involves cells rather than antibodies and has a slow onset (24–72 hours).
- Antigen-specific Th1 cells are the key mediators of DTH.
- The type IV mechanism underlies contact allergy and tuberculin testing.

CHAPTER 13

The Immune Response to Infectious Agents

OBJECTIVES

At the end of this chapter you should be able to:
- Discuss how the innate and adaptive immune system might respond to a viral infection of a mucosal surface.
- Discuss how the innate and adaptive immune system might respond to a bacterial infection of a mucosal surface.
- Discuss how the adaptive immune system might respond to a helminth infection of the intestinal tract and how this effector response relates to type I hypersensitivity.
- Discuss how the adaptive immune system might respond to an obligate intracellular protozoan infection.
- Discuss how the innate and adaptive immune system might respond to a systemic fungal infection.

INTRODUCTION

The preceding chapters of this book have described the numerous individual components of a functioning innate and adaptive immune system. In the second half of this text we will investigate how these individual components interact with each other to induce a wide range of different **protective or pathological immune responses**. The principle selection pressure for evolutionary development of the immune system was the emergence and co-evolution of an array of pathogens. The developing immune system needed to keep pace with the strategies used by these organisms to outwit it and cause disease and mortality in the host species.

Earlier (see Chapter 1) we discussed the relative roles of innate and adaptive immunity and how the dendritic APC provides a key link between these two systems. Moreover, the concept that interactions between antigen and innate immune cells determine the nature of the subsequent adaptive immune response was highlighted. The aim of this chapter is to reinforce these concepts by discussing the fundamental role of the immune system in protecting animals from infectious disease. A series of examples will be used to illustrate these points and these will be taken from the major classes of infectious pathogens: viral, bacterial, fungal, protozoal and helminth. A working knowledge of microbiology will be assumed.

THE IMMUNE RESPONSE TO VIRAL INFECTION

Viruses are a highly successful class of pathogen responsible for very significant morbidity and mortality amongst both animal and human populations. This in part relates to the ability of these organisms to evolve a range of strategies to **evade or inhibit the host immune response**. Some viruses (e.g. retroviruses such as feline leukaemia virus,

FeLV) have been able to integrate their genetic material into the host genome, others are able to alter their antigenic appearance to produce repeated epidemics or pandemics of disease (e.g. human and animal influenza viruses) and yet other viruses have been able to capture host genes and express host-related proteins that interfere with development of the protective immune response (e.g. the capture of the human IL-10 gene by Epstein–Barr virus).

As an example of a model immune response to virus infection we shall consider how the immune system might deal with a viral infection of the enterocyte lining of the intestinal tract, as might occur with, for example, an **intestinal rotavirus** infection of domestic livestock. When infectious virus particles arrive at their target surface they will encounter the array of **innate immune defences** relevant to that

surface (**Figure 13.1**). In the case of the intestinal mucosa, these will include the **enterocyte barrier**, the **secretions** that coat the luminal surface of that barrier (including mucus, antimicrobial enzymes and defensins and polyreactive immunoglobulins) and the range of **innate immune cells** that normally populate the epithelial compartment (e.g. the γδTCR T cells) and the underlying **lamina propria** (e.g. macrophages, dendritic cells and NK cells).

Virus particles generally infect host cells by binding to a **receptor molecule** expressed on the surface of the target cell. This is generally a normal surface protein that the virus uses as a receptor or co-receptor to gain entry to the target cell. In the present example, the virus interacts with receptor on the enterocyte surface to gain access to the host cell (**Figure 13.2**). Once within the cell, the aim of the virus is to **replicate** in

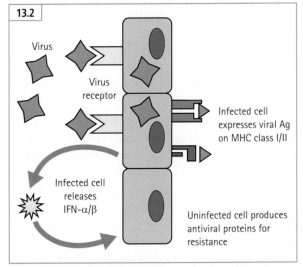

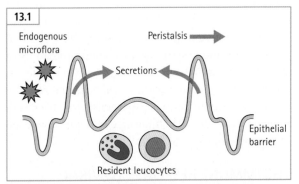

Fig. 13.1 Innate immune defences of mucosal surfaces.
Potential pathogens must initially evade the range of innate immune defences present at mucosal surfaces. In the case of the intestine, these include peristaltic movement, the luminal microflora, the mucosal secretions (mucus, enzymes, defensins, polyreactive immunoglobulins and complement molecules), the epithelial barrier, the intraepithelial γδ TCR T cells and innate immune cells of the lamina propria (dendritic cells, macrophages, mast cells and NK cells).

Fig. 13.2 Viral infection of a mucosal surface. Virus particles enter host target cells by utilizing surface receptor molecules. Within the host cell the virus replicates by mechanisms determined by the nature of the genetic material of that virus. Newly produced virus particles seek to infect new host cells. Virally infected cells secrete antiviral interferons (IFN-α and IFN-β), which confer resistance to infection on nearby uninfected cells. Virally infected cells may express viral antigen (Ag) associated with MHC class I or II molecules.

order to produce new virions that might then leave that cell (and in the process destroy the cell) to infect new targets. The means by which this is achieved depends on the nature of the virus and its genomic material. Fortunately, most virus-infected cells begin to secrete the **antiviral cytokines IFN-α and IFN-β**. These antiviral interferons bind receptors on adjacent non-infected tissue cells and stimulate the uninfected cell to produce an array of other proteins, which confer a measure of resistance to certain viral infections. The virus-infected cell may also display viral antigen on its surface membrane and if that expression is concurrent with down-regulation of MHC class I molecules, the infected cell becomes a **target for innate NK cells** in the vicinity. The antiviral interferons may also positively influence local NK cells. Alternatively, the infected cell may process and present virus antigen in the context of MHC class I or II molecules, but this may only be of significance later.

At this stage of the viral infection it would be hoped that lamina propria **dendritic cells** may be able to sample virus antigen or even become infected by virus particles, allowing classical processing and presentation by these APCs. The interaction between virus and APC is mediated by viral **PAMPs** with dendritic cell **PRRs** that may be either surface (e.g. TLR2, TLR4 and TLR13 recognize viral structural proteins) or cytoplasmic (e.g. TLR3 recognizes viral double-stranded RNA, TLR7 and TLR8 recognize single-stranded RNA and TLR9 recognizes DNA). These interactions presumptively lead to selective gene activation in the APC. In addition, the dendritic cell should enter the lymphatics and migrate to the regional **mesenteric lymph nodes**. It is also possible that virus antigen broaches the intestinal barrier through the Peyer's patch lymphoid tissue.

Once the antigen-laden APC has entered the paracortex of the mesenteric lymph node, it will aim to locate and activate recirculating antigen-specific naïve or memory T cells bearing receptors specific for viral peptides. The interaction between the T cell and the APC will be guided by the range of co-stimulatory surface molecules and cytokines that have been activated within the APC following PRR–PAMP interaction. As the most 'relevant' type of adaptive

immune response for this type of infection would be a **Th1-regulated cytotoxic effector response**, it would be hoped that the APC will activate clones of **Th1 CD4⁺ T cells** and **CD8⁺ cytotoxic T cells**. Cross-presentation of viral antigen would permit expression of viral peptides by both MHC class I and class II (**Figure 13.3**).

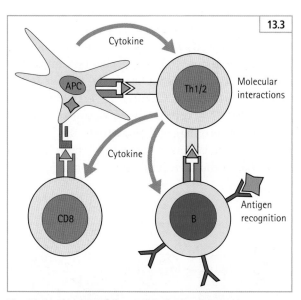

Fig. 13.3 Induction of the antiviral adaptive immune response. Virus antigen presented by dendritic cells within the lymph node paracortex activates Th1 cells, which in turn provide help for the activation of CD8⁺ cytotoxic T cells and those B cells that class switch to the subclass of IgG able to participate in cell-mediated immune responses. In the context of mucosal virus infections, activation of Th2 cells and IgA-producing B cells may also occur.

The range of Th1 and Tc cells generated must then leave the mesenteric lymph node in efferent lymph in order eventually to enter the bloodstream and 'home' to the anatomical site of viral infection (the intestinal mucosa). This will involve the interaction of **homing receptors** such as the $\alpha_4\beta_7$ integrin with the **vascular addressin** MAdCAM (see Chapter 5). Once these adaptive immune cells arrive in the mucosa, the full **effector phase of adaptive immunity** will come into play (**Figure 13.4**). Th1-derived IFN-γ will amplify the effects of NK cells and Tc, and such cell-mediated cytotoxicity is the major effector mechanism in the antiviral immune response.

There is a role for both IgG and IgA antibody in this immune response. Th1 cells stimulate IgG production, but it is also likely that some **Th2 effectors** are generated to ensure production of antiviral IgA. IgG plasma cells may largely be located within the bone marrow, producing circulating antiviral IgG that diffuses into the mucosal environment from the circulation. In contrast, IgA B cells activated in the mesenteric lymph node recirculate back to the intestine and produce IgA locally within the mucosa after differentiating to plasma cells. IgA antibodies are transported across the epithelial barrier to the mucosal surface (see Chapter 2). IgG antibodies may mediate NK cell ADCC or opsonize infected cells for macrophage phagocytosis. IgG bound to infected cells may also mediate their lysis via activation of the classical pathway of complement.

Antiviral IgA secreted across the mucosal barrier may bind virus particles and block their interaction with receptors. If this adaptive immune response is successful in containing the infection, then late stage immunosuppression (**induced Treg cells**) and the development of T- and B-cell **memory** will occur.

THE IMMUNE RESPONSE TO BACTERIAL INFECTION

To remain with the intestinal model, we will next consider the nature of the immune response that might be generated in response to an **enteric bacterial pathogen** such as *Escherichia coli* or *Salmonella* spp. On arrival in the intestinal tract these organisms will also immediately encounter the range of innate immune defences outlined in **Figure 13.1**. However, of particular importance in this context would be the presence of the **endogenous intestinal bacterial microflora**, which will compete with the pathogen for space and nutrients, making colonization more challenging. Another element of innate immunity that may have greater relevance to this class of infection is the $\gamma\delta$ **T cell** within the enterocyte layer. These cells are well situated for early interaction with bacterial pathogens and are thought to be primarily activated in response to this type of organism.

As for viruses, bacteria often require an initial **receptor-mediated interaction** with target host cells. For example, the K88 and K99 pili of *E. coli*

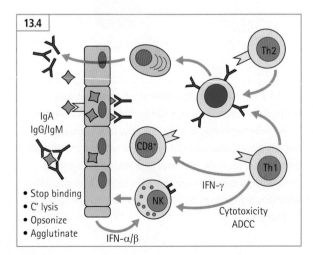

13.4

- Stop binding
- C' lysis
- Opsonize
- Agglutinate

IgA
IgG/IgM

IFN-γ

Cytotoxicity
ADCC

IFN-α/β

Fig. 13.4 The effector immune response to virus infection. CD8+ T cells destroy virus-infected target cells following recognition of MHC class I presenting virus peptide. NK cells may contribute to the cytotoxic response, but they will only kill infected targets in which there has been down-regulation of class I expression. Both cells are functionally enhanced by signalling via Th1-derived IFN-γ and NK cells may also respond to IFN-α and IFN-β. Th1 and Th2 cells enhance production of IgG and IgA virus-specific antibodies. IgG antibody may contribute to NK cell action via ADCC. IgA antibody may be actively secreted across the mucosal surface and inhibit virus–receptor interactions, while IgG antibody may diffuse from the plasma and contribute to the destruction of virus particles (e.g. by ADCC or complement-mediated lysis [C' lysis]).

permit attachment to receptors at the enterocyte interface between these bacteria and host tissue. Enteric pathogens such as *E. coli* or *S. enterica* serovar Typhimurium (*S. typhimurium*) may utilize a variety of different mechanisms to induce disease, dependent on the genetic strain of the bacterium. Some may produce locally active **enterotoxins** that bind toxin receptors and lead to osmotic imbalance and **metabolic diarrhoea** (e.g. enterotoxigenic *E. coli*). Others may attach to and disrupt the epithelial surface (e.g. enteropathogenic *E. coli*, which cause 'attaching and effacing' lesions) or **invade** the intestinal mucosa and regional lymph nodes, leading to a local **pyogranulomatous inflammatory response** (e.g. enteroinvasive *E. coli* or enterohaemorrhagic *E. coli*). Such **gram-negative rods** are also characterized by the ability to produce systemically absorbed **endotoxins** responsible for severe generalized disease (**endotoxaemia**) (**Figure 13.5**).

Once the mucosal surface is colonized, the adaptive immune response will be required to help resolve the infection. Again, mucosal dendritic cells should sample bacterial antigen and this process involves the interaction of PRRs with a range of bacterial PAMPs. APC surface PRRs involved in the recognition of bacterial PAMPs include TLRs 1, 2, 4, 5 and 6 (and in the case of gram-negative bacteria, particularly TLR4, which recognizes lipopolysaccharide and TLR5, which recognizes flagellin), while TLR9 recognizes bacterial CpG DNA within the APC. Bacterial antigen may also cross the epithelial barrier via **M cells** within the dome epithelium overlying the **Peyer's patch**, which is certainly the case for *S. typhimurium*. The activated dendritic cells will activate T cells and, in turn, follicular B cells in the Peyer's patch or **mesenteric lymph nodes**. One desired effector immune response would be the production of antigen-specific immunoglobulin, so APC signalling of the naïve CD4+ T cell would generate **Th2 effectors** (**Figure 13.6**). These, together with antigen-specific B cells, would then exit the mesenteric lymph node to home back to the mucosal surface.

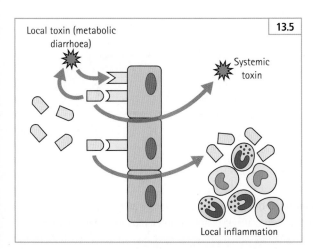

Fig. 13.5 Pathological mechanisms utilized by enteropathic bacteria. Bacteria infecting the intestinal tract (e.g. *Escherichia coli*) may cause disease via several distinct mechanisms. Some strains may secrete locally active enterotoxins that mediate metabolic diarrhoea. Others attach and efface the surface epithelium or invade into the lamina propria, inducing a pyogranulomatous inflammatory response. Some strains elaborate endotoxins that are systemically absorbed to induce endotoxaemia.

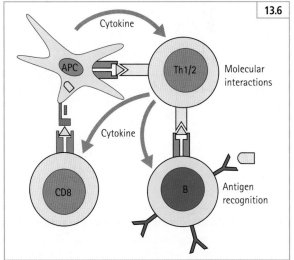

Fig. 13.6 Induction of the antibacterial immune response. Dendritic cells expressing bacterial antigen within the paracortex of the mesenteric lymph node activate Th2 lymphocytes and those B cells that will class switch to the production of antigen-specific IgA. Generation of Th1 and Tc cells is also important for intracellular pathogens such as *Salmonella typhimurium*.

The effector humoral immune response will involve the synthesis of specific **IgA and IgG antibodies**. For those organisms mediating pathology via toxin production, IgG neutralization of toxin will be important. IgG antibodies may also **opsonize** invasive organisms for phagocytosis or permit the **complement-mediated lysis** of the bacteria. Bacterium-specific IgA antibodies will be secreted to the luminal surface where they may interfere with the interaction of organism with receptor molecules (**Figures 13.7a, b**).

In the case of invasive and intracellular pathogens such as *S. typhimurium*, a protective host immune response would also require a robust cell-mediated immune response, involving activation of Th1 and CD8+ T cells (**Figure 13.6**). *S. typhimurium* has virulence genes encoded in 'pathogenicity islands' (SPI-1 and SPI-2) that are responsible for the production of a type III secretion system (a needle-like complex that conveys bacterial effector molecules into the cytoplasm of the target cell). SPI-1 encoded molecules are important for the initial interaction with the target host cell, while SPI-2 molecules are involved in the endocytosis of the bacterium and the formation of '*Salmonella*-containing vacuoles' in the cytoplasm. *Salmonella* readily invades and proliferates inside macrophages, resulting in a granulomatous inflammatory response. The innate

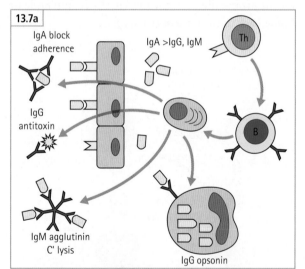
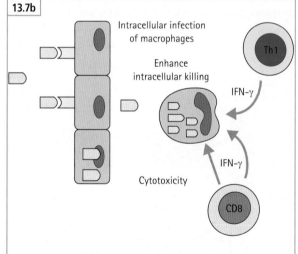

Figs. 13.7a, b The effector immune response to enteropathogenic bacteria. (a) Following homing of antigen-specific Th2 and B cells to the affected segment of intestinal mucosa, these cells mediate local production of IgA and IgG antibodies, which may be secreted (IgA) or diffuse (IgG) to the luminal surface. IgA antibodies may interfere with the receptor-mediated attachment of bacteria to the epithelial surface. IgG antibodies may cause complement-mediated cytolysis or opsonize bacteria for phagocytosis. IgG antibodies may also bind to and neutralize enterotoxins or endotoxins. (b) Th1 cells enhance the bactericidal activity of infected macrophages through IFN-γ signalling and CD8+ Tc may destroy infected targets and produce further IFN-γ.

host response to such intracellular pathogens involves an early production of reactive oxygen species (ROS) generated by nicotinamide adenine dinucleotide phosphate (NADPH) oxidase within the phagosome, in addition to production of nitric oxide synthase (NOS), characteristic of M1 macrophages. The survival of *Salmonella* within the macrophage relies on methods of evading protective responses. For example, the organism may prevent maturation of the phagosome and localization of NADPH oxidase to this compartment, may modify endosomal trafficking within the cytoplasm and may inhibit NOS production. The Th1 effector immune response, with production of IFN-γ, is crucial to enhance the bactericidal activity of macrophages. A role for CD8+ Tc is also proposed in the case of salmonellosis; by the cytotoxic destruction of infected target cells and further production of IFN-γ (**Figures 13.7a, b**).

Again, in a successful immune response, final down-regulation of the effector populations will be required together with the generation of immunological memory.

THE IMMUNE RESPONSE TO HELMINTH INFECTION

The final example of an intestinal immune response is that related to protection from **helminth endoparasitism**. The physical size of such parasites is clearly a challenge for the immune system, but a series of strategies have been devised that contribute to a protective adaptive immune response. These strategies may sometimes be particularly successful, as in the '**self-cure phenomenon**' in which there may be rapid elimination of adult *Haemonchus contortus* by sheep that mount a hypersensitivity reaction to antigens from developing larvae. So, how then might the immune system respond to the presence of a large and biologically complex parasite that might be physically attached to the intestinal mucosa and feeding on host tissue or blood?

Fortunately, such parasites release a range of antigenic molecules (**excretory–secretory [ES] proteins**), which may be sampled by APCs and processed and presented by these cells within the Peyer's patch or mesenteric lymph node paracortex and follicle. The ideal immune response in this circumstance is one in which parasite PAMPs interact with APC PRRs to permit activation of **Th2 effector** cells. Concurrently, **class switching** in antigen-specific B cells will be towards **IgE and IgG** (the latter of restricted subclass). These effector B lymphocytes enter the recirculating vascular pool. Some may differentiate to become plasma cells in lymphoid tissue and produce circulating plasma antibody, but others may home back to the intestinal mucosa to generate local IgE and IgG antibody.

The normal intestinal mucosa is rich in **tissue mast cells** and these are located immediately beneath the enterocyte layer in close association with small capillaries. In this effector immune response, parasite-specific IgE occupies Fcε receptors on the surface of these mast cells. When further parasite ES antigen is absorbed across the mucosal barrier it will **cross-link these IgE molecules**, leading to local mast cell **degranulation** and subsequent tissue oedema (**vasodilation**) and egress of serum proteins and leucocytes (**inflammation**). **Eosinophils** are prominent within these inflammatory infiltrates. This is, of course, a classical **type I hypersensitivity response** and, as discussed in Chapter 12, this adaptive immune mechanism evolved for this purpose rather than for mediating allergic diseases. One specific consequence of triggering an intense local tissue inflammatory response is that it makes the tissue a less attractive 'meal' for the parasite, such that the organisms may even detach from the mucosal surface. In combination with this detachment, infiltrating T lymphocytes are thought to secrete molecules (e.g. IL-13) that interact with **goblet cells**, causing them to increase in number, to **discharge mucus** into the intestinal lumen and to alter the chemical composition of the mucus. The mucus coats the outside of the detached parasite, making it much simpler for **peristaltic movement** to push the organisms along the intestinal tract for eventual **expulsion** (**Figure 13.8**).

In concert with these effector mechanisms, the immune system also mediates a direct attack on parasites within tissue in a 'David and Goliath' manoeuvre. IgE and IgG antibodies are able to coat the outer surface of the parasite and form an **Fc receptor-mediated bridge** to granulocytes (particularly

eosinophils) that are bought into close apposition with the outer coat of the organism. These cells are then able to **degranulate** locally and the granule mediators are thought to cause direct damage to the parasite coat in the process of '**frustrated phagocytosis**'. Local antibody may also bind and neutralize any secreted products of the parasite (**Figures 13.8**). These anti parasitic mechanisms occur when the parasite is embedded within or migrating through the mucosal tissue as opposed to simply feeding from the surface (**Figures 13.9a, b**).

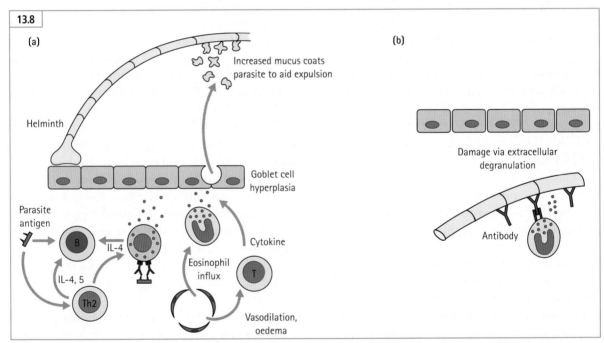

Fig. 13.8 The effector immune response to intestinal helminths. (a) Parasite ES antigens activate Th2 cells and IgG- and IgE-committed B cells within the mesenteric lymph node. Circulating parasite-specific antibody may be produced systemically by plasma cells in lymphoid tissue or locally if effector B cells home to the intestinal mucosa. IgE coats sub-epithelial mast cells, which degranulate when further ES antigen is absorbed and cross-links IgE molecules. Mast cell degranulation leads to oedema of the lamina propria and an inflammatory response characterized by recruitment of eosinophils. This inflammatory response may result in surface-feeding parasites detaching from the mucosa. T-cell-derived cytokines (e.g. IL-13) concurrently stimulate goblet cells to produce mucus that coats the parasite, and these effects combine with peristaltic movement to help expel the parasite from the intestine (the 'self-cure phenomenon'). **(b)** Parasite-specific IgG or IgE may directly coat the surface of tissue-migrating forms of helminths and create a bridge to those leucocytes expressing appropriate Fc receptors (e.g. eosinophils, neutrophils, macrophages). This has the effect of bringing granulocytes into close apposition with the parasite surface and local degranulation of these cells may cause damage to the coat of the organism ('frustrated phagocytosis'). IgG antibodies may also bind and neutralize any further excreted or secreted products from the parasite.

THE IMMUNE RESPONSE TO PROTOZOAL INFECTION

In previous chapters we have used the example of the protozoan infection leishmaniosis to explain a number of immunological concepts. Here we review these mechanisms in the context of the antimicrobial immune response. *Leishmania* spp. cause zoonotic disease of major significance to the human population in endemic areas such as Central and South America. The domestic dog is the predominant reservoir of infection, which is transmitted to both species by a range of sandfly vectors. The canine disease is now established in North America. The disease is endemic in Mediterranean countries and is of significant concern in traditionally non-endemic European countries as a consequence of the mass movement of pet dogs under EU pet travel legislation.

The bite of the sandfly transmits the promastigote stage of the organism into the cutaneous microenvironment of the dog. The organism enters dermal macrophages where it transforms and multiplies as an amastigote, which is the obligate intracellular stage of the life cycle. Eventually, parasitized macrophages may rupture and release amastigotes that establish infection in new host phagocytic cells (**Figure 13.10**).

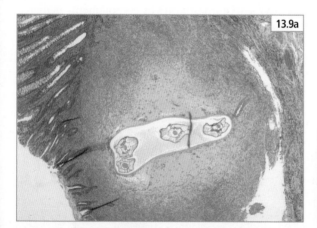

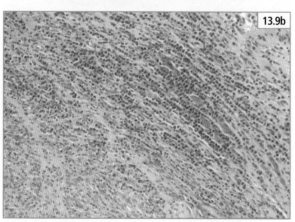

Figs. 13.9a, b Immune response to intestinal helminths.
(a) Section of large intestine from a horse with migrating strongyle larvae and an intense localized inflammatory response.
(b) Eosinophils are prominent in the inflammatory infiltrate.

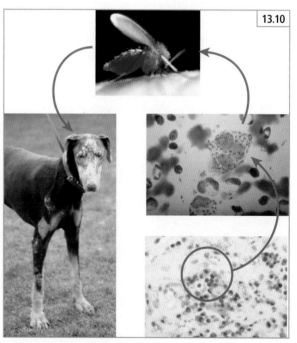

Fig. 13.10 The life cycle of *Leishmania*. An infected sandfly bites the canine or human host in order to take in a blood meal and injects promastigotes into the dermis. The promastigotes are phagocytosed by macrophages and divide within these cells to form amastigotes. Parasitized macrophages may rupture and release amastigotes, which infect other host cells locally or systemically. Infected macrophages may also be taken up by naïve sandflies as they take a blood meal, and released amastigotes transform again to promastigotes and multiply in the gut of the sandfly.

There are two main outcomes to this infection in the dog. These outcomes are **genetically controlled** and entirely reflect the nature of the host immune response to the pathogen. Dogs of the genetically 'resistant' phenotype make an appropriate immune response that controls but does not eliminate the infection. These animals do not develop clinical disease, but remain subclinically infected carriers and a source of infectious agent to sandflies. In contrast, dogs of the 'susceptible' phenotype make an entirely inappropriate, non-protective immune response, allowing dissemination of the infection and development of secondary immune-mediated sequelae. These dogs develop severe, terminal multisystemic disease if untreated.

We consider here the development of the protective immune response in a **resistant** dog. In this situation, dermal dendritic cells capture antigen for processing and presentation within the paracortex and follicle of the regional cutaneous draining lymph node. Within this lymphoid tissue, the essential immune response that must be generated is that regulated by **Th1 lymphocytes (Figure 13.11)**. The subpopulation of B cells class switched to the appropriate IgG subclass associated with cell-mediated immunity may also be activated. These effector populations then recirculate and home to cutaneous (or other) sites of infection. The effector phase of the protective immune response essentially involves the **secretion of IFN-γ by Th1 cells**. This cytokine **signals parasitized macrophages**, which then permit those cells to destroy the amastigotes proliferating within the cytoplasm. **IgG antibody** produced systemically or locally probably has an adjunctive role in binding and destroying free amastigotes by complement-mediated lysis as they exit ruptured macrophages in an attempt to infect new target cells.

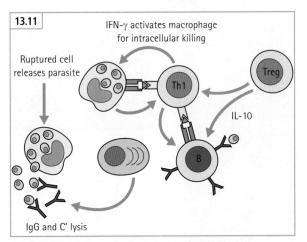

Fig. 13.11 The effector immune response to *Leishmania* in a dog of resistant phenotype. Resistant dogs mount a polarized immune response dominated by Th1 effector cells. The IFN-γ secreted by these cells activates parasitized macrophages and permits them to destroy the cytoplasmic amastigotes. Th1-related B-cell production of IgG antibody also occurs. This specific IgG may be able to bind free amastigotes as they leave a ruptured macrophage in search of new targets and lead to complement-mediated lysis of these organisms. In the late stages of the immune response, IL-10-producing regulatory populations (either induced Treg cells or switched Th1 cells) seek to limit the potential for secondary immune-mediated pathology, but permit persistence of low-grade infection.

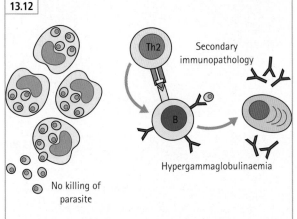

Fig. 13.12 The effector immune response to *Leishmania* in a dog of susceptible phenotype. Susceptible dogs make an inappropriate polarized Th2 response to *Leishmania*, with the generation of high concentrations of serum antibody and suppression of Th1-mediated cellular immunity. The infection is allowed to disseminate widely and the antibody response underlies the secondary immune-mediated pathology that accounts for many of the clinical signs of active disease. These humoral effects include the induction of autoantibodies and the formation of circulating immune complexes.

In most resistant animals this effector immune response is thought not to entirely kill the infectious agents (known as 'sterilizing immunity'). This leaves a **low-grade persistent infection** with the potential for that animal to still act as a reservoir of infection or for infection to recrudesce later in life. Failure to sterilize the infection is thought to relate to the **onset of a regulatory T-cell response** during the latter stages of the effector reaction. This may be mediated by **induced Treg cells** secreting **IL-10**, although there is now also evidence that Th1 cells may undergo a subsequent phenotypic shift to take on a regulatory (IL-10 producing) role. The reason for such regulation is to prevent the onset of secondary immune-mediated sequelae, as occur in susceptible animals.

In dogs of the **susceptible** phenotype, antigen presentation stimulates an inappropriate **Th2-regulated immune response**. This leads to the generation of high levels of **serum antibody** and inhibition of Th1 function, which permits uncontrolled infection. The range of **secondary immune-mediated sequelae** that characterize the clinical infection relate to the development of circulating immune complexes (e.g. polyarthropathy, glomerulonephritis and uveitis) or to the induction of autoantibodies (e.g. anti-erythrocyte, antiplatelet and antinuclear antibodies) (**Figure 13.12**).

THE IMMUNE RESPONSE TO FUNGAL INFECTION

As with helminths, many fungal pathogens provide a challenging target for the immune system because of the relative colony size of the organisms. In this final example we shall consider the immune response of the dog to colonization of the nasal sinuses and nasal cavity by the organism *Aspergillus fumigatus* (**Figure 13.13**). This fungus forms a large colony over the mucosa of these nasal tissues, but the organisms tend not to infiltrate into the lamina propria. The colonies comprise a tangled mass of **fungal hyphae** with intermittent **conidia** that represent the sites of **spore** formation (**Figure 13.14**).

In order for such a colony to establish, the organism must broach the normal innate immune barriers of the upper respiratory tract, including the antimicrobial substances found within nasal secretions. Although innate phagocytic cells (neutrophils and macrophages) are capable of phagocytosing fungal spores, they appear unable effectively to kill these elements. The fungal hyphae are simply too large a target for effective phagocytosis.

The adaptive immune response to this infection is well characterized. Recent studies have shown up-regulation of expression of genes encoding

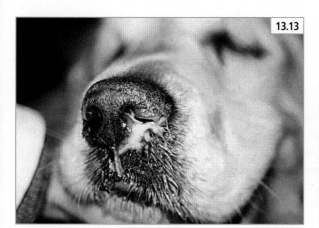
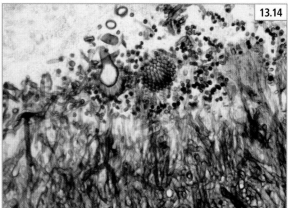

Figs. 13.13, 13.14 Canine sinonasal aspergillosis. (13.13) This dog has a nasal discharge secondary to infection of the nasal sinuses by *Aspergillus fumigatus*. **(13.14)** *A. fumigatus* fungi grow over the surface of the sinonasal mucosa as large plaques of hyphae with intermittent conidia formed of fungal spores. These structures are very large targets for the immune system.

TLRs1–4 and 6–10 and NOD2 in the mucosa of dogs with sinonasal apsergillosis. It is likely that APCs carrying fungal antigen stimulate this response in regional lymphoid tissue such as the **nasopharyngeal tonsil** or **retropharyngeal lymph nodes**. The effector phase of the mucosal immune response involves infiltration by **CD4$^+$ Th1** and probably **Th17 cells**, as determined by up-regulation of gene expression for **IFN-γ and IL-23** in inflamed tissue. There is also a marked **pyogranulomatous** element to the reaction and infiltration of IgG-bearing plasma cells. Th1-derived IFN-γ most likely provides stimulation to macrophages to permit these cells to destroy any phagocytosed fungal spores. Antibody and complement molecules are likely to coat the hyphal elements and form a bridge to FcR-bearing

granulocytes. Similar to helminth infection, these cells may **degranulate** locally and induce focal damage to the hyphae. Infected dogs generally mount a strong **serum IgG** antibody response to the organism, which is useful diagnostically. The inflammatory response itself is likely to be responsible for the extensive tissue and bone destruction that may occur in this disease. Similar to observations in leishmaniosis, there is an additional **regulatory element** to the response, as there is concurrent up-regulation of **IL-10** gene expression. Again, this is interpreted as an attempt by the adaptive immune system to prevent extensive tissue damage or the onset of systemic sequelae, but at the same time allow **persistence of infection** and development of chronic sinonasal disease (**Figure 13.15**).

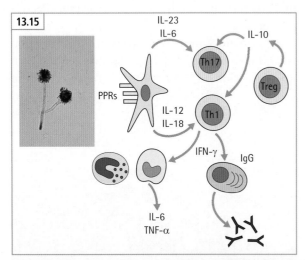

Fig. 13.15 The effector immune response in canine sinonasal aspergillosis. The mucosa underlying the fungal plaque is heavily infiltrated by CD4$^+$ and CD8$^+$ T cells, macrophages and IgG-producing plasma cells. Analysis of cytokine gene expression in these inflammatory lesions is consistent with activation of Th1 and Th17 cells. The effector immune response may therefore involve IFN-γ enhancement of macrophage function and the production of local and systemic antigen-specific IgG. Antibody and complement molecules may coat fungal elements, forming a bridge to granulocytes that may degranulate to cause damage to the organisms. Antibody may also opsonize fungal spores or hyphal fragments for macrophage phagocytosis and destruction once that phagocytic cell is signalled by IFN-γ. A regulatory process involving local IL-10 production is also recognized within these lesions. This may limit secondary immune-mediated tissue damage, but also permits persistence of the infection.

KEY POINTS

- Viruses generally enter host cells by utilizing cell surface membrane receptors.
- Virally infected cells produce the antiviral cytokines IFN-α and IFN-β.
- NK cells and cytotoxic CD8$^+$ T cells are important in the immune response to viral infection.
- Th1 cells provide help for antiviral cell-mediated and IgG humoral immunity.
- Intraepithelial $\gamma\delta$ TCR-expressing T cells may be important in the initial immune response to some bacterial pathogens of mucosal surfaces.
- Excretory–secretory antigens are important in initiating antiparasite immune responses.
- The type I hypersensitivity mechanism evolved as an antiparasitic defence mechanism.
- Parasites induce Th2-regulated immunity with generation of IgE and involvement of mast cells and eosinophils.

- The 'self-cure' phenomenon is immunologically mediated.
- Eosinophil degranulation may damage the surface coat of parasites.
- The immune response to *Leishmania* is genetically determined and may be polarized to a Th1 (resistant) or Th2 (susceptible) phenotype.
- Late-stage regulation of the immune response to infectious agents is required in order to prevent secondary immune-mediated pathology, but this may also allow persistence of infection. Regulation probably involves IL-10-producing induced regulatory T cells.
- Th17 cells may act with Th1 cells in the immune response to particular types of infectious agent.

CHAPTER 14

Cancer Immunology and Immune System Neoplasia

OBJECTIVES

At the end of this chapter you should be able to:
- Define what is meant by 'tumour antigen'.
- Discuss how the adaptive immune system responds to the presence of a tumour.
- Give an example of current approaches to immunotherapy for cancer.
- Discuss the anatomical, histological, cytological, immunophenotypic and molecular classification of lymphoma and understand why such a classification is important.

- Briefly discuss how lymphoma affects various domestic animal species.
- Distinguish lymphoid leukaemia from lymphoma.
- Distinguish plasmacytoma from multiple myeloma.
- Describe the paraneoplastic effects associated with multiple myeloma.
- Distinguish canine histiocytoma from histiocytic sarcoma.

INTRODUCTION

This chapter considers aspects of how the immune system responds to neoplastic cells and the range of tumours of cells of the immune system. Tumour cells derive from normal body cells or **tumour stem cells** during the process of **neoplastic transformation**. Neoplastic transformation and development of clinical neoplasia is largely a genetic event involving the **oncogenes** and **tumour suppressor genes** that regulate the **cell cycle** and **apoptosis**, but other factors, including failure of **immune surveillance**, contribute to the progression of malignancy. It is generally believed that the relatively higher incidence of cancer in ageing populations relates to age-related alterations in immune function (**immunosenescence**), which particularly impair the cell-mediated and cytotoxic reactions that underlie an effective anticancer immune response.

TUMOUR ANTIGENS

Tumour antigens are the targets of the antitumour immune response. They are molecules that distinguish transformed from normal body cells and are of a variety of origins. The process of neoplastic transformation may give rise to progressive **mutations in genes encoding naturally expressed self-antigens**, such that the protein products of these genes have sufficiently altered sequence and structure that they become targets of the immune response. In contrast, some tumour cells produce excessive quantities of a normal self-protein. In the case of **virally induced neoplasia** (e.g. that caused by FeLV), transformed cells might express virus-associated protein that identifies them as neoplastic. Expression of the feline oncornavirus-associated cell membrane antigen (FOCMA) is an excellent example of this phenomenon. Finally, neoplastic cells may begin to express molecules uncharacteristic of that cell type through activation of previously silent genes ('**derepression**' of these genes).

THE ANTITUMOUR IMMUNE RESPONSE

The immune response to cancer proceeds through three stages. The first of these is **elimination**, during which the immune system is able to completely destroy tissue cells that have undergone neoplastic transformation. The second stage is **equilibrium**, during which immune-resistant tumour cells emerge, but the immune system continues to destroy susceptible cancer cells. Equilibrium may last for many years in individual patients. The final stage is **escape**, at which point the tumour cells have developed strategies to evade immune detection and destruction. These strategies might include loss or downregulation of tumour antigens, the secretion of inhibitory cytokines, downregulation of MHC expression or presentation of tumour antigens to T cells without providing co-stimulatory signals, leading to **T-cell anergy** and effective tolerance to the tumour.

The most important elements of the innate immune system that may have an antineoplastic effect are the **NK cells**. The mode of action of these cells is discussed in Chapter 8. NK cells may recognize tumour antigens expressed on the membrane of target neoplastic cells, but will also require that the tumour cells downregulate expression of MHC class I to avoid the inhibitory effects of the NK cell inhibitory receptors.

The range of tumour antigens must be classically processed and presented for induction of the adaptive antitumour immune response. This necessitates shed tumour antigens or neoplastic cells being taken up and processed by APCs. Cross-presentation of tumour antigens will likely occur and antigen presentation will occur within the regional lymphoid tissue closest to the location of the tumour. Ideally, the nature of APC co-signalling will activate populations of tumour-specific **CD4+ Th1 cells** and **CD8+ Tc** within the lymph node paracortex. A humoral response to tumour antigens may also be engendered and this may preferentially involve class switching to that IgG subclass triggered by signalling via Th1 cells.

Activated cytotoxic lymphocytes will recirculate to the location of the tumour and it is widely recognized that most neoplasms have a peripheral infiltrate of lymphoid cells. Indeed, immunohistochemical studies have readily demonstrated such T-cell infiltration

(**Figures 14.1a, b**). The most relevant form of antitumour immunity will be the cytotoxic immune response mediated by CD8+ Tc and promoted by **IFN-γ** secreted by Th1 cells (**Figure 14.2**). Unfortunately, this immune response is generally unable to contain a tumour once the neoplastic lesion has reached the stage of clinical disease. The rapid division of tumour cells readily outstrips the ability of the immune system to destroy individual targets. One rare exception to this is the example of the **canine histiocytoma** presented in Chapter 8. The spontaneous regression that characterizes these tumours is known to be associated with the action of infiltrating CD8+ Tc.

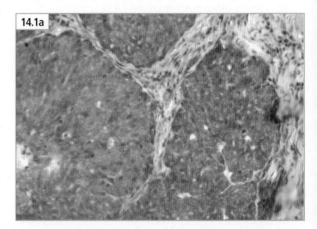

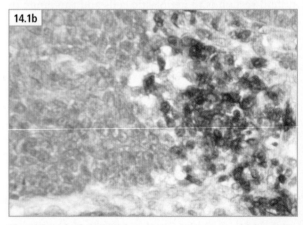

Figs. 14.1a, b The immune response to tumours. (a) A section of a carcinoma growing in the nasal cavity of a cat. **(b)** A serial section from the tumour labelled immunohistochemically shows infiltration of CD3+ T cells at the margins of the lobules of neoplastic epithelium.

TUMOUR-PROMOTING IMMUNE ACTIVITY

Despite the immunological recognition of neoplastic tissue as 'foreign' and the mounting of an adaptive immune response, the survival and metastatic spread of tumours may in part be attributed to tumour-promoting immunological activity (**Figure 14.3**). One such effect is mediated by **tumour-associated macrophages** (TAMs). These macrophages infiltrate tumour tissue and enhance the growth, infiltration and metastasis of tumour cells. TAMs are of the M2 macrophage phenotype and mediate these effects by producing tissue remodelling matrix metalloproteinases, angiogenic vascular endothelial growth factor (VEGF) and the immunosuppressive cytokine IL-10. TAMs may be recruited to neoplastic tissue following the production of chemokines (e.g. CCL2) by mesenchymal stromal/stem cells within the tumour.

In addition to the negative effects of TAMs, populations of Treg cells are also present within the inflammatory infiltrates associated with neoplastic tissue. These Treg cells may inhibit the effector function of Tc and NK cells. Such regulatory cells are identified in both human and canine cancer patients. Dogs with neoplastic disease have elevated numbers of Foxp3+ CD4+ Treg cells in blood and lymph nodes draining the site of the tumour. Both Treg cells and TAMs would appear to be appropriate targets for tumour therapy, as inhibiting or deleting these populations would allow more effective antitumour immune responses and reduce the metastatic potential of tumours. In this regard, a recent study of low-dose cyclophosphamide therapy of dogs with soft tissue sarcomas has shown a reduced number of circulating Treg cells in treated patients.

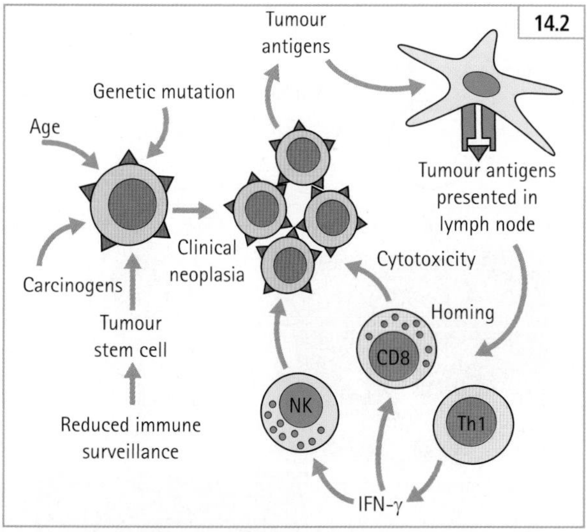

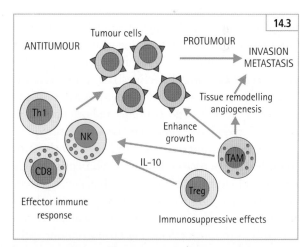

Fig. 14.2 The immune response to tumours. A series of tumour initiating and promoting events leads to transformation of a cell or tumour stem cell and proliferation of that cell to the stage of induction of tissue pathology and clinical signs (clinical neoplasia). The tumour cells display neo-antigens that are processed and presented by APCs within the regional lymphoid tissue. The antitumour immune response comprises CD4+ Th1 and CD8+ Tc cells that home to the periphery of the tumour to attempt cytotoxic destruction of the neoplastic cells. There is an additional role for NK cells, whose action may also be amplified by Th1-derived IFN-γ.

Fig. 14.3 The immune response to tumours. In addition to appropriate cytotoxic effector immune responses to tumours, there are counteractive responses that may enhance the malignant potential of the cancer. These include the presence of Treg cells within the population of tumour-infiltrating lymphocytes and the presence of TAMs of the M2 phenotype that may encourage the growth, invasion and metastasis of the tumour.

IMMUNOTHERAPY TO ENHANCE THE ANTITUMOUR IMMUNE RESPONSE

The mainstays of tumour therapy currently rely on attempts to destroy tumour cells by **chemotherapeutic** inhibition of cell division or targeted cellular damage via procedures such as **radiotherapy**. Adjunctive therapies that might enhance the systemic cellular immune response also have a role in management. These will be discussed further in Chapter 22.

Novel approaches to **tumour immunotherapy** might target three of the areas described above: (1) promotion of tumour antigen presentation by dendritic cells, (2) promotion of protective cytotoxic T-cell responses and (3) overcoming immunosuppression within the tumour itself.

There are numerous examples of such approaches, some of which have also been attempted in companion animal oncology. These techniques range from simple to complex in conception. Simple non-specific approaches include the systemic administration of recombinant cytokines that might enhance T-cell activity. A novel product (Oncept IL-2™, Merial) using this approach has just been released for the adjunct treatment of feline injection site sarcoma (FISS) (see Chapter 20). This product is a canarypox virus vector carrying the feline IL-2 gene, which is injected around the site of surgical excision of the tumour at the time of post-surgical radiotherapy. The treatment reduces the time to relapse of the tumour.

Another appproach is the generation of **'lymphokine activated killer' (LAK) cells**. In this method, blood lymphocytes from the cancer patient are cultured *in vitro* with cytokines such as IL-2 and the expanded and activated cells are re-injected into the patient to more effectively target tumour cells. Alternatively, tumour cells may be collected and genetically modified so that they are able to express surface molecules or cytokines that recruit and activate cytotoxic lymphocytes once the modified cells are injected into the periphery of the tumour. **Monoclonal antibody technology** has also been evaluated for tumour therapy. Monoclonal antibodies raised against specific tumour antigens may be used by themselves or engineered to carry an array of substances (e.g. drugs, pro-drugs or toxins) directly to a tumour when injected intravenously. Such antibodies have been referred to as **'magic bullets'** because of their selective targeting of tumour cells.

The first **'cancer vaccine'** used therapeutically for the treatment of canine malignant melanoma has been introduced recently. This is a **'naked DNA'** vaccine (see Chapter 20) comprising a bacterial plasmid into which is inserted the gene encoding the molecule tyrosinase, a tumour antigen expressed by melanoma cells. The vaccine contains the human tyrosinase gene, as the human molecule is sufficiently different to canine tyrosinase to engender an immune response (an immune response would not normally be made to a self-protein), but also sufficiently homologous to canine tyrosinase for that immune response to target the canine molecule. Transfection of dendritic cells following injection of the vaccine leads to the generation of antitumour adaptive cellular immunity. Preliminary studies have suggested that this is able to delay progression of the clinical disease (**Figure 14.4**).

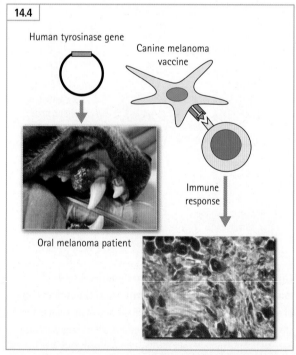

14.4

Human tyrosinase gene

Canine melanoma vaccine

Oral melanoma patient

Immune response

Fig. 14.4 Canine melanoma vaccine. This naked DNA vaccine incorporates a bacterial plasmid containing the human tyrosinase gene. When injected into a dog with oral malignant melanoma, the gene transfects dendritic cells and tyrosinase peptides are presented. This tumour antigen presentation amplifies the antitumour immune response.

TUMOURS OF THE IMMUNE SYSTEM

The cells of the immune system may undergo neoplastic transformation leading to the formation of a range of tumours. Tumours of lymphocytes (lymphoma, lymphoid leukaemia), plasma cells (plasmacytoma, multiple myeloma) and dendritic cells (histiocytoma, localized and disseminated histiocytic sarcoma) will be discussed here. There are a number of other less common variants of such tumours and for information on these you should refer to clinical texts. Some of these tumours (e.g. histiocytoma, lymphoma) are very common in animals. A detailed discussion of oncogenesis is beyond the scope of this chapter, but development of these neoplasms invariably involves genetic mutation compounded by co-factors such as age, failure of immune surveillance and the action of carcinogens or retroviruses.

Lymphoma

Lymphoma (sometimes referred to as lymphosarcoma) is probably the **most common tumour recognized in domestic animals**. The disease is most frequent in **dogs, cats and horses** because these animals generally have a longer life span and this is most often a disease of middle to older age. Sporadic cases of lymphoma are recognized in production animals and the disease is significant in poultry. Lymphoma is a solid tumour that causes nodular or diffuse enlargement of the viscera in which it grows.

Lymphoma may be classified on the basis of (1) **anatomical distribution**, (2) **histological appearance**, (3) **cytological appearance**, (4) **immunophenotype** and (5) **gene rearrangement**. In human medicine the classification scheme developed by the World Health Organization (WHO) takes all of these elements into account when defining the numerous subtypes of lymphoma. The latest **WHO classification scheme** has now been successfully adapted for canine and equine disease. The aim of such classification is to allow formulation of a prognosis and to select the optimum treatment for that specific entity.

Anatomically, lymphoma may be classified as (1) **multicentric**, (2) **thymic**, (3) **alimentary**, (4) **cutaneous** or (5) **solitary**. Multicentric lymphoma involves widespread organ involvement, most often starting in lymphoid tissue and with probable metastasis. Any organ may be involved, but those most commonly affected are lymph nodes, spleen, liver, kidney, heart, lungs and gastrointestinal tract (**Figure 14.5**). Thymic lymphoma involves the thymus and possibly also the mediastinal or cervical lymph nodes (**Figure 14.6**). Alimentary lymphoma

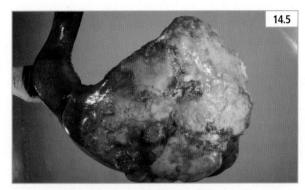

Fig. 14.5 Multicentric lymphoma. This is the spleen from a horse containing a very large (note the relative size of the author's hand) cream-coloured mass with the microscopic appearance of a lymphoma. Multiple lymph nodes were similarly enlarged and similar neoplastic tissue was present surrounding the pelvic–femoral articulation and arising from the intercostal area of the thoracic cavity. This horse presented with unilateral hindlimb lameness.

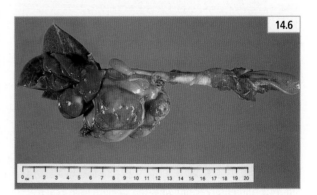

Fig. 14.6 Thymic lymphoma. This is the thoracic content from a cat infected experimentally with FeLV. The heart and lungs are to the left of the photograph and anterior to the heart is a large cream mass arising from the thymus. The mass is several times larger than the heart. The cat presented with dyspnoea, dysphagia and local subcutaneous oedema.

may arise at any level of the gastrointestinal tract and extend to the mediastinal lymph nodes and possibly the liver and other abdominal viscera (**Figure 14.7**). Alimentary lymphoma may be solitary (i.e. a single location in the stomach or intestinal tract) or there may be multiple foci of disease. Cutaneous lymphoma arises in the skin and may extend to draining lymph nodes. Two forms of cutaneous lymphoma are recognized. **Dermal lymphoma** arises within the dermis and does not extend to the epidermis and may be of T- or B-cell phenotype (see below). In contrast, **epitheliotropic lymphoma** extends into the epidermis to form small intraepidermal aggregates known as 'Pautrier's microabscesses'. Epitheliotropic lymphoma is always of T-cell type and the cells express integrins that are responsible for the epithelial localization (**Figure 14.8**). Finally, solitary lymphoma is a single tumour focus in any body organ.

The histological classification of lymphoma is made after examination of tissue biopsies and this area has recently become increasingly complex as new subtle variations of tumour growth are identified. Simplistically, neoplastic lymphocytes generally grow in one of two basic patterns. The most common is '**diffuse lymphoma**' where normal tissue structure is entirely obliterated by an infiltrating sheet of closely packed tumour cells (**Figure 14.9**). In contrast, in '**follicular lymphoma**' the neoplastic cells (generally within lymphoid tissue) grow in a pattern reminiscent of normal lymphoid follicles, but these aggregates are grossly expanded and have abnormal microanatomy (**Figure 14.10**).

The cytological classification of lymphoma relates to examination of aspirates from a tumour mass or tumour cells exfoliated into body fluids. Neoplastic lymphocytes satisfy the fundamental criteria for malignancy (e.g. cellular pleomorphism, increased mitotic rate) and are also often categorized in terms of size (e.g. small, medium or large lymphocytes), the relative proportions of nucleus and cytoplasm and the appearance of nuclear chromatin and nucleoli (**Figure 14.11**).

Lymphoma **immunophenotype** refers to the cell of origin of the tumour. **Immunohistochemical**, **immunocytochemical** or **flow cytometric** analyses (see Chapters 5 and 10) are used to determine the nature of surface molecule expression by the tumour cells. In a research setting, this may be taken to a high level of phenotyping, but in general practice it is now commonplace to determine whether lymphoma is of T- or B-cell origin (**Figure 14.12**). In dogs, this has prognostic significance when considered

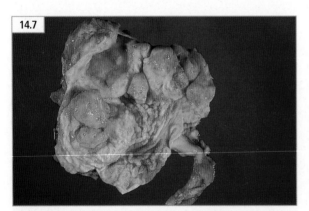

Fig. 14.7 Alimentary lymphoma. This stomach from a cat has been opened to display the mucosal surface, which is entirely replaced by a series of cream nodular masses. The cat had a chronic history of vomiting (sometimes haematemesis) and weight loss. It has been suggested that this form of lymphoma may be triggered by gastric *Helicobacter* spp.

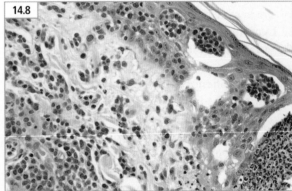

Fig. 14.8 Epitheliotropic lymphoma. Skin biopsy from a dog with epitheliotropic lymphoma. Note the clusters of neoplastic lymphocytes within the epidermis (Pautrier's microabscesses). These are always T-cell tumours and the neoplastic cells express adhesion molecules that interact with ligands on the surface of keratinocytes.

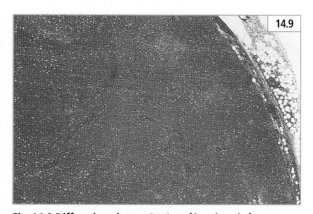

Fig. 14.9 Diffuse lymphoma. Section of lymph node from a dog with lymphoma. The normal corticomedullary structure is completely obliterated by a diffuse sheet of neoplastic lymphocytes that extends focally into the perinodal adipose tissue.

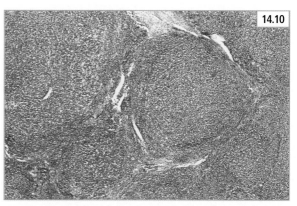

Fig. 14.10 Follicular lymphoma. Section of lymph node from a dog with lymphoma. The neoplastic cells are growing with a nodular arrangement, which is sometimes difficult to distinguish from hyperplastic cortical follicles. These are generally tumours of B-cell origin.

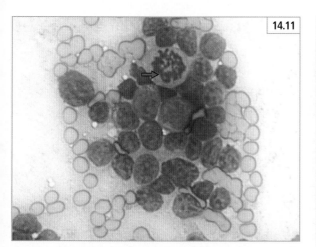

Fig. 14.11 Lymphoma cytology. A fine-needle aspirate from the lymph node of a cat with multicentric lymphoma. There is a population of lymphoblastic cells with minimal cytoplasm surrounding a nucleus with aggregated chromatin. A bizarre mitotic figure is present in one cell (arrowed).

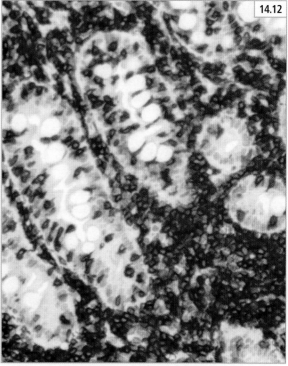

Fig. 14.12 Lymphoma immunophenotyping. It is now routine to determine whether a lymphoma is of T- or B-cell origin. This biopsy sample is from a cat with alimentary lymphoma labelled with antibody to CD3. The neoplastic lymphocytes infiltrating the lamina propria are small T lymphocytes. T cells are also present within the crypt epithelial layer, suggesting a tendency to epitheliotropism.

in conjunction with histological features. Recent studies have shown the longest median survival time (or relapse-free survival time) for low-grade T-cell lymphoma, the shortest survival time for high-grade T-cell lymphoma and intermediate survival for dogs with B-cell lymphoma.

The most recent adjunct to lymphoma diagnosis is '**clonality testing**'. This methodology utilizes PCR technology to determine whether a population of lymphocytes carries **rearrangements** in the variable or joining region elements of genes encoding **T- or B-cell receptors** (TCR β or γ chains; BCR heavy chain). Whereas in a normal or reactive population one would expect numerous clonal specificities, in a neoplastic population there is restricted receptor usage consistent with clonal expansion of the tumour cell (**Figure 14.13**).

As stated earlier, lymphoma may arise in any species, but is particularly common in dogs and cats. **Canine lymphoma** has a **genetic basis** and is more commonly recognized in certain breeds (e.g. boxers, golden retrievers). There is currently great interest in defining genetic associations in canine and feline lymphoma. Lymphoma in the dog is a disease of middle to older age and the most commonly recognized anatomical form is multicentric. Although a number of largely chemical carcinogens have been proposed as triggers of canine lymphoma, there are no definitive studies and numerous investigations have failed to provide evidence for a canine oncogenic retrovirus.

In contrast, **feline lymphoma** may be associated with **FeLV** infection and there is some evidence that co-infection with feline immunodeficiency virus (**FIV**) may also contribute to lymphomagenesis. However,

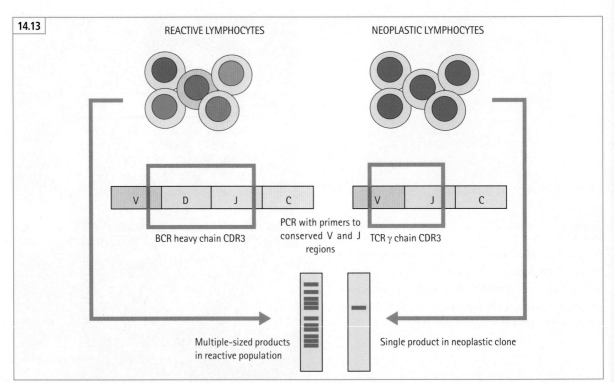

Fig. 14.13 Clonality testing. This diagnostic tool helps distinguish between a reactive population of lymphocytes of mixed antigenic specificity and a clonal population of neoplastic lymphocytes with identical receptor specificity. The complementarity determining region 3 (CDR3) of the BCR or TCR forms the antigen-binding site and is an area of high sequence variability due to differential recombination between VDJ genes and further somatic mutation in B cells. In clonality testing, a PCR reaction amplifies the CDR3 region of the BCR heavy chain (VDJ) or the TCR γ chain (VJ). The PCR employs primers directed at conserved regions of the V and J genes in each case. The amplicons are then separated by size (e.g. by polyacrylamide gel electrophoresis) and visualized. Products of multiple sizes indicate a reactive population, while a single-sized product indicates clonality and is consistent with neoplastic transformation.

since the advent of good diagnostic tests and vaccines for FeLV, the prevalence of this infectious agent in the feline population has decreased and the pattern of feline lymphoma has altered. Two decades ago, feline lymphoma was invariably FeLV associated and most commonly presented as thymic disease in a young animal of pure breed. Currently, the most common presentation of feline lymphoma is alimentary in an older cat that may be negative on current retrovirus testing. A recent study has presented the intriguing hypothesis that **feline gastric lymphoma** might be triggered by the presence of *Helicobacter* bacteria, as is the case for human gastric lymphoma.

Bovine lymphoma may also be retrovirus associated. Bovine leukaemia virus (**BLV**) may be responsible for multicentric lymphoma in adult cattle, but multicentric lymphoma in young calves or thymic lymphoma in animals under 30 months of age is not BLV associated (see Chapter 22). Lymphoma is relatively rare in pigs, sheep and goats, but is not an uncommon disease in the horse, where all anatomical variants are recognized.

Avian lymphoma is of major significance in domestic poultry and is a virus-associated disease. **Marek's disease (neurolymphomatosis)** is caused by a DNA virus (**herpesvirus**) and presents in young birds as paralysis relating to the tropism of the tumour for growth around nerve trunks. In contrast, **lymphoid leukosis (visceral lymphomatosis)** is triggered by an RNA virus (**retrovirus**) and generally affects the viscera of older birds. **Vaccines** are available that successfully control the occurrence of Marek's disease.

Lymphoid leukaemia

Lymphoid leukaemia is a form of lymphoid neoplasia that arises from the **bone marrow**, extends to the **peripheral blood** and from there colonizes vascular organs such as the spleen and liver. The diagnosis is generally made from evaluation of a blood smear in an animal with profound lymphocytosis (**Figure 14.14**). The disease is relatively **rare in animals**, but is most often recognized in dogs and cats (see Chapter 22). Feline lymphoid leukaemia may be FeLV associated. Two subtypes of lymphoid leukaemia are

reported. **Acute lymphoblastic leukaemia** (ALL) is a more severe disease with acute onset and large lymphoblastic cells within the circulation. In contrast, **chronic lymphoid leukaemia** (CLL) involves a better differentiated population of small lymphocytes and has a slower clinical course and a better prognosis.

Plasmacytoma

Plasmacytoma is a **benign** plasma cell tumour that appears as a slow-growing nodular mass most often affecting the lips, oral cavity or distal extremities of **dogs** and **cats**. These are relatively **uncommon** tumours.

Multiple myeloma

Multiple myeloma is a **malignant plasma cell tumour** that is again relatively **uncommon**, but is most often documented in dogs and, to a lesser extent, in cats (see Chapter 22). Classically, the tumour arises in the **bone marrow** of long bones or vertebral bodies where it may cause localized osteolysis; however, recent studies have shown than **feline myeloma** may be a primary disease of the **abdominal viscera**,

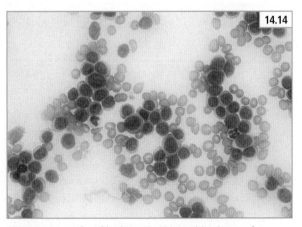

Fig. 14.14 Lymphoid leukaemia. This is a blood smear from a dog with marked lymphocytosis consistent with lymphoid leukaemia. These tumours arise from the bone marrow and spill over into the circulating blood. Neoplastic cells may then colonize vascular organs such as the spleen and liver.

particularly the liver and spleen (**Figure 14.15**). This tumour is associated with two distinct **paraneoplastic effects** (**Figure 14.16**). The first of these is the propensity of these tumours (and, incidentally, also many lymphomas) to produce a range of parathyroid hormone (PTH)-like peptides that mimic the effect of PTH and inappropriately and excessively elevate serum calcium concentration (the '**hypercalcaemia of malignancy**'). The second feature of myeloma is that these tumours continue to produce immunoglobulin, but these antibodies are produced in uncontrolled fashion and may be structurally abnormal. This results in very high serum protein concentration, which on electrophoresis presents as a sharply defined band in the gamma globulin region correlating to this clonally derived immunoglobulin (**Figure 14.17**). This situation is referred to as a **monoclonal gammopathy** and the abnormal immunoglobulin as a **paraprotein**.

Paraproteins are most often of the IgG or IgA class. IgM paraproteins are uncommon and to date IgD or IgE paraproteins have not been identified in animals. **Paraproteinaemia**, particularly of the IgM or IgA class, may be associated with **serum hyperviscosity**, which leads to a range of associated clinical signs. The abnormal nature of the serum paraprotein may be demonstrated by **immunoelectrophoresis** (**Figures 14.18a, b**) or **western blotting** (see Chapter 4), which are used diagnostically in this disease.

Histiocytoma

Histiocytoma is the most **common skin tumour of the dog** and has been extensively studied because of its propensity for **spontaneous regression** (see p.168 and Chapter 8). The most common clinical presentation is of a rapidly growing, solitary nodular

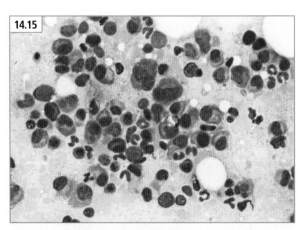

Fig. 14.15 Multiple myeloma. This aspirate from the bone marrow of a dog with multiple myeloma reveals a dominance of abnormal plasma cells, some of which are binucleate.

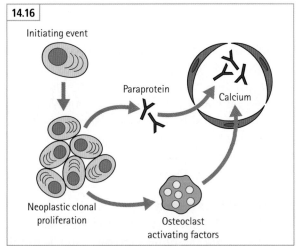

Fig. 14.16 Paraneoplastic effects in multiple myeloma. The neoplastic plasma cells produce large amounts of abnormal immunoglobulin (paraprotein) that causes a monoclonal gammopathy on serum protein electrophoresis and, in the case of IgM or IgA paraproteins, may lead to serum hyperviscosity. The production of PTH-like peptides stimulates osteoclasts to resorb bone. In combination with increased dietary absorption and reduced urinary loss of calcium, this leads to the hypercalcaemia of malignancy.

mass arising anywhere in the haired skin. Although histologically having the appearance of macrophages, immunohistochemistry has defined this as a tumour of **epidermal Langerhans cells.** The spontaneous regression that occurs over several weeks is mediated by infiltrating Tc cells.

Histiocytic sarcoma

There is a spectrum of neoplastic disease of dendritic cells in dogs and cats that includes benign canine histiocytoma (see above) and the malignant histiocytic sarcomas. **Localized histiocytic sarcoma**

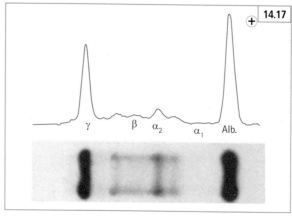

Fig. 14.17 Monoclonal gammopathy. This serum protein electrophoresis shows the presence of a restricted band of high concentration within the gamma globulin region. Such monoclonal gammopathy is typical of multiple myeloma, but may occur also in some infectious diseases.

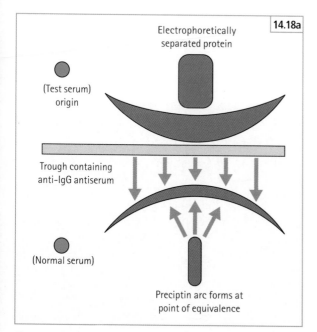

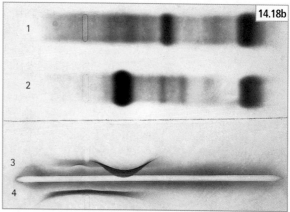

Figs. 14.18a, b Immunoelectrophoresis. (a) This immunological technique is used to define the nature of a paraprotein in multiple myeloma and to demonstrate that the protein has abnormal electrophorectic mobility consistent with altered charge. Serum proteins are first separated by standard electrophoresis. A range of antisera (specific for different immunoglobulin heavy chain and light chain types) are then added to troughs cut parallel to the separated proteins. The antiserum diffuses into the agar gel and, where it meets the serum paraprotein, forms an arc of precipitation within the gel. This can be highlighted with a protein stain. **(b)** Lanes 1 and 2 show serum protein electrophoresis with serum from a normal dog and a dog with myeloma, respectively. The trough between lanes 3 and 4 has been loaded with antiserum specific for canine γ heavy chain. Serum from the dog with myeloma is in lane 3 and from the normal dog in lane 4. Note the much denser arc produced with the myeloma serum and that this arc has more anodal migration.

most often presents as a solitary skin tumour arising particularly on the limbs and around the joints of dogs. These tumours may metastasize to regional lymph nodes. There are breed predispositions for the Bernese mountain dog, flat coated retriever, golden retriever, Labrador retriever and rottweiler. **Disseminated histiocytic sarcoma** shares the same breed predispositions, but is a multicentric disease involving a wide range of viscera, but rarely the skin (**Figures 14.19a, b**). Both tumours are of dendritic cell origin. Disseminated histiocytic sarcoma carries a poor prognosis, but non-metastatic localized histiocytic sarcoma may be treated by surgical excision and/ or radiotherapy.

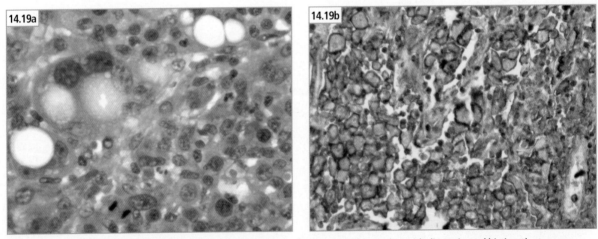

Figs. 14.19a, b Disseminated histiocytic sarcoma. (a) Section of a lung mass from a dog with disseminated histiocytic sarcoma. The neoplastic cells are highly pleomorphic and mitotic. Note the presence of large multinucleate cells with cytoplasmic vacuolation. **(b)** Canine disseminated histiocytic sarcoma showing immunohistochemical expression of CD18. This is one of the molecules used immunohistochemically to define the dendritic cell origin of these tumours.

KEY POINTS

- Oncogenesis is a complex process that involves genetic mutations, carcinogens and reduced immune surveillance.
- Tumour antigens are the targets of the antitumour immune response and may be of a variety of origins.
- The antitumour immune response is cytotoxic and involves NK cells, Tc cells and Th1 cells.
- Some elements of the immune system (TAMs and Treg cells) promote tumour growth, invasiveness and metastasis.
- A range of immunotherapeutic approaches to treating cancer is being evaluated, including the first 'cancer vaccine' for treatment of canine malignant melanoma.
- Lymphoma may be classified on the basis of anatomical distribution, histological and cytological appearance, immunophenotype and gene rearrangement.
- Lymphoma classification helps determine prognosis and therapeutic management.
- Anatomically, lymphoma may be multicentric, thymic, alimentary, cutaneous or solitary.
- Cutaneous lymphoma may be dermal or epitheliotropic.
- Histologically, lymphoma may be diffuse or follicular, but more detailed subtypes exist.
- Cytological assessment of lymphoma includes evaluation of the criteria of malignancy and the size and differentiation of the cells.
- Animal lymphoma may currently be classified as T or B cell in origin. Canine high-grade T-cell lymphoma carries a less favourable prognosis than B-cell lymphoma.
- Clonality testing determines whether a population of lymphocytes expresses multiple different TCRs or BCRs (normal or reactive) or a restricted range of receptors (lymphoma).
- Feline and bovine lymphoma may be caused by a retrovirus.
- FeLV testing and vaccination have altered the pattern of feline lymphoma, which is now most often alimentary and in older cats.
- *Helicobacter* spp. has been suggested as a possible trigger for feline gastric lymphoma.
- Lymphoma in poultry is virally induced by a herpesvirus (Marek's disease) or retrovirus (lymphoid leukosis). Vaccines are available for the control of Marek's disease.
- Lymphoid leukaemia is a rare neoplasm that arises in the bone marrow and extends to the blood.
- Plasmacytoma is a benign plasma cell tumour of the oral cavity or distal extremities of the dog and cat.
- Multiple myeloma is a malignant plasma cell tumour of the bone or viscera, most often reported in dogs and associated with the hypercalcaemia of malignancy and paraproteinaemia.
- Multiple myeloma may be diagnosed by serum protein electrophoresis, immunoelectrophoresis or western blotting.
- Histiocytoma is the most common canine skintumour; it is of Langerhans cell origin and shows spontaneous regression mediated by Tc cells.
- Localized or disseminated histiocytic sarcomas are malignant tumours of dendritic cell origin most often recognized in certain breeds of dog.

Immunological Tolerance

INTRODUCTION

The preceding chapters have shown how the adaptive immune system actively responds when foreign antigen enters the body. In contrast, there are some situations in which the immune system fails to make a response to a specific antigen and this process is known as **immunological tolerance**. This chapter outlines the various forms of tolerance and describes why they are necessary.

NEONATAL TOLERANCE

One of the earliest demonstrations of the phenomenon of tolerance was a veterinary example. **Dizygotic twin cattle** develop from two separate ova that are fertilized at the same time. The twins may be of the same or opposite sex and are likely to be genetically dissimilar. However, because these animals **share a placental circulation** they are exposed to each other's alloantigens *in utero*. Later in life it is possible to graft tissue from one twin to the other and for this graft to survive in the absence of allograft rejection. Each twin is

therefore tolerant of alloantigens from the other. This phenomenon provides a classical example of **neonatal tolerance**, whereby exposure of the developing immune system to foreign antigen either *in utero* or during early neonatal life leads to the induction of tolerance to that antigen such that antigenic challenge later in life fails to induce an immune response. This effect has been widely replicated experimentally by **immunizing neonatal laboratory rodents** with antigen and demonstrating tolerance in later life. More recently it has been possible to produce **transgenic mice** in which a foreign gene is expressed *in utero* and again leads to tolerance to the protein product of the gene. It is most likely that the mechanisms underlying such tolerance relate to intrathymic clonal deletion and the induction of natural Treg cells (see p. 183 and Chapters 8 and 11).

An important veterinary example of neonatal tolerance is that which develops to infection with **bovine viral diarrhoea virus** (BVDV), the cause of 'mucosal disease' in cattle. If a fetal calf is infected between days 42 and 125 of gestation (before immunocompetence develops in the final trimester), the animal will become persistently infected as it develops immune tolerance to that particular strain of the virus. These persistently infected (PI) animals are viraemic and continually shed virus, acting as a reservoir of infection within the herd. The PI animal remains seronegative because of the tolerant state, but other animals in the herd will develop high-titre virus neutralizing antibodies. The PI animal remains tolerant to the specific strain of virus that it carries, but it may be superinfected with a cytopathic biotype of BVDV to which it is not tolerant and this may result in fatal mucosal disease.

ADULT TOLERANCE

It has also proven possible experimentally to induce tolerance to foreign antigen in adult laboratory animals (**adult tolerance**). This effect is very much dependent on the experimental protocol employed and particularly on the dose of antigen given. Two fundamental protocols for tolerance induction are described. In **'high-zone' tolerance** the animal is injected with a single very high dose of antigen that induces paralysis of both T and B cells. In contrast, in **'low-zone' tolerance**, repeated injections of a low dose of antigen induce T-cell tolerance. As most antigens are T dependent, induction of T-cell tolerance generally leads to concomitant B-cell tolerance. Induction of adult tolerance also likely works via the activation of Treg cells.

ORAL TOLERANCE

By definition, **oral tolerance** is failure to respond to systemic immunization with an antigen where that antigen has previously been delivered orally at a particular dose. Although an interesting experimental phenomenon, oral tolerance probably has enormous biological significance in preventing the intestinal immune system from responding to absorbed dietary molecules and to the endogenous microflora of the gut lumen. In fact, **failure of this tolerance mechanism** is now recognized to underlie disorders such as **food allergy** (dietary hypersensitivity) and various forms of **inflammatory bowel disease**. It is remarkable that

the intestinal immune system is able to selectively tolerate such antigens while retaining the ability to mount an active protective immune response against pathogens (see Chapter 13).

The mechanisms underlying oral tolerance have been widely investigated. At one level the phenomenon may relate to the route by which the tolerizing antigen is absorbed across the intestinal mucosa. **Particulate antigens** to which an active immune response is induced are more likely to be absorbed by **M cells** overlying Peyer's patches. In contrast, **tolerated antigens** are more likely to be **soluble** and absorbed directly across the **enterocyte surface** (**Figure 15.1**). This tolerance may not be absolute, as most normal individuals have detectable serum IgG or IgA antibody specific for dietary antigens.

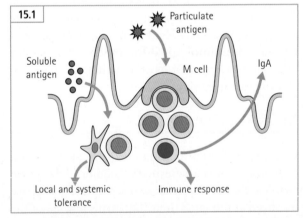

Fig. 15.1 Intestinal absorption of antigen. Particulate antigen is most likely to be absorbed by M cells overlying the Peyer's patch and this leads to induction of an active immune response. Soluble antigen may be absorbed directly across the enterocyte barrier and may trigger a tolerizing immune response.

It is now recognized that oral tolerance is probably an active immunological event. The tolerizing antigen must be processed and presented by dendritic cells, but the consequence of such presentation may be variable. Some T cells that recognize processed antigen may undergo **apoptosis** (clonal deletion) and others might recognize antigen but fail to become fully activated, as not all three signals required for T-cell activation are received. Such T cells are not deleted, but remain non-functional or **anergic** (the process is referred to as the induction of anergy). More importantly, the presentation of tolerogenic antigen may induce specific **regulatory T cells**. Although IL-10-producing Tr1 cells might be activated, the form of Treg cell thought to be most important in mediating oral tolerance is the **Th3 cell**, which is characterized by the preferential **secretion of TGF-β**. Clonal deletion and anergy might be relevant at the level of the intestinal mucosa, but the systemic aspects of oral tolerance (i.e. failure to respond to antigen subsequently injected) are likely to be mediated by these regulatory cells, which may migrate to systemic lymphoid tissues (e.g. the spleen) (**Figure 15.2**).

The phenomenon of oral tolerance is readily induced in domestic animals. In one study dogs were fed ovalbumin (OVA) over the first weeks of life and immunized systemically with OVA and Der p1 from the house dust mite *Dermataphagoides pteronyssinus*. Dogs previously fed OVA failed to develop serum antibodies to that antigen, while they mounted a classical primary serological response to the Der p1 component of the immunization (**Figure 15.3**).

ORAL TOLERANCE AS IMMUNOTHERAPY

The fact that it is possible to induce Treg cells and inhibit systemic immune responses by feeding antigen was not lost on clinical immunologists, who saw this as a means of potentially treating an array of allergic or autoimmune diseases. To that end, in recent years numerous clinical trials have been performed whereby target autoantigens have been fed to patients with autoimmune diseases in an attempt to slow the progression of their disease. For example, bovine myelin has been fed to patients with multiple

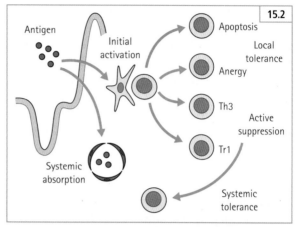

Fig. 15.2 Mechanisms of oral tolerance. Oral tolerance is an active immunological event involving processing and presentation of absorbed antigen. Antigen-specific T cells may be deleted by apoptosis or may remain anergic if they fail to receive the full range of co-stimulatory signals required for activation. These two mechanisms might be important at the level of the intestinal mucosa. Presentation of antigen might also trigger the activation of TGF-β-producing Th3 regulatory cells. The systemic migration of these cells may underlie the observed failure to respond to challenge with antigen given systemically.

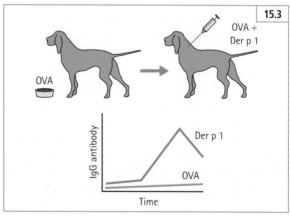

Fig. 15.3 Canine oral tolerance. In this experiment young dogs were fed with OVA for a 10-day period. Two weeks after this feeding period the dogs were injected subcutaneously with a mixture of OVA and the antigen Der p1 in adjuvant. The dogs failed to mount an effective serum IgG response to OVA, but made a normal primary immune response to Der p1.

sclerosis, chicken type II collagen to rheumatoid arthritis patients, bovine retinal S antigen to patients with uveitis and human insulin to those with type I insulin-dependent diabetes mellitus. The overall outcomes from these trials have been equivocal, although individual patients do appear to benefit.

Extending from experimental investigations of oral tolerance has been the recognition that **other mucosal surfaces** may also be used to demonstrate this effect. In fact, **intranasal tolerance** with delivery of target antigen across the nasal mucosa is a much more potent means of inducing systemic tolerance using significantly smaller doses of antigen. Significantly, the effect is even greater when small peptide fragments of antigen are delivered in this way. At present, human clinical trials of intranasal tolerance therapy are progressing for some allergic and autoimmune diseases. Intranasal delivery of myelin-derived peptides may prove an effective means of ameliorating the clinical progression of human multiple sclerosis.

SELF-TOLERANCE

Self-tolerance is the ability of the immune system to tolerate the self-antigens that comprise the tissues of the body. Failure of self-tolerance leads to an autoimmune response and autoimmune disease (see Chapter 16). In order to achieve self-tolerance, potentially autoreactive T and B lymphocytes must be brought under control.

Most is known about how self-tolerance is achieved for T cells. One mechanism that is clearly significant is the elimination of potentially autoreactive clones of T cells by **negative selection** during intrathymic maturation (**central tolerance**; see Chapter 8). However, if this process was fail-safe, there would be no such thing as autoimmune disease, so a proportion of autoreactive T cells must 'escape' clonal deletion and be allowed to enter the peripheral T-cell pool. Circulating autoreactive T cells are readily identified in man and have also been demonstrated in the dog. These cells must clearly be controlled in the

'periphery' (**peripheral tolerance**) in order to prevent autoimmunity and a range of mechanisms are probably employed to achieve this aim (**Figure 15.4**). Some autoreactive T cells may recognize antigen presented to them in peripheral lymphoid tissue. These cells may either undergo apoptosis ('**peripheral deletion**' as opposed to 'central' intrathymic deletion) or they may become **anergic** if they fail to receive appropriate co-stimulatory signals (see Chapter 8). Other autoreactive T cells may be kept away from their target autoantigens in a process known as '**immunological ignorance**'. This may work at different levels; for example, some body tissues are normally kept at a distance from the adaptive immune system behind a 'blood–brain barrier' or 'blood–testis barrier', so it is relatively difficult to induce autoimmunity to brain or testicular tissue. Alternatively, this may work at the level of the APC, which processes self-antigen but fails to present it. Although all of these mechanisms might be at play, the single most important means

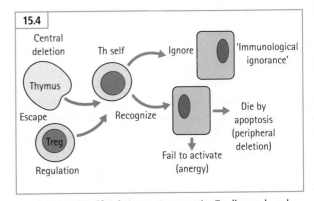

Fig. 15.4 T-cell self-tolerance. Autoreactive T cells may largely be eliminated within the thymus by the process of negative selection. Those autoreactive cells that escape to the periphery must be controlled to prevent autoimmunity. Self-antigen might be presented to these cells so that they are eliminated by apoptosis (peripheral deletion) or become anergic. Alternatively, the cells may never be exposed to self-antigen as it remains anatomically sequestered or is not appropriately presented by APCs (immunological ignorance). More importantly, natural Treg cells may maintain control over the autoreactive cells.

of controlling autoreactive T cells is via **Treg cells**, particularly the population of IL-10-producing **natural Treg cells**.

Autoreactive B cells must also be kept in check in order to prevent those autoimmune diseases caused by autoantibody production. The development of B lymphocytes is less well defined than that for T cells, but also involves a form of clonal deletion (see Chapter 9). The control of autoreactive B cells within the periphery likely relies on the regulation of those autoreactive T cells that would normally be required to provide help for activation of the B-cell response. Lack of T-cell help renders the autoreactive B cell **anergic**. Autoreactive B cells within the periphery may also be 'ignorant' of their cognate antigen if these antigens are normally kept sequestered away from the immune system.

FETOMATERNAL TOLERANCE

In 1953, the immunologist Sir Peter Medawar recognized that the state of **pregnancy is an immunological paradox** as the fetus expresses paternally derived antigens equivalent to an incompatible allograft. This should mean that the maternal immune system would by default act to target and destroy the maternal–fetal interface, leading to abortion. It is now well-recognized that the decidua of women who undergo spontaneous abortion does contain increased numbers of NK cells and CD8+ cytotoxic T cells that might be expected to mediate fetal loss. The immune system also plays an intrinsic role in the abortions of domestic livestock induced by pathogens such as *Toxoplasma gondii*, *Neospora caninum*, *Chlamydophila abortus*, *Listeria monocytogenes* and BVDV. For example, in ovine enzootic abortion caused by *Chlamydophila abortus*, replication of the organism in placental tissue leads to an inflammatory response and activation of both fetal and maternal inflammatory cells. The effects of fetal macrophages (producing TNF-α) and maternal macrophages and T cells (producing IFN-γ) contribute to disruption of the placental interface and fetal loss.

In order to prevent maternal immune destruction of the placental interface, a number of adaptations must be in place to enable the mother to 'tolerate' the fetal allograft. Placental tissue has **upregulation of immunosuppressive cytokines** such as IL-10 and TGF-β and parallel inhibition of TNF-α and IFN-γ. There may be **reduced MHC expression** within this location, with the exception of expression of 'non-classical' MHC class I molecules of minimal polymorphism, which will act to inhibit activation of NK cells (see Chapter 8). Additionally, the **Fas ligand** may be expressed within placental tissue such that infiltrating T cells expressing Fas receive signals for apoptotic death. Human studies show significantly more induced Treg cells within the placenta of women undergoing induced abortion than in the placenta of women undergoing spontaneous abortion, suggesting that **active maternal immune regulation** is a key event in survival of the fetus. This effect has been modelled in mice, in that there are significantly more induced Treg cells in the decidua of female mice mated with allogeneic (genetically dissimilar) males than in the decidua of female mice mated with males of the same strain (syngeneic).

This state of maternal immunomodulation has systemic as well as local influence. In order to protect the fetus, the maternal immune system undergoes a shift towards Treg cells and Th2 activity. The most convincing manifestation of this immune deviation occurs in women with the Th1-mediated autoimmune disease rheumatoid arthritis. During pregnancy, the polyarthritis goes into clinical remission as a result of the altered T-cell balance and disease recurs after parturition. The systemic Th2 bias in the mother extends to the fetus, and it has been clearly shown that newborn mice, human infants and canine puppies have an immune system skewed towards Th2 reactivity (referred to as the 'neonatal Th2 bias'). In contrast, foals appear to have the reverse pattern with a Th1 bias in neonatal life.

KEY POINTS

- Immunological tolerance is failure to respond to an antigen delivered via a protocol that would normally be expected to induce an immune response.
- Neonatal tolerance refers to exposure to antigen *in utero* or during early neonatal life such that challenge with that antigen later in life fails to trigger an immune response.
- Adult tolerance involves induction of tolerance to a foreign antigen during adulthood by giving a single high dose (high-zone tolerance) or multiple lower doses (low-zone tolerance) of that antigen.
- Oral tolerance is failure to respond to systemic immunization with an antigen that has been previously delivered orally.
- Breakdown of oral tolerance may lead to the development of food allergy or inflammatory bowel disease.
- Oral tolerance is an active event involving the induction of apoptosis, anergy or regulatory Th3 cells.
- Self-tolerance is the ability of the immune system to ignore self-antigens.
- Failure of self-tolerance leads to autoimmunity and autoimmune disease.
- T-cell self-tolerance likely involves a combination of central deletion, peripheral deletion, anergy, immunological ignorance and the effects of natural Treg cells.
- B-cell self-tolerance follows the absence of help provided by regulated autoreactive T cells.
- Fetomaternal tolerance involves suppression of the maternal immune response to paternal alloantigens expressed by the fetus by diverse mechanisms including the action of induced Treg cells.

CHAPTER 16

Autoimmunity and Autoimmune Disease

OBJECTIVES

At the end of this chapter you should be able to:
- Discuss the immunological basis for autoimmunity.
- Describe the spectrum of autoimmune diseases.
- Discuss the genetic basis of autoimmune disease.
- Discuss the effects of age and gender on autoimmune disease.

- Discuss how infectious agents may have a role in the development of autoimmune disease.
- Describe the principle and interpretation of the Coombs test, antinuclear antibody (ANA) test, rheumatoid factor (RF) test and thyroglobulin autoantibody test.

INTRODUCTION

Autoimmunity results from a **failure of self-tolerance** allowing activation of self-reactive T and B lymphocytes, which may produce tissue pathology and clinical **autoimmune disease** (**Figure 16.1**). The mechanisms that normally control autoreactive lymphocytes and maintain self-tolerance have been described in Chapter 15. In this chapter we explore the basis for autoimmunity in man and domestic animals.

Autoimmunity is a **multifactorial** process involving a range of interlinked **predisposing and triggering factors**. A certain number of these factors must be in place before autoimmune disease becomes manifest. The key elements of the autoimmune response are:
- An **immunological imbalance** with reduced function of natural Treg cells permitting the activation of autoreactive Th1, Th17 or Th2 cells and autoreactive B cells.
- An appropriate **genetic background**.
- **Predisposing factors** including age, gender, lifestyle and diet.

- **Environmental factors** such as exposure to UV irradiation (for some diseases), chemicals (including drugs and vaccines) or infectious agents that may act as triggers for the autoimmune process.

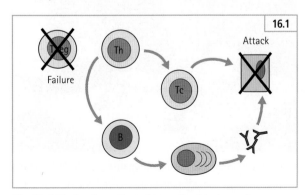

Fig. 16.1 Mechanism of autoimmunity. Autoimmunity occurs when deficient natural Treg cell activity permits inappropriate activation of autoreactive T and B lymphocytes. Autoreactive Th cells may amplify both cell-mediated cytotoxic and autoantibody-mediated destruction of self-cells.

AUTOIMMUNE DISEASE

A wide spectrum of autoimmune diseases exists as there are a large number of self-antigens that may potentially become targets for an autoimmune response. Virtually any body system can be affected by autoimmune disease. Most autoimmune diseases are '**organ specific**' and target autoantigens related to a single body system or organ, but some are '**multisystemic**' and involve two or more body systems.

Human autoimmune diseases are of major medical and economic significance. They are most common in the Western world and may be **increasing in prevalence** as lifestyle alters (see Chapter 17). Examples of human autoimmune diseases include juvenile diabetes mellitus (type I diabetes), rheumatoid arthritis, systemic lupus erythematosus (SLE), myasthenia gravis, Hashimoto's thyroiditis, Grave's disease, pemphigus, and multiple sclerosis.

In veterinary medicine autoimmune diseases are **most prevalent in the dog**. They occur with less frequency in cats and horses and are only sporadic in production animals, most likely due to the fact that these latter species generally do not live to the age at which autoimmunity often becomes manifest.

Some examples of canine autoimmune diseases include autoimmune haemolytic anaemia (AIHA), autoimmune thrombocytopenia (AITP), autoimmune neutropenia (AINP), the spectrum of pemphigus disorders, bullous pemphigoid, cutaneous lupus erythematosus (CLE), autoimmune polyarthritis (e.g. rheumatoid arthritis), myasthenia gravis, lymphocytic thyroiditis, Addison's-like disease, diabetes mellitus, exocrine pancreatic insufficiency (EPI) and SLE.

The canine autoimmune diseases are **close mimics of the equivalent human disorders**, with a similar immunological basis, tissue pathology and clinical presentation. For this reason there is currently great interest in the study of canine autoimmune disease as a spontaneously arising model of the same human disorder. These diseases involve a number of different immunopathological mechanisms, which include **types II, III and IV hypersensitivity reactions** (see Chapter 12). For example, AIHA involves the destruction of erythrocytes mediated by IgG or IgM autoantibody and the classical pathway of complement (type II hypersensitivity), and lymphocytic thyroiditis involves the destruction of thyroid follicular epithelium by cytotoxic T lymphocytes (type IV hypersensitivity) (**Figures 16.2, 16.3**).

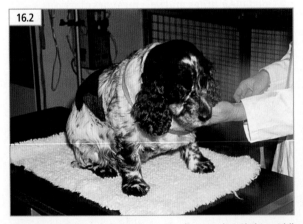
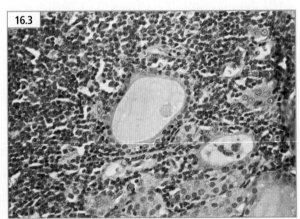

Figs. 16.2, 16.3 Canine autoimmune disease. (**16.2**) This middle-aged cocker spaniel dog has obesity and lethargy secondary to hypothyroidism. In this idiopathic autoimmune disease (also called lymphocytic thyroiditis) the immune system targets self-antigens associated with thyroid follicular epithelial cells or proteins within the colloid (e.g. thyroglobulin). (**16.3**) There is an infiltration of cytotoxic T cells into the thyroid gland, which mediates follicular destruction and atrophy, and a range of serum autoantibodies to thyroid proteins are recognized.

THE GENETIC BASIS FOR AUTOIMMUNITY

There is a clear **genetic predisposition** to autoimmune disease in a number of species. Some autoimmune diseases have greater prevalence in certain human races and are inherited within families. Inbred lines of laboratory mice and rats show particular susceptibility to the spontaneous development of autoimmune disease. For example, non-obese diabetic mice develop type I diabetes mellitus and New Zealand black mice develop AIHA and a lupus-like syndrome. Similarly, particular **breeds of dog** are susceptible to autoimmune diseases and these often occur within pedigree lines (**Figure 16.4**). Canine autoimmune diseases are often perpetuated within **pedigree groups** because of line breeding. The same breed susceptibility is often recognized internationally due to the **'founder effect'** whereby related breeding stock is disseminated to different countries to form the basis for a breed group in that geographical area. This stock may have been selected for optimum breed phenotype, but may also carry disease-associated genes that are then perpetuated in the population. A classical example of a predisposed breed is the cocker spaniel, which is recognized internationally as susceptible to autoimmune cytopenias (AIHA, AITP).

Given that for some time we have had access to both the human and canine genome, the genes that underlie the inheritance of autoimmune disease should be well characterized. This is not yet the case, but candidate susceptibility genes are recognized. The genes most strongly linked to the occurrence of autoimmunity are those of the MHC. **MHC disease associations** in man and dogs have been discussed in Chapter 6. The reason for such close associations between autoimmunity and MHC genotype might be explained if the specific MHC molecules involved were the most effective at presenting self-antigenic peptides in order to activate autoreactive T cells. Alternatively, the inheritance of other genes, perhaps more directly involved in autoimmune pathogenesis, may be closely associated with the inheritance of particular MHC types (a phenomenon known as 'linkage disequilibrium').

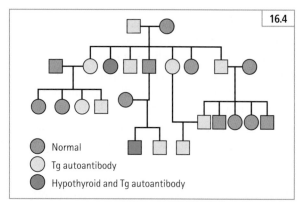

Fig. 16.4 Inheritance of canine autoimmunity. This pedigree shows the inheritance of serum autoantibody to thyroglobulin through three generations of a family of Great Danes. In addition to inherited susceptibility to this autoimmune response, individual dogs develop clinical evidence of hypothyroidism (lymphocytic thyroiditis). (Data from Haines DM, Lording PM, Penhale WJ (1984) Survey of thyroglobulin autoantibodies in dogs. *American Journal of Veterinary Research* **45**:1493–1497.)

A second genetic association with autoimmunity is that with **IgA deficiency**. An inherited inability to produce sufficient IgA (see Chapter 19) results in a weakened mucosal defence and greater susceptibility to infection. As will be described below, infectious agents may commonly trigger autoimmunity, thus accounting for the association between IgA deficiency and autoimmune disease. This association has also been documented in the dog.

The publication of the canine genome in 2005 has permitted the development of molecular techniques enabling screening of individual dogs for single nucleotide polymorphisms (SNPs) across tens of thousands of genes across the genome (see Chapter 17). Populations of dogs with breed-associated autoimmune diseases are now being compared with control healthy dogs of the same breed in **'genome-wide association studies'** (GWAS) to identify genes associated with the disease. One of the first studies identified a strong association between SNPs in genes related to T-cell activation in Nova Scotia duck tolling retrievers with multisystemic autoimmunity.

Although genetic background strongly determines susceptibility to autoimmune disease, it is not the sole determinant. This is well documented in studies of human identical twins that are separated at birth and raised in different families, in different environments and sometimes in different geographical areas. Often only one twin will develop autoimmune disease, indicating that environmental influences have a major role in autoimmune pathogenesis.

AGE SUSCEPTIBILITY TO AUTOIMMUNE DISEASE

In both man and dogs, autoimmune disease most commonly occurs in **middle to older age**. There are some notable exceptions (e.g. juvenile rheumatoid arthritis and type I diabetes mellitus often occur in childhood). The reason for this (and the increased susceptibility to cancer discussed in Chapter 14) likely relates to age-related changes in immune function (**immunosenescence**). Older people (as well as older dogs, cats and horses) retain the ability to make humoral immune responses and often have elevated IgG production. In contrast, there is a reduction in cell-mediated immune function and a shift in the balance of blood T cells, with relatively more CD8+ cells and fewer CD4+ T cells. If the declining population of CD4+ cells includes natural Tregs, this could clearly account for an increased onset of autoimmune reactivity.

HORMONAL INFLUENCE ON AUTOIMMUNITY

In human medicine there is a clear **female gender predisposition** to autoimmune disease. This does not appear to be the case for most canine autoimmune diseases, where there is little evidence to support either a male or female bias. This may in part relate to the fact that many companion animals are neutered. A recent epidemiological study of 40,000 dogs within a combined university teaching hospital database suggested that neutered dogs are more likely to die from immune-mediated diseases than sexually intact dogs. The hormonal influence on autoimmunity has

been studied in experimental rodent models. For example, particular genetic strains of laboratory rat will develop lymphocytic thyroiditis and diabetes mellitus if they are thymectomized early in neonatal life and then irradiated. These rats have a disturbed balance of T cells, which is likely to be related to the onset of these diseases. The incidence of thyroiditis is much higher in female compared with male rats. If female rats are ovariectomized and then injected with oestrogen, the incidence of thyroiditis significantly decreases, but when ovariectomized rats are injected with progesterone the incidence of disease becomes even greater than in an intact animal.

PRIMARY VERSUS SECONDARY AUTOIMMUNE DISEASE

Although genetic background, age and gender may influence the development of autoimmune disease, other factors might more directly act as triggers for the autoimmune event. These factors are described below. It is therefore possible to distinguish clinically between a **primary and a secondary autoimmune disease**. Primary idiopathic autoimmune disease arises in a genetically susceptible individual in the absence of any identifiable trigger factor. In contrast, secondary autoimmune disease occurs in a patient that has a recognized underlying trigger factor.

Confusingly, some autoimmune diseases are often referred to as '**immune-mediated diseases**'. Therefore, a primary immune-mediated disease is equivalent to a primary idiopathic autoimmune disease, whereas a secondary immune-mediated disease is precipitated by a known trigger factor. For example, a dog in which IMHA is triggered by a distinct factor (e.g. drugs, vaccine, neoplasia or infection) has secondary IMHA. In contrast, a dog with IMHA in which no underlying trigger is identified may be described as having either primary IMHA or AIHA.

Cancer or inflammation as a trigger for autoimmunity

There are numerous clinical examples of situations in which an autoimmune disease might arise concurrently with or subsequent to neoplasia or the presence of a chronic inflammatory disease. For example, immune-mediated cytopenias might arise secondary to a range of tumours (lymphoma, splenic haemangiosarcoma, myeloproliferative disease of the bone marrow) or to chronic pancreatitis or inflammatory bowel disease. The precise mechanisms underlying these associations are poorly defined.

Environmental triggers for autoimmunity

The nature of the environment appears to be a factor predisposing to autoimmunity. In human populations, factors such as lifestyle, affluence, stress and diet may have a role in the development of autoimmune disease. Although it is possible that similar factors may contribute to the onset of canine autoimmunity, it is difficult to characterize these. Dogs developing AIHA may have disease precipitated by **stressful factors** such as oestrus, whelping or kennelling. One simple environmental influence is that of **exposure to UV light** on the development of canine nasal CLE (**Figure 16.5**). It is proposed that UV light might in some way modify the antigenic structure of target autoantigens within the skin.

Drugs and vaccines as triggers for autoimmunity

There is little doubt that particular **drugs and vaccines** may be able to precipitate autoimmunity. Antimicrobial drugs are most implicated and in canine medicine the **trimethoprim–sulphonamides** (TMSs) are particularly recognized as triggers of IMHA, thrombocytopenia and neutropenia. In these cases the drug may be acting as a **hapten** (see Chapter 2), which by binding to the membrane of the target cell directly forms a target for an immune response. Alternatively, by modifying the structure of a self-protein the drug forms a novel drug–protein structure that is also capable of inducing an immune response. Dobermann dogs are particularly predisposed to this effect, but TMSs may induce immune-mediated cytopenia in a range of other breeds. In feline medicine the drugs used to manage hyperthyroidism medically (carbimazole/methimazole) are also recognized triggers for IMHA, IMTP and serum ANA production. A recent study reported a series of dogs that developed pemphigus foliaceus (an autoimmune skin disease) after topical application of a combination antiparasitic drug containing metaflumizine and amitraz.

There is a great deal of interest in both human and veterinary medicine as to whether vaccines might also trigger autoimmune diseases (see Chapter 20). Although there is little doubt that this can happen in individual patients, it has proven difficult to define the immunological mechanisms that might explain the association. It is clear that some dogs might develop immune-mediated cytopenias or polyarthritis 1–2 weeks post vaccination, but such events are relatively rare in the vaccinated population. A more common occurrence would appear to be the induction of serum autoantibodies to a range of connective tissue or epithelial proteins following vaccination. There is no evidence that these antibodies are a cause of clinical disease and they probably arise because of the incorporation into vaccines of small quantities of serum or tissue protein used in manufacture.

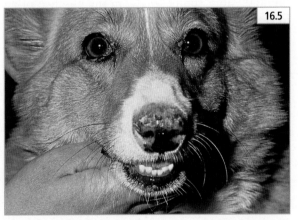

Fig. 16.5 Environmental triggers of autoimmunity. This dog has nasal CLE, a complex immune-mediated disease targeting the skin of the planum nasale. Immunological mechanisms involved in this disease include a lymphocytic infiltration of the junction between epidermis and dermis and immune complex deposition at the basement membrane zone of the epidermis. UV light is thought to act as one trigger for the occurrence of this disease.

Infectious triggers of autoimmunity

The most significant trigger factor for autoimmunity is **infection**. There is growing evidence that many diseases once considered to be primarily idiopathic (autoimmune) in nature might actually be triggered by infection. These infections might occur immediately before the onset of autoimmune disease or there might be a long lag period between active infection and the autoimmune sequela. The types of infectious agents associated with autoimmune disease are those that are **difficult to identify** by traditional methods (i.e. are unculturable and may require techniques such as PCR diagnosis) or those that induce **chronic infection** with sequestration of the organism in a body reservoir. In human medicine, viral infections are often considered to be triggers of autoimmune disease.

There is also strong experimental evidence that infectious agents can trigger autoreactivity. There are numerous rodent models in which infection, or challenge with a peptide derived from an infectious agent, is able to induce clinical autoimmunity in a susceptible strain. Such animals may have serum autoantibody or autoreactive lymphocytes readily demonstrated in splenocyte cultures. The autoimmune disease may be inhibited by immunosuppressive therapy. More compellingly, in the absence of an infectious agent, adoptive transfer of T cells from animals with infection-induced autoimmunity will lead to the same autoimmune disease in the recipient animal. One example of this phenomenon is the experimental infection of mice with an attenuated strain of the lymphocytic choriomeningitis virus. Shortly after infection these mice become anaemic due to the triggering of an erythrocyte autoantibody that mediates red cell destruction.

Infectious agents might trigger autoimmune responses by a variety of different mechanisms:

- One well-recognized consequence of viral infection is the **polyclonal activation of numerous clones of B lymphocytes**, with serum polyclonal hypergammaglobulinaemia and peripheral lymphadenopathy. Some of these B cells may be virus specific, but some viral antigens are able to non-specifically activate any B cell in a mitogenic fashion. If these non-specifically activated cells are autoreactive, then autoantibody production might ensue.

- A second possibility relates to the action of some microbially derived substances as '**superantigens**'. Classical examples of superantigens are the toxins produced by certain staphylococci, but a wide range of infectious agents can elaborate superantigenic substances. A superantigen is able to non-specifically activate a range of different T or B cells and if these targets are autoreactive, then autoimmunity might result. Superantigens non-specifically activate T cells by cross-linking the variable region of the TCR β chain with the α chain of MHC class II in the absence of interaction with any peptide. Superantigenic activation of T cells involves binding to the outer region of the antigen-binding fragment of the BCR (**Figure 16.6**).

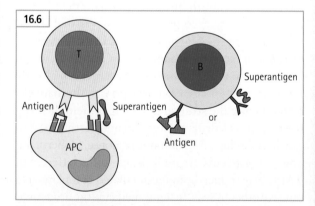

Fig. 16.6 Superantigens. A superantigen (generally derived from an infectious agent) can non-specifically activate quiescent autoreactive T or B cells and initiate autoimmunity. The superantigen cross-links the TCR β chain with the MHC class II α chain or binds to the BCR external to the antigen-binding site of the molecule.

- The third possible mechanism involves a microorganism that attaches to the membrane of a host cell or infects that cell, leading to expression of microbial antigen on the cell surface. An appropriate adaptive immune response is made to the infectious agent, but this also non-specifically destroys the host cell that carries the organism (**Figures 16.7, 16.8**). This is known as the '**innocent bystander**' effect. This effect may be important in diseases such as feline infectious anaemia where circulating erythrocytes are parasitized by the surface membrane-dwelling organism *Mycoplasma haemofelis*. Cats with this disease are generally Coombs test positive (i.e. have antibody associated with the surface of RBCs) and the infection and anaemia precede the development of these erythrocyte-bound antibodies. Although it is possible that the antibodies target the infectious agent, there are two alternative hypotheses. The first hypothesis suggests that the infection triggers the production of true autoantibodies and the second suggests that by binding to an autoantigen, the infectious agent changes the structure of that antigen, making it a target for an immune response (the '**modified self**' hypothesis, as may also occur with the binding of a drug as discussed above).

- Some autoimmune diseases involve circulating **immune complex deposition** in antigen-excess type III hypersensitivity. A fourth possibility for infection triggering autoimmunity is that the antigenic component of such complexes (which is rarely characterized) is derived from a microorganism.

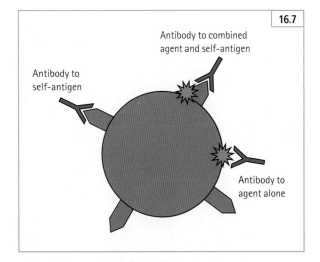

Figs. 16.7, 16.8 The 'innocent bystander' effect. (16.7) An infectious agent or drug that attaches to the surface of a host cell (e.g. an RBC) directly provides a target for the adaptive immune response or combines with a self-antigen to form a novel target ('modified self'). The immune response, in this case antibody and classical complement, will destroy the host cell in addition to the specific target in a process known as 'bystander destruction'. **(16.8)** An example of such an infection might be feline infectious anaemia in which *Mycoplasma haemofelis* parasitizes the surface of circulating erythrocytes. Cats with this infection become Coombs test positive. The red cell-bound antibody might be specific for the parasite, an erythrocyte membrane protein (autoantigen) or a novel epitope formed through the infection.

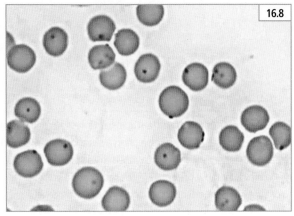

- Any infection may induce a local tissue inflammatory response with an adaptive immune response characterized by infiltration of effector cells producing cytokine. If the inflammatory response includes IFN-γ production, this cytokine might lead to the **induction of non-professional APCs** (e.g. epithelial, stromal or endothelial cells) that may express MHC molecules containing self-peptides and thereby trigger autoreactive T cells.
- A sixth possibility for infection-associated autoimmunity is that this appropriate immune response to an infectious agent extends inadvertently to self-tissue through the phenomenon of '**bystander activation**'. This might work in different ways. For example, the inflammatory response might lead to damage to self-tissue, with release of self-antigens that are processed and presented to allow activation of self-reactive lymphocytes. The inflammatory milieu might also simply provide sufficient cytokine signalling and MHC class II upregulation to permit non-specific activation of autoreactive lymphocytes. Finally, the inflammatory response may alter the way in which APCs deal with self-antigen. In normal circumstances some self-antigens ('**cryptic epitopes**') may not be presented by an APC in order to prevent autoreactivity. In an inflammatory context, expression of these hidden epitopes might occur, thereby allowing activation of self-reactive lymphocytes (**Figure 16.9**).

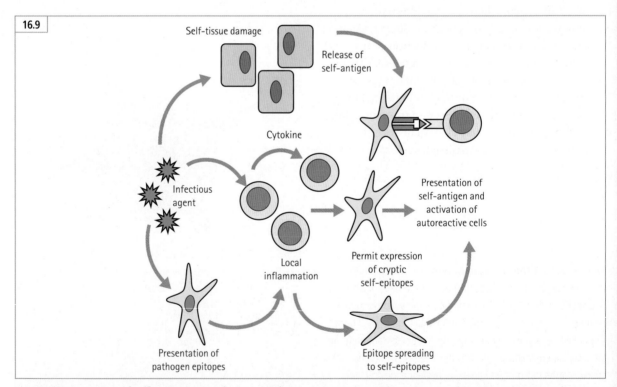

Fig. 16.9 Presentation of self-antigens. An infectious or inflammatory response within a tissue involving tissue damage and infiltration of pathogen-specific lymphocytes and local cytokine production may lead to secondary autoimmunity. Damaged tissue may release self-antigen, which can be processed and presented for activation of autoreactive lymphocytes. Alternatively, the inflammatory milieu may alter the activity of APCs to allow them to present previously 'cryptic' (hidden) self-antigenic peptides. The immune response to pathogens might extend to self-antigens via the process of 'epitope spreading'.

- The final mechanism is that of '**molecular mimicry**'. This suggests that microbial antigens and self-antigens might share regions of peptide sequence. Presentation of a microbially derived peptide as an attempt to induce a legitimate adaptive immune response to infection might inadvertently provide the means for activation of autoreactive T cells that have a TCR that can bind the cross-reactive molecular mimic. Activation of autoreactive Th cells in this fashion might also provide co-stimulatory signals for autoreactive B cells that directly recognize the molecular mimic expressed by the microbe (**Figure 16.10**).

In addition to feline haemoplasmosis, there are a number of other examples of companion animal autoimmune disease that might be triggered by infectious agents. Some years ago it was found that dogs with rheumatoid arthritis had synovial deposits of canine distemper virus (CDV) antigen, with antibody to CDV found in synovial fluid. In this instance the virus might act as a trigger for what ostensibly presents clinically as an idiopathic autoimmune disease. A recent study has shown increased bacterial load (as detected by PCR) in the joints of dogs with rupture of the cruciate ligament and it was proposed that these environmentally derived antigens might trigger immunological dysregulation within the affected joint. The best examples of this phenomenon relate to the group of arthropod-transmitted infectious agents (e.g. *Babesia*, *Ehrlichia*, *Leishmania*, *Borrelia*, *Anaplasma* and *Rickettsia*). The complex interplay between these infectious agents, the arthropods that transmit them and the host immune system often leads to **secondary immunopathology** in the chronic stages of infection. These infections are often associated with clinical signs such as polyarthritis, uveitis, glomerulonephritis, anaemia and thrombocytopenia and the presence of autoantibodies specific for RBCs or platelets, or the presence of serum circulating immune complexes or ANA (**Figure 16.11**).

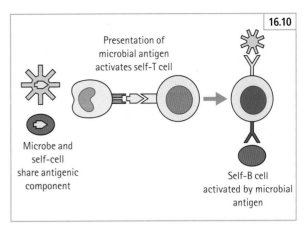

Fig. 16.10 Molecular mimicry. An infectious agent may bear an epitope (or peptide sequence within an epitope), which is shared with an epitope (or peptide sequence) within a self-antigen. Presentation of the peptide during the immune response to the infectious agent may lead to activation of quiescent autoreactive Th cells that provide help to quiescent autoreactive B cells that are able to recognize the shared epitope. In this instance, what starts out as an appropriate immune response to an infectious agent becomes an inappropriate autoimmune response. In the case of T-cell epitopes, the molecular mimic need only share key 'contact residues' with the self-peptide.

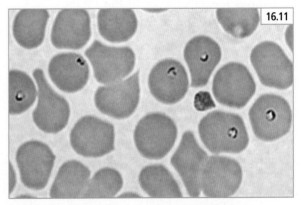

Fig. 16.11 Autoimmunity in canine babesiosis. The erythrocytes from this dog are parasitized by one of the small forms of *Babesia*. Such dogs may become Coombs test positive and it is suggested that the antibodies associated with erythrocytes are true autoantibodies with specificity for red cell membrane antigens. It is conceivable that a *Babesia* antigen carries an epitope that acts as a molecular mimic for an epitope within a red cell protein.

IMMUNODIAGNOSTIC TESTS FOR AUTOIMMUNITY

Wherever possible, clinical suspicion of an autoimmune disease should be supported by immunodiagnostic testing aimed to demonstrate the presence of an autoantibody or autoreactive T-cell population with specificity for cells of the target tissue or organ. In veterinary medicine there are relatively few commercially available tests relevant to the diagnosis of autoimmune disease and these are mostly designed to detect circulating (serum) or cell-bound autoantibody. These tests include:

- The Coombs test (or direct antiglobulin test, DAT) for the detection of erythrocyte-bound autoantibody.
- Tests for the detection of antiplatelet or antineutrophil antibody.
- Radioimmunoassay for the detection of antibody to the neuromuscular acetylcholine receptor (AchR) in myasthenia gravis.
- ELISA for the detection of thyroglobulin, T3 or T4 autoantibodies.
- Indirect immunofluorescence, immunoprecipitation or ELISA for the detection of serum ANA.
- Indirect agglutination or ELISA for the detection of serum or synovial fluid rheumatoid factor (RF).
- Tissue immunofluorescence or immunohistochemistry for the detection of cell-associated autoantibody or immune complex *in situ*; for example, interepithelial adhesion molecule autoantibody in pemphigus foliaceus or glomerular immune complex in membranous glomerulonephritis.

Although a range of other autoantibody detection methods is documented, the tests are not widely available in clinical practice. Examples of the most commonly performed tests are given below.

Coombs test

The Coombs test (or DAT) is named after Robin Coombs, a veterinarian whose contribution to clinical immunology has been described in Chapter 12. The test aims to demonstrate the presence of antibody and/ or complement attached to the surface of circulating erythrocytes in primary or secondary IMHA. The Coombs test relies on the principle of **agglutination** discussed in Chapter 4. When erythrocytes coated by antibody are incubated with antiserum specific for the antibody, the antiserum will cross-link molecules of antibody. This results in the suspended red cells being held in a lattice-like arrangement, which is seen visually as agglutination (**Figure 16.12**).

An EDTA anticoagulated blood sample is collected from the patient that is thought to have IMHA. The sample is centrifuged and the plasma and buffy coat removed by pipette. The pelleted erythrocytes are resuspended in phosphate buffered saline (PBS) and re-centrifuged. This process is repeated to 'wash' the red cells of plasma protein. A suspension of washed erythrocytes is made in PBS at known concentration (typically 2.5% v/v).

The antiserum generally used in the Coombs test is known as the '**polyvalent Coombs reagent**' and it has multiple specificities for IgG, IgM and complement C3. The test may also be performed with individual antisera specific for these three immunoreactants. The Coombs test is performed in the U-bottomed wells of a plastic microtitration plate. Each antiserum is double diluted (from 1/2 or 1/5 starting dilution in PBS) across the rows of the plate. A set of negative control wells containing only PBS is also included (**Figure 16.13**). An equal volume of the red cell suspension is added to the wells of serially diluted antiserum and PBS control. The reactants are then mixed and the plate incubated at an appropriate temperature, most often 37°C, although a duplicate plate may be incubated at 4°C.

Following incubation the plate is examined for the presence of agglutination and the titre of reaction with each antiserum is determined. The titre obtained does not necessarily correlate with the severity of anaemia, but the pattern and temperature of reactions may correlate with the clinical presentation and pathogenesis of haemolysis. When performed correctly, false-negative results are uncommon. An alternative methodology, whereby red cell-bound antibody is detected by antiserum with a fluorescent label and the flow cytometer (see Chapter 10), is also described and simple in-house, rapid, tube-based tests have been produced for the dog and cat.

Antinuclear antibody test

The ANA test aims to demonstrate the presence of serum autoantibody specific for one or more of the constituents of the cellular nucleus. A range of antigenic material is present within the nucleus and although it is possible to determine the fine specificity of the reaction by techniques such as gel precipitation or ELISA, the ANA test performed most widely simply seeks evidence for the presence of any nuclear autoantibodies. A proportion of normal animals or animals with chronic disease may have low-titre serum ANA as a reflection of cell turnover in the body. In the context of autoimmune disease, only a high-titre ANA is regarded as significant. The presence of **high-titre serum ANA** is one of the diagnostic criteria for the rare multisystemic autoimmune disease **SLE**, but this autoantibody might also be present in animals with a range of other autoimmune disorders.

The most widely used methodology for detection of serum ANA is the **indirect immunofluorescence assay** (see Chapter 4). A nucleated cell line is grown over the wells of a sectored glass microscope slide and fixed to the glass surface (such slides are prepared commercially). Serial dilutions of patient serum are added to individual wells of the slide and if ANA is present, it will bind to the nucleus of the cells.

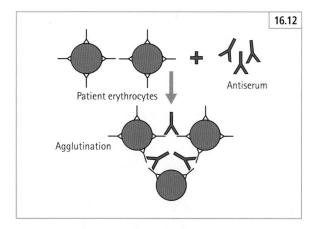

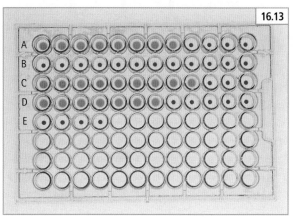

Figs. 16.12, 16.13 Coombs test. (**16.12**) Erythrocytes from an animal with IMHA are coated by antibody and/or complement *in vivo*. Incubation of these cells with antiserum specific for the immunoreactants leads to agglutination of the cells, which may be identified visually. (**16.13**) A canine Coombs test performed in a microtitration system. Four antisera are used in this test: Row A, polyvalent canine Coombs reagent; Row B, anti-dog IgG; Row C, anti-dog IgM; and Row D, anti-dog complement C3. Each antiserum is double-diluted in PBS across the plate from a starting dilution of 1/5 in well number 1 to a final dilution of 1/10,240 in well number 12. Row E contains only PBS. An equal volume of a 2.5% suspension of washed patient red cells is added to all the wells and the plate is mixed and incubated at either 4° or 37°C. Agglutination is seen as a mat of cells spread over the base of the well. This dog is Coombs test positive. The red cells are coated by IgM (titre 1,280) and complement C3 (titre 320).

Positive and negative control sera are also included. This immunological reaction is then visualized by the use of a secondary antiserum (e.g. to dog IgG), which is conjugated to a fluorochrome (most often fluorescein isothiocyanate) (**Figure 16.14**). When the slide is viewed under UV light of appropriate wavelength, the cellular nuclei appear apple-green on a black background (**Figure 16.15**). It is also possible to perform this test using an enzyme–substrate visualization system. The titre of autoantibody is determined from assessment of the dilution series and the pattern of nuclear labelling (diffuse, rim, speckled or nucleolar) should also be reported.

Rheumatoid factor test

RF is an autoantibody that is classically associated with the autoimmune disease rheumatoid arthritis, but it may also occasionally occur in other forms of autoimmune polyarthritis. **Canine rheumatoid arthritis** was once a relatively common disease; however, it is now rarely diagnosed so this assay is not widely requested. RF is classically an IgM (or sometimes IgA) autoantibody that binds to IgG as its target autoantigen. The target IgG molecule may be conformationally altered by itself binding to some form of antigen. RF may be found in both serum and synovial fluid and may have a role in the pathogenesis of the arthritis.

The classical means of detecting serum or synovial fluid RF is by the **Rose–Waaler test**, which is a simple **agglutination** reaction (see Chapter 4). In this test, a suspension of RBCs (often SRBCs) is first pre-coated with an IgG anti-SRBC antiserum at a dilution that is insufficient to cause agglutination of the cells. This IgG becomes the target for the RF. When serial dilutions of patient serum or synovial fluid are incubated with the antibody-coated SRBCs, any RF present will bind the IgG and lead to agglutination of the indicator cells. Positive and negative control sera are included and the titre of the RF is determined by assessing agglutination in the dilution series.

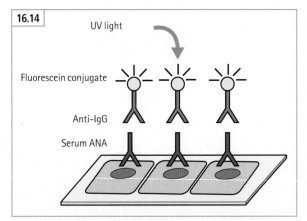

Fig. 16.14 Antinuclear antibody test. Serial dilutions of patient serum are added to individual wells of a sectored glass microscope slide on which a nucleated cell line has been grown. ANA binds to the nucleus and in turn a secondary antiserum binds the patient's autoantibody. The antiserum is conjugated to a fluorochrome, which emits light when the slide is viewed with a microscope that produces UV light of appropriate wavelength.

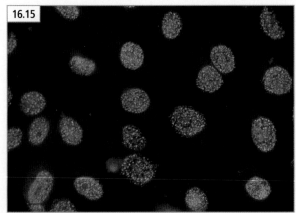

Fig. 16.15 Antinuclear antibody test. The appearance of a positive ANA test. The nuclei of these cells emit apple-green fluorescence in a speckled pattern when viewed under UV light of appropriate wavelength. The cell cytoplasm cannot be seen.

Antithyroglobulin autoantibody

Autoimmune thyroiditis (**lymphocytic thyroiditis**) is a relatively common canine disease that mimics human Hashimoto's thyroiditis. Although the hypothyroidism is largely due to cell-mediated destruction of thyroid tissue, a range of serum autoantibodies to components of the colloid are also identified and provide a useful diagnostic tool. The most widely available assay is that for detection of autoantibodies specific for thyroglobulin (Tg). **Tg autoantibodies** are most readily identified by an ELISA. The wells of microtitre trays are first coated with purified canine Tg. Appropriately diluted patient serum is then added and if autoantibody is present, it will bind to the Tg. This reaction must be visualized by a secondary antiserum (e.g. anti-dog IgG) conjugated to an enzyme such as alkaline phosphatase (ALP). Addition of substrate will lead to a colour change in positive wells, which may be measured spectrophotometrically (see Chapter 4).

KEY POINTS

- Autoimmunity results from failure of self-tolerance.
- Autoimmunity is multifactorial.
- Autoimmunity involves immunological imbalance, particularly insufficient natural Treg cell activity.
- Autoimmunity may lead to clinical autoimmune disease.
- Autoimmune disease may be organ-specific or multisystemic.
- Autoimmune disease in animals is most common in dogs.
- The immunopathology of autoimmunity may involve type II–IV hypersensitivity mechanisms.
- Autoimmune disease has a genetic basis and occurs in particular breeds and pedigrees of dogs.
- MHC genes are most closely associated with susceptibility or resistance to autoimmune disease.
- IgA deficiency is linked to autoimmune disease. Weakened mucosal immune defence may predispose to exposure to infectious triggers of autoimmunity.
- Autoimmune disease occurs in middle to older age, likely due to immunosenescence.
- Autoimmune disease has a female gender predisposition in humans, but not in dogs.
- Primary autoimmune disease has no recognized underlying trigger.
- Secondary autoimmune disease has a recognized underlying trigger.
- Triggers for autoimmune disease include cancer, stress, UV light and administration of drugs or vaccines.
- Infection is a major trigger of autoimmune disease.
- Infectious agents associated with autoimmunity may be unculturable or sequester in body reservoirs.
- Infection may precede the onset of autoimmunity by some time.
- Infectious agents may trigger autoimmunity by inducing non-specific polyclonal activation of lymphocytes or non-specific superantigenic stimulation of autoreactive cells.
- An infectious agent attached to a host cell may cause bystander destruction of that cell.
- Infectious agents may induce immune complex formation and tissue pathology associated with deposition of complexes.
- Epitopes of infectious agents may act as molecular mimics of self-epitopes.
- A range of immunodiagnostic tests are available for the detection of autoantibodies. These are most often used in canine patients.

CHAPTER 17

Allergy

OBJECTIVES

At the end of this chapter you should be able to:
- Define allergy.
- Review the immunopathological mechanisms involved in allergic disease.
- Discuss factors predisposing to allergic disease.

- Discuss the 'hygiene hypothesis'.
- Give examples of allergic diseases in animals.
- Describe the methods used in diagnosis of allergic disease.

INTRODUCTION

The immunological basis for allergy has been discussed in Chapter 12. **Allergy** is the pathological manifestation of hypersensitivity and may be defined as 'a state of **immunological sensitization** to an **innocuous environmental antigen** that leads to an **excessive** (symptomatic) **immune response** on **re-exposure** to the antigen'. Although allergy may theoretically involve any of the four hypersensitivity mechanisms described in Chapter 12, most clinically significant allergic diseases are manifestations of **type I or IV hypersensitivity**. The word 'atopy' is used to describe the genetically-mediated propensity of an individual to become sensitized to environmental allergens by producing **allergen-specific IgE antibodies**, which mediate immediate hypersensitivity reactions. Such individuals are referred to as being 'atopic' and probably have **overactive Th2 immunity** as a consequence of **impairment of Treg cell** function (**Figure 17.1**).

Allergic diseases with a type I hypersensitivity basis are of major significance in human medicine. Diseases such as **hay fever**, **asthma** and **atopic dermatitis** (AD) have high morbidity in populations within the Western world. Such diseases have greatest prevalence amongst children, and it is

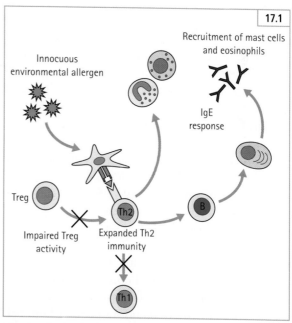

Fig. 17.1 **Basis of allergic disease.** In a genetically susceptible individual with impaired Treg cell function, exposure to innocuous environmental allergen leads to an expanded Th2 immune response that mediates production of allergen-specific IgE antibody and recruitment of mast cells and eosinophils. In the initial phases of such an aberrant immune response there is inhibition of Th1 activity, but in chronic disease with secondary infection Th1 cells become an important contributor to pathogenesis.

universally recognized that the incidence of AD has markedly increased in such populations over the past five decades. This range of diseases is also of great importance in companion animal medicine, affecting dogs, cats and horses. **Contact dermatitis**, involving type IV hypersensitivity, is less frequently recognized in animals than in humans.

FACTORS PREDISPOSING TO ALLERGIC DISEASE

As is characteristic of many immune-mediated diseases, allergic disease has a **multifactorial** basis. One of the strongest predisposing factors is **genetic background**. In human families there is no doubt that allergic disease is highly heritable (e.g. in the author's family, asthma has affected at least four generations). Despite this very strong genetic predisposition to IgE responsiveness, the precise molecular basis for allergy is not yet clearly defined. Genomic studies have shown association with numerous polymorphic candidate genes, including those of the **MHC** and a **cytokine gene cluster** including loci encoding a number of Th2-related molecules. These genetic associations most likely relate to the elements of immunoregulation that are imbalanced in allergic disease (i.e. impaired Treg cells and excessive Th2 activity).

Similar genetic influences are recognized in veterinary medicine. There are clear **breed predispositions** to canine allergic disease. The heritable risk for AD is well defined in dogs of the Labrador, golden retriever and West Highland white terrier breeds and recent studies have suggested that there are breed-specific patterns in the nature of the disease (e.g. lesion distribution). Huskies show increased susceptibility to the asthma-like disease eosinophilic bronchopneumopathy (EBP). Experimental lines of beagles have been selected for their propensity to develop IgE responses ('**high IgE responder beagles**') when sensitized to a variety of dietary allergens or aeroallergens. As with human

allergic disease, the precise molecular associations for canine allergic disease remain undefined. One **gene expression microarray study** (**Figure 17.2**) indicated a number of candidate genes that were upregulated in skin biopsies from atopic dogs. Several **genome-wide association studies** (GWAS) compared genomic sequences between atopic and non-atopic dogs of susceptible breeds (**Figure 17.2**). Although a wide range of genetic associations has been highlighted, the results from different studies are inconsistent, likely reflecting differences in breed, geographical location (breed pool) and environment between the populations investigated.

There are similar genetic influences on the development of allergic disease in horses. Ponies, and particularly Icelandic ponies, are susceptible to developing hypersensitivity to the saliva of *Culicoides* midges ('**sweet itch**' or '**insect bite hypersensitivity**', **IBH**). Of note is the fact that the incidence of this allergy is greatest in adult Icelandic ponies born in Iceland (which lacks midges) and subsequently exported to countries in which the midge is present. The prevalence of disease increases with increasing time since export. There are also genetic influences on the development of **recurrent airway obstruction** (**RAO**) in the horse. Although hypersensitivity disease occurs in cats, there are, in contrast, no recognized breed associations.

Age influences on the development of allergic disease are also apparent. The fact that many human allergic diseases have an onset in early childhood may be related to the 'hygiene hypothesis' discussed below. There is also a clear age predisposition for canine AD, with up to 75% of cases being diagnosed at less than 3 years of age.

Allergen exposure is an obvious factor predisposing to the development of these disorders. Environmental exposure is required in order to sensitize the allergic individual and to trigger the hypersensitivity response. Humans, dogs and cats share reactivity to common indoor environmental allergens (e.g. house dust

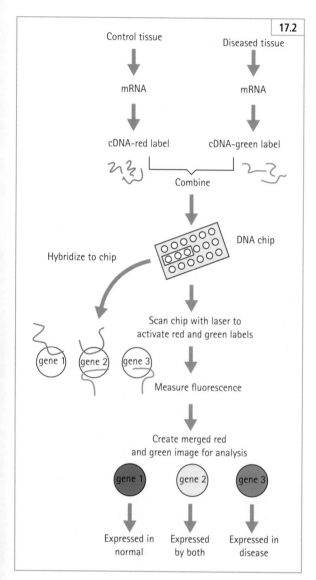

Fig. 17.2 Gene microarray. There are two types of gene microarray study. The first of these seeks to determine which genes within the genome might be up- or downregulated within diseased cells or tissue relative to normal cells or tissue. In such an experiment, mRNA is isolated from the tissues of interest and reverse transcribed to cDNA. The cDNA from test and control tissue is labelled by different fluorochromes and then both cDNAs are hybridized to a DNA chip that typically contains up to 40,000 gene sequences. The chip is scanned with a purpose-built laser and fluorescence emission is recorded. In this way it is possible to determine genes that are transcribed only in disease, only in normal tissue, or in both sample types. The second form of microarray aims to determine the presence of particular single nucleotide polymorphisms (SNPs) within the genome of an individual animal. In this instance, DNA from that animal is hybridized to a chip containing up to 200,000 canine SNPs and the SNP genotype of the dog determined. This methodology is employed in a genome-wide asociation study in which the genomes of groups of diseased and normal dogs (of one breed) are compared in order to identify disease-associated SNPs.

mites, human dander) and pollens, although there may be differences in the precise epitopes leading to sensitization in different species. There are often geographical differences in the relative significance of particular allergens. Exposure to haemophagous arthropods (e.g. fleas, flies, mosquitoes) is also clearly required for the onset of diseases such as **flea allergy dermatitis** (FAD). Repeated ingestion of dietary antigen is generally required in order to develop a **food allergy**. Coupled with allergen exposure may be a **reduction in mucocutaneous barrier function** in susceptible individuals. Such biomechanical defects may allow increased penetrance of inhaled, ingested or percutaneously absorbed allergens. It is of note that some of the genes recently associated with canine AD were those encoding molecules related to cutaneous barrier function.

Intercurrent disease may also impact on the development or clinical flares of allergy. For example, cutaneous infection with *Staphylococcus* bacteria or *Malassezia* yeasts may increase the severity of AD by enhancing pathogenic Th2 immune responses or providing a source of **superantigens**. Allergic diseases also are often associated (e.g. the presence of both allergic rhinitis and EBP, or AD and FAD, in the dog).

THE HYGIENE HYPOTHESIS

The '**hygiene hypothesis**' has gained favour as an explanation for the observation that in the human population, allergic diseases have progressively increased in prevalence over the past 50 years. Although initially developed to account for this change in allergic disease, the hypothesis was later modified to include an explanation for the parallel rise in some autoimmune disorders (e.g. juvenile type I diabetes mellitus), inflammatory bowel disease (IBD), neuroinflammatory diseases, atherosclerosis, depression and some forms of neoplasia over the same time period.

There are a number of interconnected strands to the hygiene hypothesis. The first of these relates to the immunological paradox that is pregnancy (see Chapter 15). Newborn human infants and animals are born with an immune system deviated towards Th2 immunity and so there is a requirement in early life that the newborn immune system must be 'rebalanced' by exposure to antigens capable of expanding the populations of Th1 and Treg cells. Such antigens are infectious agents, so the hygiene hypothesis proposes an obligate requirement for exposure to microbes in early life to 'reset' the immune balance in that infant. If this fails to occur, then that newborn has a persisting imbalanced immunity with lack of Treg cells and overactivity of Th2 cells that might lead to the development of allergic or autoimmune disease in childhood.

The hygiene hypothesis therefore proposes that what has changed over the period since 1960, and that may account for the increasing prevalence of allergic and some autoimmune diseases, is lifestyle and in particular the way that children are raised. Children now lead a more '**sanitized' lifestyle** that fails adequately to redirect the developing immune system towards Treg cell and Th1 cell activity. Such influences include factors such as:

- A more sedentary indoor lifestyle with more solitary computer- or television-based activity.
- A centrally heated and carpeted indoor environment that may contain more allergens but fewer microorganisms than in previous decades because of widespread use of antimicrobial cleaning agents.
- Smaller families with low sibling numbers.

The hygiene hypothesis therefore clearly indicates that exposure to **infectious agents** that **promote the expansion of Treg cells** is a crucial part of early life development. The hypothesis helps explain numerous epidemiological observations; for example, the protective effects (from developing allergic disease) if children are raised on farms, are part of multi-sibling families, have pets, are permitted contact with other children through nurseries or receive Th1 promoting vaccinations (e.g. with mycobacteria).

It also appears that **helminths** have a much more potent effect on the **induction of Treg cells** than do many bacteria or viruses. For many years an inverse relationship between intestinal parasitism and allergy has been recognized, despite the fact that both situations involve a Th2-dominated immune response (see Chapter 13). The endogenous parasitism that occurs in human populations within developing countries appears to have a protective effect, as such individuals are rarely affected by allergy or autoimmunity but most likely succumb to infectious disease. The concept that a certain low level of endogenous parasitism confers immunological benefit has now been demonstrated in human medicine. Deliberate establishment of an intestinal parasitic infection in human patients with allergy or IBD has led to marked clinical improvement in these individuals.

Similar benefits have been attributed to **probiotic bacteria**, which are also thought to expand intestinal Treg cell populations and lead to amelioration of such diseases. Organisms such as helminths, *Mycobacterium* and *Lactobacillus* have been described as 'old friends' that have co-evolved with the human population and tend to induce tolerance responses mediated by Treg cells. This is known as the '**old friends hypothesis**'.

It is an intriguing thought that the strict control of endoparasites in companion animals (which is done for the most appropriate of public health reasons) might actually underlie an increasing prevalence of allergic and immune-mediated diseases in these species. A recent pilot study evaluated the effect of deliberately establishing an endoparasitic infection in dogs with AD. Twelve dogs with AD were given embryonated eggs of *Trichuris vulpis* or L3 larvae of *Uncinaria stenocephala* monthly for 3 months and there was reduction in the clinical severity of their disease as assessed by the canine AD extent and severity index (CADESI). However, a second larger placebo-controlled study of 21 atopic dogs given *T. vulpis* eggs or physiological saline failed to replicate the significant effect of the pilot study. The dogs in the placebo-controlled study generally had milder clinical disease than those in the pilot study and so it might be that this type of therapy produces greater clinical effect in more severely affected animals. Although this novel approach to treating human and animal immune-mediated disease shows promise, the more important step forward will be in identifying the specific parasite-associated immunomodulatory molecules that underlie the effects and formulating them in a more practical manner.

ALLERGIC DISEASES IN ANIMALS

Allergic diseases are of major clinical and economic significance in companion animal medicine. These disorders are investigated most often in the dog, where a spectrum of allergic disorders is reported. A relatively uncommon manifestation of type I hypersensitivity in this species is the presence of the related conditions of **urticaria**, **angioedema** and **anaphylaxis**. These all involve sensitization to a range of possible allergens including drugs, vaccines, incompatible erythrocytes, food, plants and biting or stinging insects. All have acute onset, as is characteristic of a type I hypersensitivity reaction. Urticarial lesions are most often cutaneous and involve the formation of **localized or generalized wheals** that may be **pruritic**. In angioedema there is involvement of subcutaneous tissue and **facial swelling** is a common manifestation (**Figure 17.3**). These lesions are generally **transient** and resolve spontaneously, but angioedema may become life-threatening if the process extends to involve the larynx and upper respiratory tract. The most severe of this group of disorders is anaphylaxis in which there is **acute systemic vasodilation** leading to generalized oedema, reduction of blood pressure and shock that may progress to death. In the dog this process particularly affects the liver, whereas in most other species the '**shock organs**' are the lung and intestine.

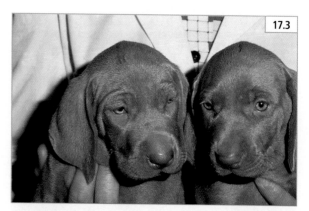

Fig. 17.3 Angioedema. These two pups were vaccinated and the pup on the left developed facial swelling due to subcutaneous oedema within 15 minutes of vaccination. The pup is sensitized to a component of the vaccine and this reaction might be expected to occur again when the animal is next vaccinated.

The most highly prevalent canine allergic disease in many parts of the world is **FAD**. The causative allergens are proteins within the saliva of *Ctenocephalides felis*, which have now been cloned and sequenced. The immune response to these antigens has been well characterized and FAD has a classical type I hypersensitivity pathogenesis with a late-phase response. The cutaneous lesions may become chronic due to **self-trauma** and **secondary infection** and typically involve the skin of the tail base and hindlimbs (**Figures 17.4, 17.5**). Intriguingly, some dogs that are chronically exposed to fleas appear to develop a tolerance response rather than hypersensitivity. Dogs may also develop allergic reactions following sensitization to the bites of other arthropods (e.g. ticks) or as part of the pathogenesis of mite infestation (e.g. *Sarcoptes scabei*).

Canine **AD** has received a great deal of research attention and has numerous similarities to the disease in man (see Chapter 22). A wide spectrum of causative allergens may be involved, but internationally these are most often '**indoor allergens**' and particularly those derived from **house dust mites** (*Dermatophagoides pteronyssinus* and *D. farinae*). The most significant allergen is a molecule known as Der f15, which is a 98 kDa chitinase enzyme found within the cells lining the digestive tract of the mite. In contrast, the major mite allergens in human AD are of lower molecular weight and are components of mite faecal particles.

The immunology of canine AD is well characterized and involves numerous elements discussed in previous chapters:

- A classical **type I hypersensitivity** reaction.
- **Th2** cytokine driven with increased expression of genes encoding IL-4, IL-5 and IL-13 in lesional skin.

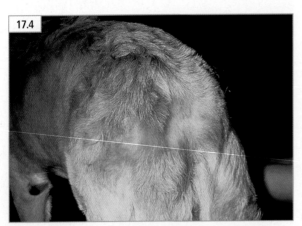

Fig. 17.4 Flea allergy dermatitis. This dog has acutely self-traumatized the skin over the base of the tail. This area is classically involved in the pruritic response triggered by flea allergy.

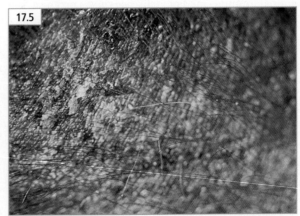

Fig. 17.5 Flea allergy dermatitis. In this more chronic case of FAD there has been prolonged self-trauma leading to alopecia and thickening and hyperpigmentation of the skin.

- Production of **IgE**, IgG1 and IgG4 allergen-specific antibodies.
- **Impairment of Treg cell function** with reduction in IL-10 production.
- Recognition of the role of epidermal Langerhans cells in allergen capture.
- Increased expression of MHC II and CD23 (FcεR) by Langerhans cells and dermal dendritic cells.
- CD4⁺ T-cell infiltration of lesional dermis.
- CD8⁺ T-cell infiltration of lesional epidermis.
- Expression of cutaneous lymphocyte antigen (CLA) homing receptors by lesional T cells.

- A **late-phase response**.
- A progression to **Th1 immunity** with IFN-γ production **with chronicity and secondary infection**.

Canine AD has **breed and age predispositions** (discussed above) and presents as erythematous and pruritic lesions that particularly affect the **face and feet** (**Figures 17.6**, **17.7**), but may become generalized. The lesions progress following chronic self-trauma and **secondary bacterial and yeast infection**.

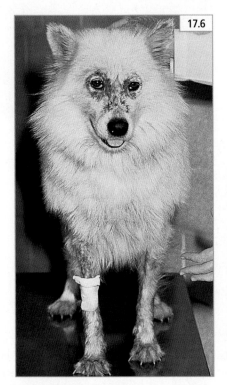

Fig. 17.6 Canine atopic dermatitis. This Samoyed has AD. There is erythema and pruritus affecting the face and forelimbs.

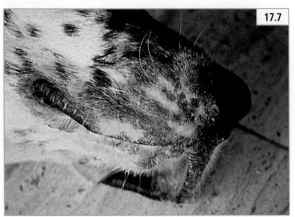

Fig. 17.7 Canine atopic dermatitis. Facial erythema in a dog with AD.

Dietary hypersensitivity or **food allergy** is, in contrast, poorly characterized in the dog. Affected animals develop IgE antibodies to dietary components, most commonly beef, chicken, milk, eggs, corn, wheat and soy. The disease may be reproduced experimentally and colonies of spontaneously affected dogs have also been studied. Most dogs with dietary hypersensitivity present with a pruritic cutaneous disease that may mimic AD, but fewer animals may present with primary gastrointestinal disease (vomiting, diarrhoea and weight loss). A recent study suggested that the immunological features of lesional skin from dogs with dietary hypersensitivity differ from those of AD by having a dominant CD8+ T cell infiltration with elevated expression of genes encoding IL-4, IL-13, IFN-γ and Foxp3.

All of these allergic disorders also occur in the **cat**, but their immunopathogenesis is less well investigated and there are some species differences. The anaphylactic response in the cat more often involves the respiratory and gastrointestinal tracts, which are the primary 'shock organs'. The clinical presentation of cutaneous type I hypersensitivity disease (FAD, AD or food allergy) is more variable, with a series of 'cutaneous reaction patterns' including **ulcerative facial dermatitis**,

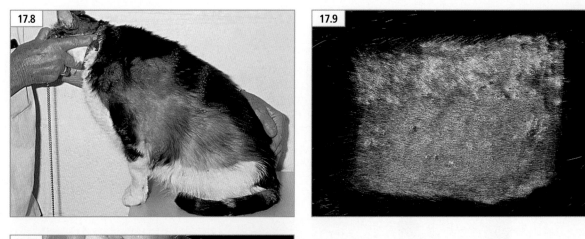

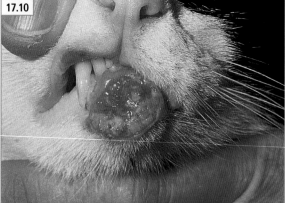

Figs. 17.8–17.10 Feline allergic skin disease. The cat may develop one of a series of 'cutaneous reaction patterns' in response to allergic skin disease. Symmetrical alopecia in a cat with AD (**17.8**), miliary dermatitis in a cat with flea allergy (**17.9**) and collagenolytic granuloma in a cat with atopy (**17.10**) are shown. The lesion in **17.10** is one of those that comprise the feline 'eosinophilic granuloma complex'.

symmetrical alopecia (**Figure 17.8**), **papular** ('miliary') **dermatitis** (**Figure 17.9**) or the complex of **'eosinophilic granuloma'** lesions (**Figure 17.10**). Some immunological features of feline allergic skin disease are similar to those described for the dog; for example, lesional skin is infiltrated by IL-4-producing T cells and dendritic cells upregulate MHC class II expression. However, the role of allergen-specific IgE in feline AD is less clear, as clinically normal cats may have significant levels of such antibodies. Cats may also develop sensitization to the bites of arthropods other than fleas, and mosquito bite hypersensitivity is well documented.

The **horse** may also be afflicted with a range of allergic disorders. Urticarial reactions may develop following sensitization to agents such as drugs (**Figure 17.11**). The most significant allergic skin disease of the horse is **IBH** in which there is sensitization to salivary proteins injected by the biting midges of the genus *Culicoides*. This leads to pruritic skin disease with self-trauma of the mane and tail regions and secondary infection (**Figure 17.12**). The disease is most prevalent during the summer when the midge is active. The immunology of this disease is now becoming well documented. The causative salivary antigens are being characterized and the serum

IgE response to these proteins has been measured. Lesional skin from affected Icelandic ponies displays an increased number of CD4$^+$ T cells, increased IL-13 gene expression and decreased Foxp3 and IL-10 gene expression relative to normal or non-lesional skin. These findings are consistent with elevated Th2 and depressed Treg cell activity. Icelandic ponies with IBH also have fewer CD4$^+$CD25$^+$Foxp3$^+$ Treg cells in their circulating blood than control animals.

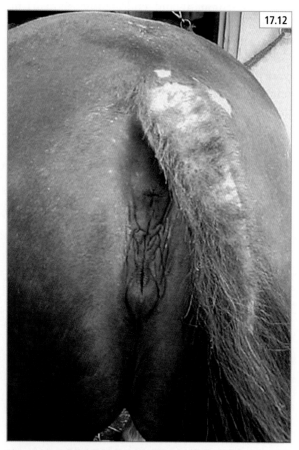

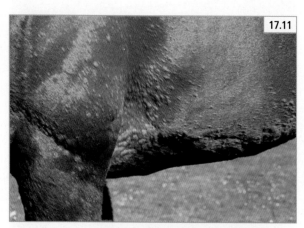

Fig. 17.11 Equine urticaria. Within minutes of being exposed to an allergen this horse has developed multiple oedematous wheals over most of its body. These lesions are mild and transient and will resolve spontaneously.

Fig. 17.12 Insect bite hypersensitivity. This horse has lesions related to self-trauma over the mane and tail base regions. The lesions develop in summer with exposure to bites of *Culicoides* midges. (Photograph courtesy D. Wilson)

RAO (or 'heaves') is also important, particularly in hay-fed **stabled animals**, which become sensitized to organic aeroallergens (e.g. moulds, dusts) within this environment. Inhalation of airborne **endotoxin** also plays a role in pathogenesis. RAO affects middle-aged horses, which develop coughing, dyspnoea and exercise intolerance due to bronchospasm and accumulation of mucus and neutrophils in the airways. The immunology of RAO is not clearly defined, but there is evidence suggesting a mixed Th2-mediated type I hypersensitivity and type III hypersensitivity response (see Chapter 12).

In contrast to companion animal species, allergic disease is rarely documented in domestic livestock. This may relate to factors such as life span, environment and endogenous parasitism, all of which differ significantly when compared with companion animal populations. **Milk allergy** (directed against the α casein of milk) is recognized in cows during periods of milk retention and generally relates to the drying off period. The increased intramammary pressure forces milk proteins into the circulation, allowing sensitization to occur. This disease may recur in the same cow during subsequent drying off periods and is thought to have a genetic basis in Channel Island breeds. The clinical presentation of milk allergy may include cutaneous urticaria (facial or generalized), muscle tremor, dyspnoea, restlessness, self-licking or even extreme behavioural changes such as charging or bellowing.

The major allergic diseases of animals all appear to involve an underlying Th2-regulated type I hypersensitivity response, at least in the initial stages. Other forms of allergy are less common, but **contact allergy** caused by **Type IV** hypersensitivity is documented in the dog (**Figure 17.13**). Contact sensitizers in this species include allergens derived from plants, topical drugs and shampoos, carpet dyes, polishes and cleaners, rubber, plastic, leather and metal.

DIAGNOSIS OF ALLERGIC DISEASE

Diagnosis of the allergic diseases described above proceeds through several stages. Most important is a detailed **clinical history** taking into account the age and breed of the animal, the environment, diet and the management of ecto- and endoparasites. The initial stages of diagnosis generally involve excluding contact with known allergens to determine whether there is clinical improvement. Response to a simple course of animal and environmental **flea control** would be consistent with a diagnosis of FAD. Placing the animal on a **restricted protein home-cooked diet** or a **commercial hypoallergenic or hydrolyzed protein diet** should lead to alleviation of the clinical signs of dietary hypersensitivity. These diets work on the principle of feeding a source of protein to which the animal has not been previously exposed (restricted protein) or protein fragments that are too

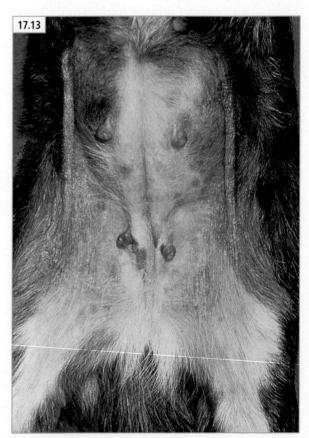

17.13

Fig. 17.13 Contact allergy. The erythematous reaction on the ventral abdomen of this dog developed repeatedly within 72 hours of contacting a particular plant.

small to enable cross-linking of mast cell-associated IgE (hydrolyzed protein). Gradual reintroduction of elements of the previous diet will then identify the causative allergen/s, but once disease is in remission such dietary challenge is rarely performed. Similarly, for diseases such as contact allergy, removal from the home environment often leads to remission and phased reintroduction to areas of the environment can identify the causative allergen.

Diagnosis of AD involves undertaking these initial steps in order to rule out FAD or food allergy. Subsequently, it is necessary to identify the causative aeroallergen/s responsible for disease in that individual. This may be achieved by the use of an **intradermal skin test (IDST)**, where a small quantity of a panel of test allergens is injected intradermally into the skin of the patient. The presence of dermal mast cells coated by allergen-specific IgE will be indicated by the development of an oedematous **wheal** at the site of injection within **20 minutes** of the injection being given (**Figure 17.14**). An alternative methodology involves the detection of allergen-specific IgE in circulating blood, most often by **ELISA**. A wide range of commercial serodiagnostic tests are now marketed for the diagnosis of allergic diseases in dogs, cats and horses. These diagnostic tests underpin the application of allergen-specific immunotherapy (ASIT), which will be discussed in Chapter 21.

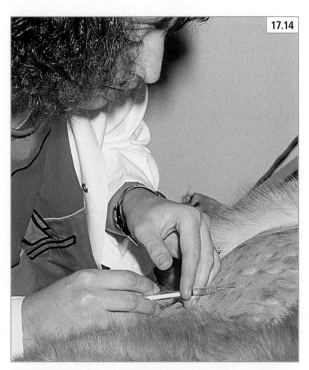

Fig. 17.14 Intradermal skin test. This atopic dog is receiving a series of intradermal injections of allergens into the clipped skin over the flank. The development of a wheal within 20 minutes of injection of similar magnitude to that induced by local injection of histamine (as positive control) indicates that the dog is allergic to that allergen and has cutaneous mast cells coated by allergen-specific IgE.

KEY POINTS

- Allergy is a state of immunological sensitization to an innocuous environmental allergen that leads to an excessive immune response on re-exposure to the allergen.
- Atopy is the genetically-mediated propensity of an individual to become sensitized to environmental allergens by producing allergen-specific IgE antibodies mediating type I hypersensitivity reactions.
- Atopy involves excessive Th2 and insufficient Treg cell activity.
- Allergy has a genetic basis, but the precise genes involved are not yet defined.
- There are breed predispositions for allergic disease in dogs and horses.
- Canine AD has onset at a young age.
- Secondary infection may complicate allergy.
- The hygiene hypothesis explains the increased prevalence of allergic, autoimmune and other diseases in the human population over the past 50 years.
- The hygiene hypothesis proposes that changes in lifestyle have reduced contact with the infectious agents that drive expansion of Treg cells.
- Intestinal helminths are particularly effective at Treg cell expansion.
- Major allergic diseases of animals include urticaria, angioedema, anaphylaxis, FAD, AD and food allergy of dogs and cats, and urticaria, IBH and RAO of horses.
- These diseases are thought to have an underlying Th2-regulated type I hypersensitivity immunopathogenesis.
- Contact allergy is uncommon in animals, but is documented in the dog.
- Diagnosis of allergic disease involves clinical history, ruling-out ectoparasite or food allergy by exclusion and an IDST and serology for AD.

CHAPTER 18

Immune System Ontogeny and Neonatal Immunology

OBJECTIVES

At the end of this chapter you should be able to:
- Briefly describe the progressive development of the immune system *in utero*.
- Describe the general composition of colostrum and milk.
- Discuss the absorption of colostrum.
- Discuss how passive transfer of maternal immunity interferes with vaccination of young animals.
- Describe the causes and effects of failure of colostral transfer.

- Understand why primary immunodeficiency disease becomes clinically manifest after loss of maternal immunity.
- Describe the pathogenesis of neonatal isoerythrolysis and list the species in which this disease is most commonly manifest.
- Understand that development of the immune system continues during the early life of animals.

INTRODUCTION

This chapter considers a range of diverse aspects of immunology related to the *in-utero* development of the immune system and to the range of specific immunological diseases that are unique to newborn animals.

IMMUNE SYSTEM ONTOGENY

During embryological development *in utero* there is progressive expansion of the different elements of the immune system. This is variably well characterized for different domestic animals, but follows a general pattern. For example, in species with a relatively long gestation, such as cattle, development of **primary lymphoid tissue** (thymus and bone marrow) occurs within the first trimester and **T and B cells** appear within the fetal circulation at that time. During the second and third trimesters there is development of

secondary lymphoid tissues (e.g. MALT) and from this time onwards the fetus is capable of mounting a **humoral immune response** to a range of potential pathogens that might be encountered *in utero*. As will be discussed below, newborn animals are born without appreciable levels of blood immunoglobulin, but such *in-utero* antigenic challenge would mean that the newborn might have detectable antigen-specific immunoglobulins.

PASSIVE TRANSFER OF MATERNAL IMMUNE PROTECTION

A basic facet of animal husbandry is the absolute requirement for newborn animals to take in maternal **colostrum** during a narrow window of opportunity immediately after parturition. This transfer of maternal immunoglobulin (together with other proteins, lymphocytes and cytokines) confers **temporary immune protection** upon the newborn animal until it is capable of activating its own endogenous immunity. This fundamental feature of the early life of domestic animals is directly related to the range of placentation that occurs in these species (**Figure 18.1**).

Colostral immunoglobulin is not essential for human and other primate neonates because the **haemochorial placentation** of these species permits transfer of maternal immunoglobulin across the chorionic epithelium, such that the neonates are born with serum IgG concentrations approaching those of the adult. In contrast, in dogs and cats the additional barrier of the maternal endothelium in **endotheliochorial placentation** permits transfer of only a small quantity of IgG. Therefore, pups and kittens may be born with only 5% or less of the level of serum immunoglobulin present in the adult. Even greater barriers characterize the **syndesmochorial placentation** of the ruminant and the **epitheliochorial placentation** of the horse, such that there is no possibility for maternal transfer of immunoglobulin *in utero* in these species. As a consequence, the colostrum of animals has significantly different composition to that of the milk.

There are species differences, but some general principles apply. The most important proteins within these secretions are **immunoglobulins**. These may broadly originate from the **maternal blood** or from **local production** by plasma cells within the mammary tissue. Colostrum is immunoglobulin rich and the majority of these molecules (particularly IgG) derive from the circulation, with relatively lower input from local plasma cells (for IgM and IgA). Colostrum is also relatively **enriched in IgG**, with lower concentrations of IgM and IgA. In contrast, milk has a considerably reduced total concentration of immunoglobulin and this may largely derive from local plasma cells rather than the maternal circulation. The relative proportion of immunoglobulin classes may also change; for example, bovine colostrum and milk are both dominated by IgG, but in non-ruminant species the concentration of IgA in milk is greater than that of IgG or IgM.

Recent studies have characterized the non-immunoglobulin components of colostrum. Bovine **colostrum contains CD4+, CD8+ and γδTCR+**

T cells and the CD8+ subset is the source of the significant concentration of **IFN-γ** within this secretion. Studies comparing calves that received entire colostrum with calves that received cell-free colostrum showed that the transfer of these maternal lymphocytes has a beneficial effect on the development of the neonatal immune system. Calves receiving entire colostrum had a greater number of blood monocytes, with more effective antigen presenting capacity and increased MHC class I expression on circulating lymphocytes. A study in piglets from sows vaccinated with keyhole limpet haemocyanin (KLH) demonstrated colostral transfer of antigen-specific lymphocytes found in the blood and mesenteric lymph nodes of the piglets. **Complement components** are also contained within colostrum and passively absorbed, but are thought to be non-functional within the neonate.

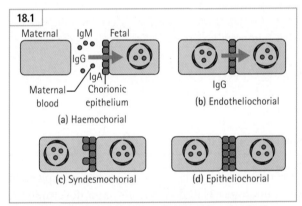

Fig. 18.1 Placentation in man and domestic animals. The absolute requirement of domestic animal neonates for maternal colostrum is defined by the nature of placentation in these animals. (**a**) The haemochorial placentation in women and other primates allows maternal IgG to pass directly to the fetal circulation so that the newborn of these species have a serum IgG concentration similar to that of the mother. (**b**) The endotheliochorial placentation of the bitch and queen provides a greater barrier (maternal endothelium and chorionic epithelium) so that only a small quantity of IgG is able to transfer *in utero*. (**c**) The syndesmochorial placentation of the ruminant means that the maternal and fetal circulations are separated by the uterine connective tissue and chorionic epithelium. (**d**) The mare and sow have epitheliochorial placentation with both uterine and chorionic epithelium providing an impenetrable barrier to maternal immunoglobulin.

The process of absorption of these colostral components is made possible by a series of modifications that are in place from approximately **6–24 hours after birth**. The colostral proteins would normally be rapidly degraded within the intestinal lumen, but they are protected by the relatively **low proteolytic activity** in this environment during this window of time together with the action of **colostral enzyme inhibitors**. Maternally-derived IgA has the additional protection conferred by the secretory piece (see Chapter 2). Immunoglobulin transfer across the neonatal intestine is mediated by the transient expression of specific receptors (**FcnR**) by **enterocytes**. Absorbed immunoglobulin may pass directly into the vascular circulation, but a proportion of this protein may first be absorbed into lacteals and subsequently transfer from the lymphatic to the vascular circulation (**Figure 18.2**). Absorption of maternal immunoglobulin results in elevation of neonatal serum immunoglobulin concentration, with a peak level between 12 and 24 hours. A proportion of this absorbed immunoglobulin is lost into the urine as the glomeruli of the neonate have increased permeability during the first 24 hours of life. This results in a **transient proteinuria** in the neonate. There are again species differences in the nature of this passive transfer. For example, in ruminants, IgG, IgM and IgA are all absorbed, but a proportion of IgA is re-secreted to the intestinal lumen to afford protection to this mucosal surface. In contrast, in horses and pigs the colostral IgA largely remains within the intestinal tract and the principle absorption is of IgG and IgM. In all of these species the 'window of opportunity' for absorption of colostral immunoglobulin is up to 24 hours after birth, but for pups and kittens this period may extend for up to 48–72 hours.

Chicks also require maternally derived immunity for protection in neonatal life. **Maternal IgY** is transferred from blood to the **yolk** of developing eggs in the ovary and is highly concentrated in this fluid. The embryonic chick absorbs this IgY, which is found in its circulation. As the egg passes through the oviduct the albumin acquires IgM and IgA from local secretions and these immunoglobulins enter the amniotic fluid to be swallowed by the embryo to provide local intestinal immunity.

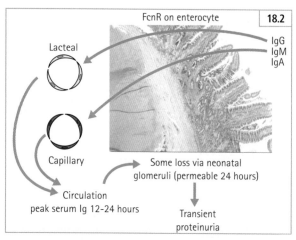

Fig. 18.2 Absorption of colostral immunoglobulin. Uptake of colostral immunoglobulin is mediated by the FcnR expressed by intestinal enterocytes. The immunoglobulin may be directly absorbed to the circulation or taken up initially into the lacteals and passed from the lymphatic to the vascular circulation. Serum immunoglobulin concentration in the neonate peaks between 12 and 24 hours of life. The renal glomeruli of the newborn are relatively permeable, so some immunoglobulin is lost in the urine during the first 24 hours of life.

NEONATAL VACCINATION

Although vaccination is considered in detail in Chapter 20, it is appropriate to consider the principles of vaccination of young animals at this point. While passive transfer of colostral immunoglobulin is crucial for the survival of the neonate, it is a 'double-edged sword' and poses a specific problem to these vulnerable animals in that this antibody **inhibits an endogenous humoral immune response** until such time as it has been sufficiently degraded. The consequences for the neonate are that these animals are unable to make humoral immune responses to the majority of currently available vaccines until such time as this has occurred. There is then a period of 'cross-over' while the young animal begins to synthesize its own immunoglobulin as the last of the maternal protein is lost. This period is often termed the '**window of susceptibility**' or the '**immunity gap**' and is defined as the period of time when there is no longer sufficient maternal immunoglobulin to afford protection from infection, but when there is still enough of this maternal protein to prevent the young animal from mounting its own protective immune response to a vaccine (**Figure 18.3**).

The timing and duration of the 'window of susceptibility' may **vary widely between individual animals** and even between **animals within the same litter**. This relates to factors including the amount of antibody in maternal colostrum and the amount of colostrum ingested and absorbed by individual young animals. For example, one animal within a litter may have a 'window of susceptibility' between 10 and 12 weeks of age, but another, which took in less colostrum or colostrum of lesser quality, may lose maternal protection earlier and have a 'window of susceptibility' between 6 and 8 weeks of age (**Figure 18.4**). The consequences of this are that within a litter or between different litters, individuals may **respond to vaccination at different ages**. The inability to define and quantify the 'window' in individual newborns has led to the development of vaccination protocols whereby **young animals receive multiple vaccinations** in order that **at least**

one may stimulate the immune response. In fact, for pups and kittens, current recommendations are for three such immunizations, typically at 8, 12 and 14–16 weeks of age, as it is recognized that a percentage of these animals will still have blocking levels of maternal immunoglobulin at 12 weeks of age with a late 'window of susceptibility'. The **booster vaccine given one year after the last of this primary series** (or at one year of age) is a crucial element in such a protocol, because if an immune response is not stimulated at 14–16 weeks, it may not occur until 'boosting' 12

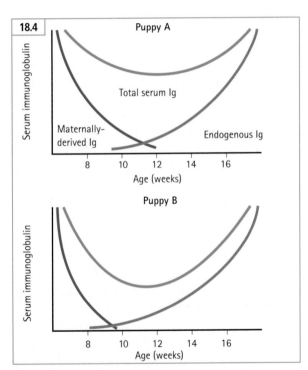

Fig. 18.4 Inter-animal variation in the 'window of susceptibility'. The two puppies in this example are from the same litter, but each took in a different amount of colostrum. Puppy A received more colostrum so has a 'window of susceptibility' between 10 and 12 weeks of age. In contrast, puppy B received less colostrum and so maternal immunoglobulin is lost earlier, with a 'window of susceptibility' between 8 and 10 weeks of age. If these pups received only a single primary vaccination at 10 weeks of age, pup A would not respond. For this reason, administration of a primary course of vaccines at 8, 12 and 16 weeks of age will ensure a primary response in all pups in the litter. This primary response must be 'boosted' with a further injection 12 months after the 16 week immunization or at 12 months of age.

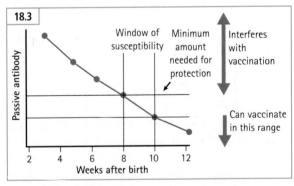

Fig. 18.3 The 'window of susceptibility'. Maternal immunoglobulin degrades over time and once this blocking antibody is lost the young animal is able to make its own endogenous humoral immune response. The 'window of susceptibility' ('immunity gap') is the time during which there is insufficient maternal immunity remaining to provide full protection, but still sufficient maternal immunity to block the ability of the animal to make its own protective immune response. In the example shown the 'window of susceptibility' is between 8 and 10 weeks of age.

months later. Such vaccination protocols give all young animals the maximum chance of responding to protective vaccination. Current recommendations also endorse the practice of determining whether pups have responded to early life vaccination by **serological testing** in order to determine whether there is a **'protective titre'** following immunization with core vaccine components such as CDV and canine parvovirus. Such tests are readily justified as there is excellent correlation between serum antibody titre and protection for such virus infections (see Chapter 4).

FAILURE OF PASSIVE TRANSFER

Despite the importance of passively acquired maternal immunity, some neonatal animals fail to receive adequate colostrum and are thus highly **susceptible to infectious disease**. Reasons for failure of passive transfer include:

- **Premature birth** such that the dam has not formed colostrum.
- **Premature lactation** with loss of colostrum.
- Production of **poor-quality colostrum** (determined by maternal nutritional and vaccinal status).
- **Failure of the neonate to suckle** within the first 24 hours of life.
- **Failure of the neonate to absorb** colostrum due to loss of the adaptive mechanisms described above.

For valuable animals (e.g. Thoroughbred racehorses) it is routine to test for the serum immunoglobulin concentration after 24 hours to determine if there has been adequate colostral uptake. This testing might involve a precise measurement by methods such as **SRID** (**Figure 18.5**) or the use of rapid semi-quantitative **commercially produced kits** that may be used 'animal side' (see SNAP® tests, Chapter 4). Simple turbidometric precipitation methods have also been widely employed in studies of newborn calves.

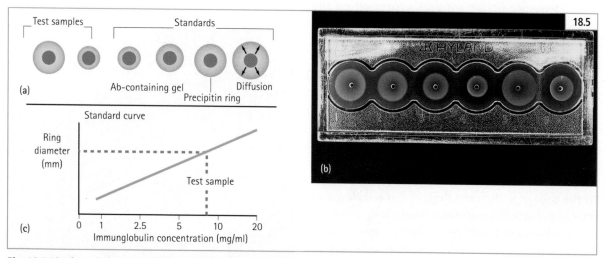

Fig. 18.5 Single radial immunodiffusion. (a) SRID is a precipitation test used to quantify the amount of protein within a sample, in this context the amount of IgG within the serum of a newborn foal after receiving colostrum. Antiserum specific to equine IgG is mixed with agarose and the gel allowed to set on a plastic plate. A series of wells is cut into the gel. A set of IgG standards of known concentration are loaded into four of the wells and test samples from two foals are loaded to the remaining wells. The gel is incubated for 24 hours during which time IgG diffuses from the well to precipitate with the antiserum impregnated into the gel. **(b)** The precipitation is seen as a visible ring surrounding each well and the diameter of the ring is proportional to the concentration of Ig in each sample. **(c)** The standards are used to plot a standard curve on a semi-logarithmic scale and the concentration of IgG in the foal serum can be determined by interpolation from the curve.

PRIMARY IMMUNODEFICIENCY

A complete discussion of primary immunodeficiency follows in Chapter 19, but it is again appropriate to consider this subject briefly here. Primary immunodeficiencies are **genetic diseases** involving a specific **mutation in a gene encoding a particular immunological molecule**. Such disorders mean that the affected individual has an **impaired immune system** rendering that animal susceptible to infectious disease. The clinical severity of the disease is determined by the nature of the gene affected. Primary immunodeficiency will generally become clinically manifest at the time colostral immunity wanes and the young animal would normally develop its own immune response.

NEONATAL ISOERYTHROLYSIS

Neonatal isoerythrolysis (NI) (or **isoimmune haemolytic anaemia**) is an immunological disorder affecting newborn animals and an uncommon deleterious effect of maternal transfer of passive immunity. In this disease the colostrum contains antibodies specific for antigens expressed on the surface of the erythrocytes of the newborn animal. Absorption of these antibodies therefore leads to **IMHA** (see Chapters 12 and 16). The dam may have such **isoantibodies**, which arise **spontaneously**, perhaps due to exposure to cross-reactive environmental antigens. Alternatively, the dam may be actively sensitized to foreign erythrocyte antigens. This most often occurs when the **blood groups of the dam and sire differ** so that the fetus expresses a blood group antigen that is foreign to the mother. At the time of parturition there is some **leakage of fetal blood into the maternal circulation**, which can immunologically **sensitize** the dam. Consequently, NI is a disease that generally affects animals born to **second and subsequent pregnancies**. Finally, it is also possible to sensitize the dam by **prior transfusion of incompatible blood**, further emphasizing the need for blood typed and cross-matched transfusions (see Chapters 4 and 22).

    NI is most common in **foals and kittens** and much less common in other species. In the horse the disease occurs when a mare that lacks expression of the Q and

A blood group antigens (Q⁻A⁻) is mated to a stallion that is Q⁺A⁺ or receives a transfusion of Q⁺A⁺ blood. The clinical presentation is of anaemia with jaundiced mucous membranes (**Figure 18.6**). The affected foal will be **Coombs test positive** (see Chapter 16). It is possible to determine the likelihood of NI before parturition by performing a simple agglutination test with serum from the mare and washed erythrocytes from the stallion. Alternatively, incubation of mare serum with washed newborn foal erythrocytes will provide the same information, but this would need to be undertaken before the foal suckled colostrum. NI can be simply prevented by **stopping access of the newborn foal to the dam's colostrum**, but an **alternative source of colostrum** must be provided for that animal.

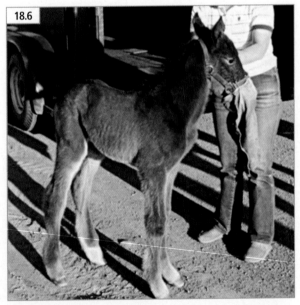

Fig. 18.6 Neonatal isoerythrolysis. This foal is at risk for the development of NI. The nose-bag is a means of ensuring that the foal does not receive colostrum, but it will not be necessary after 24 hours of life.

NI in kittens also relates to the nature of the feline blood group antigens. Simply, cats may be of blood groups A, B or AB (see Chapter 4). Type A cats may occasionally have low-titred anti-B isoantibodies, but type B cats invariably have high-titred anti-A antibodies (and type AB cats have neither). NI therefore occurs when a type B queen with anti-A antibody gives birth to kittens of type A or AB. As the type B blood group is more prevalent in particular breeds (e.g. Birman, Rex, British shorthair, Abyssinian, Persian and Somali), the disease **more frequently arises within these breeds**. Feline NI may also present clinically as a severe haemolytic anaemia with icterus, haemoglobinuria, weakness and lethargy, failure to suckle and death within the first week of life. A milder, subclinical form is recognized where agglutination of erythrocytes by antibody leads to occlusion of peripheral capillaries and ischaemic necrosis (e.g. of the tail tip) within the first few weeks of life. Affected kittens are Coombs test positive.

Breeders of susceptible breeds are very aware of this condition and will often routinely **blood type their breeding stock** to avoid at-risk matings. Testing serum from the queen with washed erythrocytes from the tom cat will provide an antenatal diagnosis. Prevention is by denying access to colostrum from the dam, but providing an **alternative source of colostrum is challenging for kittens**. Allowing kittens to suckle a type A foster mother may be performed, although feline milk is now known to be not as immunoglobulin rich as colostrum. Alternatively, artificial colostrum may be prepared by mixing cat serum (from an appropriate well-vaccinated and blood-typed donor) with commercial milk replacer.

Canine NI is uncommon, but occurs when a DEA1$^-$ bitch is sensitized by mating to a DEA1$^+$ dog or receives an inappropriate transfusion of DEA1$^+$ blood.

A newly emerged disease in Europe related to colostral antibodies is **bovine neonatal pancytopenia** (BNP) or 'bleeding calf syndrome'. Affected newborn calves develop bone marrow depletion and pancytopenia, expressed clinically as haemorrhages secondary to thrombocytopenia. The disease is thought to occur following ingestion of colostrum containing alloantibodies that bind to neonatal circulating leucocytes and, presumably, to bone marrow precursor cells. These antibodies have specificity for MHC class I molecules. The dams of affected calves have often been vaccinated against BVDV and it is suggested that antigens derived from the bovine cell line used in manufacturing this inactivated vaccine (the Madin–Darby bovine kidney cell line) may trigger antibody production in the vaccinated dams.

EARLY LIFE IMMUNE DEVELOPMENT

The immune system of young animals undergoes significant development within the first months of life and in most species immunity is not fully developed until around 12 months of age. As noted above, this development might be influenced by proteins and cells derived from colostrum. The number of blood lymphocytes increases over the first few months of life and the relative proportions of lymphocyte subsets changes. For example, in pups and kittens the CD4:CD8 ratio gradually decreases as the number of CD8$^+$ T cells expands. The responsiveness of these cells to mitogen stimulation (see Chapter 10) increases over this time. In one study, blood lymphocyte proliferation and cytokine production were monitored in pups between 4 and 10 weeks of life. Initial cytokine profiles were dominated by IL-10, which progressively declined with replacement by IFN-γ over time. The same dominance of IL-10 was seen in cultures taken from the dams of these pups during pregnancy, suggesting an immunosuppressive environment *in utero* with gradual switch to Th1 immunoregulation with increasing exposure to environmental antigens during early life (see Chapter 17). Once maternal immunoglobulin has waned it may take up to 12 months for adult levels of endogenous serum IgG, IgM and IgA to be achieved. The process of thymic involution begins at around 6 months of age and there is a progressive decline over the following 1–2 years. Tests of immune function in young and adolescent animals should always be interpreted in light of these changes.

KEY POINTS

- There is progressive development of the immune system *in utero* and the fetus is capable of an immune response if challenged.
- Newborn domestic animals must receive colostrum within the first 24 hours of life to protect them from infectious disease.
- The nature of placentation of domestic animals prevents transfer of maternal immunoglobulin *in utero*.
- Colostrum is enriched in immunoglobulin; milk contains less immunoglobulin, but the proportions of IgG, IgM and IgA in these secretions vary between different species.
- Colostrum also contains lymphocytes and cytokines and these confer benefit to the neonate.
- Colostral protein is protected by low proteolytic activity in the neonatal gut and the presence of colostral enzyme inhibitors.
- The enterocyte FcnR mediates uptake of colostral immunoglobulin.
- Some absorbed colostral immunoglobulin is lost through the glomerulus in the first 24 hours of life.
- Maternal immunoglobulin inhibits the ability of the neonate to mount its own immune response.
- The 'window of susceptibility' or 'immunity gap' is the time between the point when there is insufficient maternal immunoglobulin remaining to provide protection from infectious disease and the point when the neonate can mount a fully protective immune response.
- The 'window of susceptibility' varies between individual neonates and between animals within a litter.
- Neonates must therefore receive multiple vaccinations to ensure that at least one of these primes the immune response.
- The 12-month booster vaccine is an integral part of the young animal vaccination schedule, as it 'boosts' the primary immune response.
- Failure of passive transfer of colostral immunoglobulin renders the neonate susceptible to infection, so serological testing after 24 hours of life is justified in valuable animals.
- Primary congenital immunodeficiency becomes clinically manifest after loss of maternal immunity.
- NI occurs when the colostrum contains antibody to erythrocyte antigens expressed by the newborn; these antibodies cause IMHA.
- Isoantibodies may arise spontaneously or be induced following first parturition or incompatible blood transfusion.
- NI is most common in foals and kittens.
- NI can be predicted and prevented by denying access to the dam's colostrum; an alternative source of colostrum must be provided.
- The immune system of young animals continues to develop until adolescence.

CHAPTER 19

Immunodeficiency

OBJECTIVES

At the end of this chapter you should be able to:
- Define primary and secondary immunodeficiency.
- List the clinical features that might indicate the presence of an underlying primary immunodeficiency disease.
- Review the broad spectrum of primary immunodeficiency diseases in animals.
- Discuss the specific gene mutations that give rise to SCID, cyclic haematopoiesis, canine leucocyte adhesion deficiency (CLAD) and the trapped neutrophil syndrome of border collies.

- Describe novel experimental therapies that have been tested in canine models of primary immunodeficiency for the benefit of human patients.
- List the characteristics of immunosenescence.
- Describe how secondary immunodeficiency may be induced by chronic infectious, inflammatory or neoplastic disease.
- Discuss the clinical and immunological changes that occur in feline immunodeficiency virus infection.

INTRODUCTION

Immunodeficiency may be simply defined as **impairment** in function of part or parts of the immune system that renders the immunodeficient patient more **susceptible to infectious disease**. Two broad types of immunodeficient state are recognized. **Primary immunodeficiency** occurs when there is a **mutation in a gene** encoding a molecule of the immune system. Such diseases are **inherited** and **congenital**, with clinical signs often becoming apparent in early life. There is a spectrum of such disorders, with some mutations consistently leading to increased mortality and others related to only mild and chronic clinical presentation. In contrast, **secondary immunodeficiency** occurs in an **adult** animal that

has previously had normal immune function and may be related to age, infection, medical therapy or the presence of chronic disease.

PRIMARY IMMUNODEFICIENCY

A range of primary immunodeficiency disorders is recognized in animals and homologues for many of these exist in man. These diseases are generally **breed associated**, clearly **inherited** and have clinical and immunological abnormalities consistent with **immune dysfunction**. However, for the majority of animal immunodeficiencies the precise genetic mutation has not been established and many of these disorders remain **putative immunodeficiencies** until such evidence is provided. Primary immunodeficiency disorders are **relatively rare** and, with some exceptions, lack of available case material and lack of research funding has made these disorders difficult to study. There are, however, some very well studied animal immunodeficiencies for which the precise genetic basis is known. These diseases sometimes serve as animal models for the equivalent human disorders and colonies of affected animals (most often dogs) are kept for the purpose of developing curative therapies. It has proven possible to reverse immunodeficient states by the use of **gene therapy** in such models. Gene therapy will never be used to treat individual animal patients, but the molecular knowledge can be used successfully to develop **diagnostic tests** to identify homozygous affected and heterozygous carrier animals (many of these diseases are inherited in an **autosomal recessive** fashion) so as not to breed from these animals and gradually eliminate the trait. In fact, this approach has already proven successful with regard to one canine immunodeficiency disease (see CLAD, p. 226).

The primary immunodeficiency diseases can affect immune system development at different levels (**Figure 19.1**). A mutation that inhibits the development of both T and B lymphocytes (e.g. SCID) will have much more severe consequences for the animal than a mutation that selectively impairs the production of complement factor C3 or IgA. Some of the genetic mutations that give rise to immunodeficiency are linked to **other congenital abnormalities**, one of the best recognized being the association between the absence of a full hair coat and thymic aplasia (see p. 242). Immunodeficiency disease might also be associated with concurrent autoimmunity, allergy or immune system neoplasia.

There are certain clinical and historical features of disease that might suggest the presence of an underlying primary immunodeficiency in any animal. These include:

- Disease affecting a particular **breed**.
- Disease occurring in **young littermate animals** with onset shortly after the expected time of loss of maternally derived immunity (see Chapter 18).
- **Chronic recurrent infection**.
- **Infection of multiple body sites**.

- Failure of infection to respond to standard antimicrobial therapy.
- Infection with **environmental saprophytes** (e.g. *Aspergillus*, *Pneumocystis*).
- **Persistent lymphopenia** or **hypogammaglobulinaemia**.
- **Failure to respond to vaccination**.

The diagnosis of primary immunodeficiency disease provides particular challenges for the veterinarian. The various 'flags' described above might be recognized, but it is often very difficult to progress the diagnosis in terms of defining a specific immunological defect. This relates simply to the lack of availability of appropriate diagnostic testing. Although in animals it is entirely possible to perform the range of tests of immune function described in Chapters 4 and 10, such tests are rarely commercially available. For a small number of conditions **PCR-based diagnostic tests** are available that should provide a definitive diagnosis.

Immunodeficiency diseases are recognized in a wide range of domestic animals and have been exploited in several **inbred strains of laboratory rodent** for research purposes. Spontaneously arising primary immunodeficiencies are most common and best described in **dogs and horses**. There are about 30 canine immunodeficiency diseases, but only four of these are defined to the molecular level. It is not possible to cover the full spectrum of primary immunodeficiency disorders in this chapter, but the more common and better understood diseases are discussed below.

Severe combined immunodeficiency

SCID is recognized in both dogs and horses and because children may be afflicted by the same disorder, the animal diseases have received much research attention. **Canine SCID** is recognized in the bassett hound, Cardigan Welsh corgi and Jack Russell terrier and the genetic basis for the disease is different in each breed. SCID in the **bassett hound** is X-linked and involves a **mutation in the common γ chain** of the **receptors for the cytokines IL-2, IL-4, IL-7, IL-9 and IL-15 (Figure 19.2)**. The same gene is affected in X-linked SCID in the **Welsh corgi**, but the mutation is different. Inhibition of the action of these key cytokines means that the T-cell response to antigen is inhibited and consequently no immune response is generated. SCID in the **Jack Russell terrier** involves a distinct **mutation in the DNA protein kinase gene** involved in the recombination of VDJ regions in the formation of TCRs and BCRs. Failure to develop these receptors again inhibits the production of any immune response. The clinical consequences of SCID involve bacterial and viral infection after loss of maternal immunity. Affected animals are lymphopenic and have hypoplasia of lymphoid tissue.

They have defective blood lymphocyte mitogenic responses and profound lack of serum IgG and IgA antibodies. Experimentally, this disease can be treated by approaches such as **bone marrow transplantation, transplantation of heterologous stem cells** following partial myeloablation by irradiation, or **gene therapy** in which affected dogs are given a retrovirus vector containing the canine cytokine γ chain gene. In one study, three of four dogs receiving gene therapy developed normal numbers of blood T and B cells, normal serum IgG concentration and were able to seroconvert following vaccination.

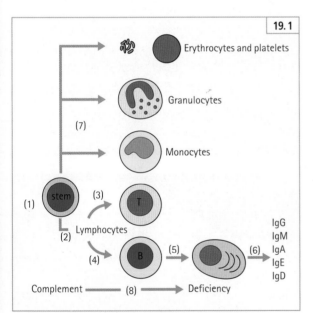

Fig. 19.1 Levels of primary immunodeficiency. The development of immune and haemopoietic cells involves progressive maturation from bone marrow stem cell precursors. Genetic mutations underlying primary immunodeficiency can involve molecules involved in different stages of this maturation process. The range of immunodeficiency disorders encompasses (1) failure of the pluripotent stem cell, (2) failure of committed stem cells, (3) failure of T-cell development, (4) failure of B-cell development, (5) failure of B-cell maturation to plasma cells, (6) failure of production of selected immunoglobulin class/es, (7) failure to produce functional phagocytic cells, or (8) failure of production of one or more complement molecules.

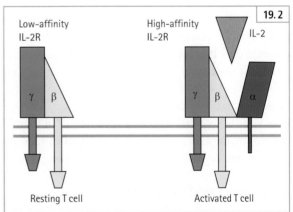

Fig. 19.2 SCID in basset hounds and Welsh corgis. Resting T cells express a low-affinity form of the IL-2 receptor composed of a β and a γ chain. On activation of this cell, expression of the α chain leads to formation of a high-affinity receptor that permits IL-2 binding and signal transduction. The γ chain is shared by receptor molecules for the cytokines IL-4, IL-7, IL-9 and IL-15. In the form of SCID affecting these two canine breeds, a (different) mutation in the γ chain means that these receptors are non-functional and there is failure of the immune response.

An experimental breeding colony of SCID dogs bearing the DNA protein kinase mutation has been developed. The Jack Russell mutation was bred into beagle dogs that could be successfully engrafted with donor bone marrow, allowing them to be kept in a normal environment. These dogs develop signs of premature ageing including intestinal malabsorption due to pancreatic insufficiency and the onset of tumours of the CNS.

SCID is also well described in **Arab horses**, where the disease also reflects a small base pair deletion in the **DNA protein kinase gene**. Equine SCID will be described further in a case study (see Chapter 22). A single Angus calf with lymphoid tissue hypoplasia, low serum IgG (of maternal origin) and absent serum IgM and IgA was also suggested to have a form of SCID.

Thymic aplasia

As mentioned above, **thymic aplasia**, with consequent **lack of T lymphocytes**, is often linked to failure of development of the hair coat. **'Nude' rats and mice** have proven useful immunological tools, as the absence of T-cell immunity means that they (similar to SCID mice) can be repopulated with lymphoid subsets to observe the interaction of these cells *in vivo*. The **hairless canine breeds** (Mexican hairless dog, Chinese crested dog) may have impaired thymic development, and a single litter of **Birman kittens** was once reported to be hairless and athymic.

Zinc-associated disorders

Two traits involving lymphocyte dysfunction and subnormal plasma zinc levels are described. **Lethal acrodermatitis of bull terrier dogs** is proposed as an autosomal recessive disease in which affected dogs have stunted growth, severe cutaneous parakeratosis and skin and respiratory infections (**Figures 19.3a, b**). There is reduced T-cell mitogen responsiveness and low serum IgA concentration. **Lethal trait A46 in black pied Danish and Friesian cattle** is also proposed as a defect in T-cell immunity related to a reduced ability to absorb dietary zinc. Affected animals have selective impairment of T-cell function

and develop cutaneous disease with alopecia and parakeratosis and hypoplasia of secondary lymphoid tissue.

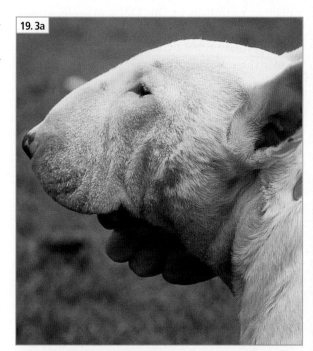

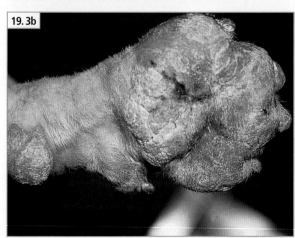

Figs. 19.3a, b Lethal acrodermatitis in bull terriers. This bull terrier dog has stunted growth, submandibular lymphadenopathy (**a**) and hyperkeratosis of the footpads (**b**), a combination of signs typical of the disorder termed lethal acrodermatitis. These dogs are also thought to be immunodeficient and the pathogenesis of the disease may involve subnormal levels of plasma zinc.

Cyclic haematopoiesis

Canine **cyclic haematopoiesis** (cyclic neutropenia or the 'grey collie syndrome') occurs in **collie pups** that are poorly grown and have diluted ('grey') coat colour. They have a cyclic (every 12 days for approximately 3 days) neutropenia, monocytopenia, thrombocytopenia and reticulocytopenia (**Figure 19.4**) that is associated with episodes of infection (pyrexia, diarrhoea, conjunctivitis, gingivitis or arthritis), epistaxis and gingival haemorrhage. The disease has **autosomal recessive** inheritance and is known to involve a **mutation in the gene encoding the α subunit of the neutrophil adaptor protein complex 3**, which disrupts the intracellular movement of neutrophil elastase. A similar disease occurs in man, but the genetic mutation is different. Experimental studies of affected dogs have shown that the disease may be treated by administration of **granulocyte colony-stimulating factor** (G-CSF) or **stem cell factor** and by **bone marrow transplantation**. **Gene therapy** has been conducted at the *in-vitro* level with viral vectors used to transfer the functional gene into haemopoietic progenitor cells from affected dogs. A lentivirus vector containing the G-CSF gene has also been used successfully to treat the disorder.

Neutrophil disorders

A range of additional disorders affecting neutrophils is recognized. The **Pelger Huët anomaly** presents as **reduced segmentation of neutrophil nuclei**, but no consistent functional consequence of this has been documented. Affected animals have normal blood neutrophil counts and other immunological parameters and are generally **clinically normal**. The anomaly is recorded in the American foxhound, cocker spaniel, Boston terrier, Australian shepherd dog and basenji and it also occurs in domestic shorthair cats where there are additional anomalies of monocytes and megakaryocytes.

The **Chediak Higashi syndrome** presents as **abnormal granulation of the neutrophil cytoplasm**. This autosomal recessive disorder is associated with defective neutrophil function and increased susceptibility to infection and is caused by a mutation in the *LYST* gene, which encodes a molecule involved in the fusion of lysosomal membranes. The disease occurs in the blue smoke Persian cat, in Hereford, Japanese black and Brangus cattle, Aleutian mink, white tigers, killer whales and man. Affected animals may have diluted coat colour and poorly pigmented irises due to fusion of the melanosomes (melanin granules), which are related to lysosomes. Haemorrhages may occur following trauma as the mutation also affects lysosomes within platelets. Birman cats are also reported with a neutrophil granulation abnormality that has no apparent clinical consequence.

The **'trapped neutrophil syndrome'** (TNS; myelokathexis) of **border collie** dogs (see Chapter 22) is an **autosomal recessive** disease that appears widespread in this breed internationally. TNS presents as a neutropenia due to **failure to release neutrophils from the bone marrow**. Affected dogs may have stunted growth and be pyrexic,

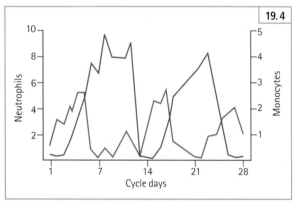

Fig. 19.4 Cyclic haematopoiesis in the grey collie. The graph shows the typical 12-day cycle in blood neutrophils (blue line) and monocytes (red line) that characterizes this immunodeficiency syndrome. (Redrawn after Benson KF, Li F-Q, Person RE *et al.* (2003) Mutations associated with neutropenia in dogs and humans disrupt intracellular transport of neutrophil elastase. *Nature Genetics* **35**:90–96.)

with vomiting, diarrhoea, inappetence, poor coat condition, lameness and joint swelling. Affected dogs have a four base pair deletion in exon 19 of the *VPS13B* gene (vacuolar protein sorting 13 homologue B), which encodes a transmembrane protein that is involved in vesicle-mediated transport and sorting of proteins in a cell. A mutation in the same gene occurs in human Cohen syndrome, which is characterized by developmental and morphological abnormalities in addition to intermittent neutropenia. A commercial diagnostic PCR test is available for dogs.

Leucocyte adhesion deficiency

Leucocyte adhesion deficiency (LAD) is best described in dogs (canine leucocyte adhesion deficiency; CLAD) and cattle (bovine leucocyte adhesion deficiency; BLAD). **CLAD** is an **autosomal recessive** disease that primarily affects the **red Irish setter** (and less commonly the red and white Irish setter). The **mutation is in the gene encoding the α_2 leucocyte integrin CD18**. Failure to express CD18 leads to failure to express CD11b and this defect means that circulating blood neutrophils cannot adhere to vascular endothelium and therefore migrate into tissues (see Chapter 5). Consequently, affected dogs develop a marked **neutrophilia** and can become susceptible to severe **multisystemic infections** in the **absence of recruitment of these cells into tissue**. The clinical presentation is of combinations of pyrexia, omphalophlebitis, metaphyseal osteopathy, craniomandibular osteopathy, osteomyelitis, infective arthritis, interstitial pneumonia, dermatitis, conjunctivitis and gingivostomatitis.

CLAD is a major success story in veterinary medicine. The definition of the genetic basis for the disease led to the general availability of a **PCR diagnostic test** able to detect affected and carrier dogs. With the co-operation of Irish setter breed societies in many countries, a programme of testing and controlled breeding was undertaken, with the result that this disorder has been **virtually eliminated** from the breed. LAD is also recognized in man and the canine disease has provided an opportunity to investigate therapeutic possibilities. One recent

experimental study has demonstrated the potential for stem cell therapy in the treatment of the disorder. A dog affected by CLAD received whole body irradiation before a transplant of donor CD34[+] **bone marrow stem cells**. This dog became a 'chimera' with haemopoietic cells of donor origin that expressed normal levels of CD18. Another recent study has reported a disease with the clinical features of CLAD in mixed breed dogs, but although these animals had downregulation of CD18 gene transcription, there was no mutation in the sequence of this gene.

The pathogenesis of **BLAD in Holstein-Friesian cattle** is similar to that described for the dog, but involves a different mutation in the gene encoding CD18. Affected calves have stunted growth, multisystemic infection and marked neutrophilia and they generally die by 7 months of age. There is autosomal recessive inheritance and carriers can be identified by a molecular diagnostic test.

Selective immunoglobulin deficiency

Deficiency in production of a single class of immunoglobulin is recognized in a number of species including man. **Relative IgA deficiency** is the most common human primary immunodeficiency disorder affecting approximately one in every 700 people in Western countries. IgA-deficient patients may lead relatively normal lives with mild chronic recurrent mucosal infections or they may have associated autoimmune, allergic or neoplastic diseases. The disease is not clearly a mutation in genes encoding the IgA molecule, but may be a **functional deficiency in IgA production**. IgA deficiency is also regarded as relatively common in the dog and is again a relative and not absolute deficiency (with consistently subnormal serum IgA concentration). IgA deficiency is suggested to underlie the susceptibility to infection of canine breeds such as the **shar pei** and **German shepherd dog** (Figure 19.5), but there is no clear understanding of the mechanisms by which this might occur.

Consistently subnormal concentrations of **serum IgG** are thought to play a role in the pathogenesis of the complex disorder of young **weimaraner dogs** (Figure 19.6) and have been recognized in young

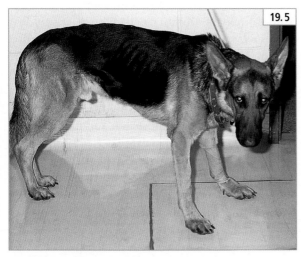

Fig. 19.5 IgA deficiency. This German shepherd dog has a disseminated infection with the fungus *Aspergillus terreus*. The susceptibility of dogs of this breed to infectious, inflammatory and immune-mediated diseases has long been thought to reflect an underlying immunodeficiency. The most studied candidate for such a defect is IgA deficiency, but the evidence for this abnormality is inconsistent.

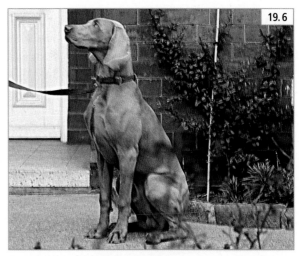

Fig. 19.6 Weimaraner immunodeficiency. This weimaraner dog has a history of chronic recurrent infections with profound neutrophilia. The dog has consistently subnormal serum IgG concentration and similarly affected siblings are found within the pedigree. This poorly characterized disease appears often to be triggered by vaccination and may develop following the initial of the puppy series of vaccines or after the 12 month booster.

cavalier King Charles spaniels with *Pneumocystis carinii* pneumonia. **Pneumocystosis** is a hallmark infection of immunodeficient people and animals and is a major cause of mortality in human acquired immune deficiency syndrome (AIDS). Selective **IgG2 deficiency** is also reported in **red Danish cattle** and is associated with pneumonia and gangrenous mastitis.

Equine selective **IgM deficiency, IgG deficiency** (in one foal) and **primary agammaglobulinaemia** (absence of B cells and lack of all immunoglobulins) is also reported. Affected foals develop recurrent infections of mucosal surfaces. Adult horses (less than 3 years old) with **common variable immunodeficiency** are recognized. These animals have recurrent infections, low to undetectable concentrations of serum immunoglobulin (in different combinations) and undetectable B cells (but normal numbers of T cells). The **Fell pony syndrome**, which is inherited in an autosomal recessive fashion, is a major immunodeficiency disorder of that breed. Clinical signs of anaemia and respiratory and enteric infections develop following loss of maternally-derived antibody and affected foals generally die by 3 months of age. There is a deficiency of B cells and plasma cells, but CD4+ and CD8+ T cell numbers are normal. Serum immunoglobulin concentrations may not be subnormal due to the presence of maternal antibody. The genetic basis for the disease is an active area of research and a recent genome-wide association study has identified a mutation on chromosome ECA26.

Complement deficiency

Selective deficiency of individual components of the complement pathway is recognized in a range of inbred laboratory animal species, but complement C3 deficiency is recognized in the **Brittany** breed. The affected Brittanys were part of an experimental colony kept for research into hereditary spinal muscular atrophy. These dogs have a single base deletion in the C3 gene, which is inherited in an autosomal recessive manner. The absence of C3 means that these animals are **susceptible to infection** and may sometimes develop **renal pathology** (immune complex glomerulonephritis or renal amyloidosis). **Yorkshire pigs** have been identified with an autosomal recessive **Factor H deficiency**. Affected animals are unable to regulate the production of C3b, which is produced in an excessive fashion and deposits within the renal glomerulus causing **membranoproliferative glomerulonephritis** and eventual death from **renal failure**.

SECONDARY IMMUNODEFICIENCY

In contrast to the rarity of primary breed-associated immunodeficiency, secondary immunodeficiency can affect animals of any breed and is relatively common. Secondary immunodeficiency affects adult animals that have had normal immune function until they undergo some form of physiological or pathological change. Causes of secondary immunodeficiency are reviewed below.

Immunosenescence

Immunosenescence is the term used to describe **age-related decline** in immune function and is a normal physiological change in older animals and people. Due to advances in veterinary healthcare, companion animals are enjoying an increasingly longer life span and an entire discipline of **geriatric medicine** has recently developed. The age-related decline in immune function has been reasonably well characterized in dogs, cats and horses and similar trends are apparent. In general, there is a relative **decrease in circulating CD4+ T cells** and a relative **increase in CD8+ T cells**, with an overall reduced CD4:CD8 ratio. These circulating T cells are predominantly **memory cells** with relatively **few naïve cells** remaining in older animals. T-cell function *in vitro* (e.g. mitogen-induced proliferation) and the ability to mount a cutaneous DTH response both decline in the elderly. In contrast, older animals have **persistent titres of serum antibody** (e.g. to vaccinal antigens) and **elevation of serum and mucosal IgA** concentration. Older animals are perfectly capable of mounting recall immune responses to antigens, but it may be more difficult to induce primary responses (e.g. to vaccines) in this population. It is suggested that immunosenescence is one factor underlying the increased susceptibility of older animals to infection, autoimmune disease and neoplasia.

Medical immunosuppression

Secondary immunodeficiency might be deliberately induced by the veterinarian when **immunosuppressive therapy** (see Chapter 21) is used to control autoimmune disease or when **chemotherapy** is used in the management of cancer. Although these procedures may counteract the pathological process, the major side-effect of such treatments is secondary immunosuppression and increased susceptibility to infection (**Figure 19.7**).

Specific infections

The single best example of infection-associated secondary immunodeficiency is **FIV** infection. FIV is a **T lymphotropic retrovirus** that infects lymphocytes and APCs and has been extensively investigated as an **animal model for human immunodeficiency virus (HIV) infection** (Figure 19.8). Infected cats have an acute phase of mild illness during which there is a progressive **decline in blood CD4+ T cells**. The cat will then become asymptomatic, but during this second phase of disease there is continued decline in circulating CD4+ T cells, which may occur over several years. During the third stage of disease there is a recurrence of mild illness, which progresses to more severe terminal stage 4–5 disease. The terminal illness is similar to human AIDS and is a **chronic, multisystemic disease** that may include gingivostomatitis, respiratory tract infection, enteritis, dermatitis, weight loss, pyrexia and lymphadenomegaly. Neurological disease and lymphoma may also develop and a range of secondary infections have been identified. FIV infection may be diagnosed by direct demonstration of virus in circulating lymphocytes, PCR-based amplification of viral nucleic acid or by demonstration of FIV serum antibody with a range of commercially available in-house test kits (see Chapter 4). **Concurrent FeLV infection** should also be considered and FeLV may be immunosuppressive in its own right due to depletion of infected T cells.

Chronic disease

Any animal afflicted by chronic infectious, inflammatory or neoplastic disease is likely to have a degree of secondary suppression of the immune system and increased susceptibility to infection. Some **infectious agents** (e.g. CDV, canine and feline parvovirus, FIV and FeLV, porcine circovirus-2 as the cause of post-weaning multisystemic wasting syndrome (PWMS) in this species, equine herpesvirus-1, bovine viral diarrhoea virus) may cause **direct depletion of lymphoid tissue**. Other infections are associated with the production of circulating **immunosuppressive factors** that appear to inhibit lymphocyte blastogenic responses. Such inhibition of lymphocyte function has been demonstrated in diseases such as demodicosis, deep pyoderma, pyometra and disseminated aspergillosis in the dog.

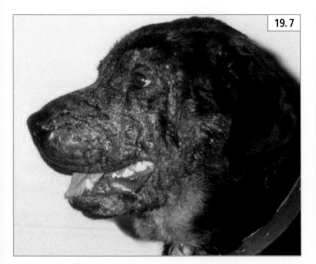

Fig. 19.7 Medical immunosuppression. This dog has been treated with immunosuppressive doses of glucocorticoid for immune-mediated disease. The immunosuppression has permitted emergence of a severe secondary *Demodex* infection. (Photo courtesy Susan Shaw)

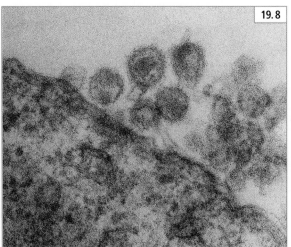

Fig. 19.8 Feline immunodeficiency virus. This transmission electron microscope image shows FIV particles budding from the cell membrane of an infected lymphocyte. FIV infection represents the best example of secondary retrovirus-induced immunodeficiency in domestic animals.

Stress

Chronic stress is also immunosuppressive and follows an elevation in endogenous glucocorticoid production. A similar effect is seen is **hyperadrenocorticism** in which there is circulating lymphopenia and increased susceptibility to secondary infection. Stress-induced immune suppression is likely to play a major role in susceptibility to infectious disease in intensively reared livestock. Animals housed indoors in high density rearing units or animals transported for long distances in close confines are considered at risk for such immune suppression. **High-intensity exercise** is also immunosuppressive, although milder exercise can enhance a range of immune functions. Young untrained horses have a range of changes in *in-vitro* immune parameters after intensive exercise including reduced proliferative responses of blood lymphocytes, reduced neutrophil function, reduced CD4:CD8 ratio and reduced NK cell function. These effects are associated with elevated plasma cortisol. Interestingly, these effects are not as marked in older horses that may have lower stress responses.

Malnutrition

Severe malnutrition leads to increased susceptibility to infection due to **impairment of T-cell function**, but with sparing of B-cell activity and immunoglobulin production. These effects are thought to be related to **leptin**, an adipokine (cytokine produced by adipocytes) related to body fat mass. An animal suffering malnutrition will have loss of body adipose tissue reserve and reduced concentrations of leptin. As leptin is also immunostimulatory (macrophage and Th1 function) and pro-inflammatory, starvation is associated with immune suppression.

KEY POINTS

- Primary immunodeficiency involves a mutation in a gene encoding a key immunological molecule; such diseases are inherited and congenital.
- Secondary immunodeficiency occurs in an adult with previously normal immune function that is now affected by advancing age, medical therapy or chronic disease.
- Most animal immunodeficiencies have a poorly defined pathogenesis and are considered 'putative' immunodeficiency disorders.
- Primary immunodeficiency is rare.
- Primary immunodeficiency in animals may model equivalent human disorders.
- Primary immunodeficiency may affect the immune system at different levels of development and consequently have a range of clinical presentation from mild to severe life-threatening disease.
- Primary immunodeficiency may be suspected clinically when dealing with chronic recurrent multisystemic infection in related littermate animals of a particular breed.
- Diagnosis of primary immunodeficiency is challenging in the absence of a specific molecular diagnostic test for the precise gene mutation.
- Primary immunodeficiency is most common in dogs and horses.
- SCID occurs in dogs and horses. The disease involves mutation in a cytokine receptor gene (bassett hound, Welsh corgi) or the DNA protein kinase gene (Jack Russell terrier, Arab horse).
- Thymic aplasia and impaired CMI may be associated with hairlessness.

- Cyclic haematopoiesis of the grey collie is a mutation in a gene encoding a molecule related to neutrophil function (cytoplasmic elastase movement).
- The 'trapped neutrophil syndrome' of the border collie involves blood neutropenia due to failure of bone marrow release of neutrophils.
- Leucocyte adhesion deficiency (LAD) occurs in dogs (CLAD) and cattle (BLAD). Affected animals have marked neutrophilia, as these cells cannot migrate into tissues because of a mutation in the gene encoding an integrin (CD18) that mediates the leucocyte–endothelial interaction.
- Selective deficiencies of immunoglobulin classes are recognized in dogs, horses and cattle.
- Complement C3 deficiency occurs in the dog and pig.
- Immunosenescence is an age-related decline in immune function.
- Key features of immunosenescence are reduced CD4 T cells, increased CD8 T cells, reduced CD4:CD8 ratio and preservation of humoral immune responsiveness.
- Medical immunosuppression or chemotherapy leads to secondary immunodeficiency.
- FIV is a T lymphotropic retrovirus that gradually depletes immune cells, leading to terminal chronic multisystemic disease akin to human AIDS.
- Any chronic infectious, inflammatory or neoplastic disease can lead to secondary suppression of immune function.
- Malnutrition and high-intensity exercise are immunosuppressive.

CHAPTER 20

Vaccination

OBJECTIVES

At the end of this chapter you should be able to:
- Discuss the difference between passive and active immunization.
- List the requirements of an ideal vaccine.
- Discuss the difference between infectious and non-infectious vaccines.
- Give examples of genetically engineered vaccines.
- Define the term 'marker vaccine'.

- Understand why it is necessary to give multiple vaccines to neonates.
- Define 'core' and 'non-core' vaccines.
- Define the term 'duration of immunity'.
- Understand the difference between a vaccine data sheet and vaccination guidelines.
- List some possible vaccine side-effects and understand why it is important to report these to an appropriate authority.

INTRODUCTION

Vaccination is the single most common application of immunology to clinical veterinary practice. Although founded on basic immunological principles, the technology and practice of vaccination has changed significantly in recent years. It is crucial that practising veterinarians keep up-to-date with current knowledge in vaccinology in order to provide the best standards of care for their patients. This chapter reviews the fundamentals of vaccination.

PASSIVE IMMUNIZATION

Passive immunization is rarely performed in veterinary medicine; it involves the administration of **preformed antibodies** specific to a particular antigen in order to provide **immediate immunological protection**. The best examples of this process are the use of tetanus antitoxin or the range of antivenoms

developed to counteract snake, arthropod or insect bites. Such antisera are traditionally raised in a large animal species such as the horse or sheep. Serum is collected from hyperimmunized animals and the immunoglobulin harvested from the serum (**Figure 20.1** *overleaf*). These immunoglobulins are antigenic when injected into heterologous species and repeated administration of antitoxins can **sensitize** the recipient for a future **hypersensitivity reaction**. The immunogenicity of the foreign immunoglobulin can be reduced by cleaving the Fc region from the protein and using just the Fab'$_2$ component of the molecule. A further consideration with the use of antitoxins is that their administration will inhibit the ability of the recipient to mount their own endogenous antibody response to the target antigen. For these reasons, the use of passive immunization should be carefully considered and the minimal possible administration undertaken.

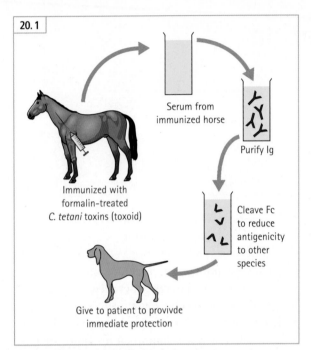

20.1

Serum from
immunized horse

Purify Ig

Immunized with
formalin-treated
C. tetani toxins (toxoid)

Cleave Fc
to reduce
antigenicity
to other
species

Give to patient to provivde
immediate protection

Fig. 20.1 Passive immunization. In this process a large animal species (e.g. horse or sheep) is hyperimmunized with the antigen of interest (e.g. tetanus toxin). The immune serum is harvested and the immunoglobulin fraction purified. This may be further treated to render it less immunogenic in the recipient animal in order to reduce the likelihood of inducing a hypersensitivity response on repeated administration.

ACTIVE IMMUNIZATION

The far more common form of vaccination involves **active immunization** in which an antigen is administered to an individual in order to **induce an immune response** and, most importantly, **immunological memory** of that antigenic exposure. At this time, active immunization of animals is mostly used to generate immune responses to **infectious agents**; these will protect the individual in the case of natural exposure to that organism. The level of protection afforded by different vaccines may vary. Some vaccines induce a very strong protective immunity, which prevents the vaccinated animal being infected by the organism. In other cases the vaccinated animal might become infected but remain clinically well, or develop only a mild form of disease caused by the agent. These levels of protection form the basis of the '**claim**' for the vaccine and will be clearly defined on the **data sheet** (or in Europe the 'summary of product characteristics', SPC) that accompanies the product.

No vaccine currently marketed is perfect and consistently able to afford the highest level of protection to every single animal that receives it. The **properties of an ideal vaccine** should include:

- Being **inexpensive** to produce in large quantity.
- Being **consistent in formulation** with minimal variation between batches.
- Being **stable** without a requirement for specialized storage conditions (e.g. refrigeration).
- Having a **long shelf-life**.
- Being able to induce the most **appropriate type of immune response** to afford protection from infection with the specific organism under consideration.
- Incorporating a **range of immunodominant epitopes** from the target organism in order to activate multiple clones of antigen-specific T and B lymphocytes.
- The ability to induce a **long-lived immune response**.
- The ability to induce **immunological memory**.
- Having **no adverse side-effects**.

Current advances in vaccine technology rely on a clear understanding of the immunological principles expounded earlier in this text. The finding that has most revolutionized vaccine development has been that of the functional dichotomy in CD4⁺ T-cell subsets and the fact that for particular infections either a Th1/Th17 or Th2 response might provide optimal protective immunity (see Chapters 8 and 13). Modern vaccines seek to **replicate the optimum T-cell and cytokine response** that is best able to eliminate a specific infectious agent. For example, vaccines currently under development for canine leishmaniosis (see Chapter 13) aim to preferentially trigger a Th1-regulated response with active production of IFN-γ.

The range of different veterinary vaccines is reviewed below, but fundamentally these may be considered as **infectious** or **non-infectious** vaccines. The most effective vaccines are those that retain the ability to infect an animal (without causing disease). Providing an animal is immunocompetent and vaccinated at the correct age, a single dose of such an infectious vaccine effectively protects that animal. In contrast, non-infectious vaccines are generally less efficacious and require up to three doses to be given several weeks apart. In the case of non-infectious vaccines the first dose **primes** the immune system, the second dose **immunizes** and the third dose **boosts** that immunity. The nature of infectious vaccines (see below) means that priming, immunization and boosting may all be achieved through a single exposure. A range of vaccine formulations are currently marketed for domestic animals. These range from relatively old and crude preparations (which are still highly effective) through to modern genetically engineered products.

INFECTIOUS VACCINES

Live virulent vaccines

Vaccines incorporating the **live and virulent form** of an infectious agent are relatively **uncommon** due to the obvious risk of inducing clinical disease rather than protection. The best example of such a product is that designed to protect sheep from the zoonotic parapoxvirus infection orf (contagious ecthyma). This vaccine is administered by scarification into the skin of the sheep.

Live attenuated vaccines

This class of vaccine is the single **most commonly used** in veterinary medicine. These vaccines are based on the use of an **intact and viable organism** that has been 'attenuated' to reduce its virulence. Live attenuated organisms are capable of inducing

low-level infection and replicating within the animal, but **do not induce significant tissue pathology or clinical disease**. Traditional means of attenuation might involve passaging the organisms multiple times through cell cultures or **heating** the organisms to develop temperature-sensitive mutants. An alternative approach might be to use an antigenically related organism that is able to induce immunity but not cause disease or an adverse reaction. An example of this approach is the use of canine adenovirus (CAV)-2 to protect against disease caused by both CAV-1 and CAV-2 without the risk of the dog developing 'blue eye' (corneal oedema secondary to immune complex uveitis) as a side-effect of vaccination with CAV-1 (see Chapter 12). A more refined means of attenuation is to use molecular techniques to produce genetically modified organisms from which **virulence genes have been deleted or modified**. An example of this approach has been the development of vaccines for pseudorabies (Aujeszky's disease) in pigs in which the thymidine kinase gene has been deleted from the causative herpesvirus.

However, there are specific safety issues related to live attenuated vaccines. These carry a theoretical risk of '**reversion to virulence**' whereby the attenuated vaccine strain might 'recapture' virulence genes from field organisms by recombination, allowing them to induce clinical disease rather than protection. Some live attenuated vaccines intended for injection (e.g. feline herpesvirus, FHV) may **induce disease** if they are accidentally aerosolized during administration or groomed by the animal from the cutaneous site of administration. The nature of large-scale manufacture of live attenuated vaccines also carries a theoretical risk that a particular vaccine might become **contaminated** with another unrelated organism if the production line used to produce both products is not adequately disinfected between production runs. Finally, live attenuated vaccines are **less stable** than killed products and require more specialized storage conditions (i.e. they are often formulated as freeze dried pellets that require refrigeration).

Heterologous vaccines

A heterologous vaccine incorporates an organism that is **antigenically related** to the target infectious agent, but is **adapted to another host** species. The best example of such an approach is the use of human measles virus to protect against the related morbillivirus CDV. The measles virus vaccine can be used to immunize pups 2–4 weeks earlier than with CDV vaccine, when the pups may still have maternally derived CDV antibody. The measles virus vaccine provides only transient immunity and the pups must still receive CDV vaccine when they are older. This procedure is no longer widely practised.

Recombinant organism vaccines

One of the most recent developments in veterinary vaccinology is the use of **recombinant organism vaccines**. In this technique a **benign 'carrier organism'** is genetically modified to incorporate a gene from an unrelated pathogen. The carrier organism expresses the gene within the host. This method has the advantage of the carrier organism being more readily taken up by APCs and triggering a more effective (often Th1 or cell-mediated) protective immune response (**Figure 20.2**). Experimentally, a range of **carrier viruses** (e.g. vaccina virus or adenovirus) have been studied and for mucosal delivery **bacteria** may be used as carriers (e.g. an attenuated strain of *Salmonella*). In veterinary medicine, the **canarypox virus** has been successfully employed as a carrier for genes derived from FeLV, CDV, rabies virus, West Nile virus and equine influenza virus. These vaccines induce very potent protective immune responses and are even capable of inducing **immunity in the face of levels of maternally derived immunoglobulin** that would block the effect of traditional live attenuated virus vaccines (see Chapter 18). The avian virus is unable to induce disease in the mammalian host and the vaccinated animal appears not to make a significant immune response to the canarypox, permitting repeated use of the vaccine. These vaccines have the added advantage of **not requiring adjuvant**, which

makes them attractive alternatives to adjuvanted FeLV or rabies vaccines. Finally, recombinant vaccines cannot **revert to virulence** as they do not contain live target virus.

Marker vaccines

A further recent advance is the development of 'marker vaccines'. Many infections are diagnosed by the detection of serum antibody as evidence of exposure (e.g. Lyme borreliosis, FIV), but as

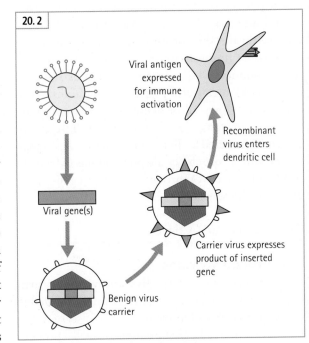

Fig. 20.2 Preparation of a recombinant organism vaccine. The gene of interest encoding an immunodominant antigen known to induce a protective immune response is taken from the pathogen and inserted into a carrier organism (e.g. canarypox virus). On injection, the carrier organism is taken up by an APC. The protein of interest is therefore ideally placed to enter the processing pathways of that cell and there is very effective presentation of peptides associated with MHC molecules. The APC relocates from the site of injection to the regional lymphoid tissue for induction of the T-cell response.

vaccination also induces serum antibody, it has traditionally been difficult to **discriminate between vaccinal and exposure titres**. Marker vaccines have now been developed to make this distinction possible. An excellent example of such a product is the marker vaccine for infectious bovine rhinotracheitis (IBR). The virus contained in this product has deletion of the gene encoding surface glycoprotein E; therefore, if a cow has serum antibody to glycoprotein E, this must have been generated by exposure to field virus rather than by vaccination (**Figure 20.3**). Development of a marker vaccine requires parallel development of an **appropriate diagnostic test**. Marker vaccines are also known as DIVA (differentiating infected from vaccinated animals) vaccines.

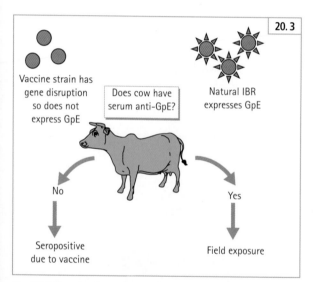

Fig. 20.3 Preparation of a marker vaccine. A marker vaccine permits discrimination between a vaccinal and an exposure immune response. The IBR vaccine incorporates a genetically modified virus that does not express glycoprotein E. A serological test is developed in parallel with the vaccine. Any cow that has serum antibody to glycoprotein E must have been exposed to field virus.

NON-INFECTIOUS VACCINES

Killed whole organism vaccines

A killed whole organism vaccine includes an organism that is **antigenically intact** but clearly **unable to replicate or induce pathology or clinical disease**. There are various means of producing killed vaccines, most often by treating the vaccinal organisms with **chemicals** such as formalin, alcohol or alkylating agents.

Differences between infectious and non-infectious whole organism vaccines

These two broad classes of vaccine have distinct properties related to the nature of the product. In general, a **live attenuated vaccine will induce more effective immunity** than a killed product containing the same organism. The reasons for this include:

- The limited **replication** of a live vaccine means an increase in antigen concentration during the immediate period following vaccination.
- Live vaccine organisms may be able more readily to **move to anatomical sites relevant** to the route of natural infection.
- Live vaccines may contain both **structural and expressed (secreted) antigens**.
- Live vaccine organisms are more likely to **replicate intracellularly** and to be presented in such a fashion that a **cytotoxic T-cell** response is induced.

As live vaccines have greater efficacy, **fewer doses** may be required in order to induce the same level of protective immunity compared with a killed vaccine. Live vaccines may also have **greater safety** than a killed product, as most **killed vaccines require an adjuvant** (see Chapter 2) in order to stimulate an adequate immune response. Vaccines containing adjuvants are generally regarded as more likely to induce adverse events. **Adjuvanted vaccines** are also more likely to induce **Th2-mediated humoral immune responses** compared with live attenuated products.

Subunit vaccines

A subunit vaccine does not contain an entire intact organism, but rather specific **immunogenic structural proteins or metabolites derived from that organism**. A good example of a subunit vaccine is the FeLV vaccine that incorporates glycoprotein 70 (gp70) extracted from the virus grown in cell culture. It is also possible to produce **synthetic peptides** based on knowledge of the structure of the antigenic protein of interest, but synthetic peptide vaccines require an adjuvant and produce immune responses of very restricted antigenic specificity.

Another means of producing a subunit vaccine is through the use of **recombinant DNA technology**. The gene encoding an immunogenic molecule of interest (able to induce a protective immune response) is inserted into a **bacterial plasmid** (generally *Escherichia coli*) so that there is expression by the organisms and the **recombinant protein** can be harvested from cultures and incorporated into a vaccine (**Figure 20.4**). Recombinant protein vaccines also require an adjuvant to induce optimum immunity. Examples of such products are the FeLV vaccine that incorporates a recombinant version of the p45 antigen mixed with adjuvant and the *Borrelia* vaccine for dogs, which includes a recombinant version of the immunodominant outer surface protein (OSP)-A of the organism.

Naked DNA vaccines

The current forefront of vaccine development is that of the **naked DNA vaccine**. In this instance a gene of interest from the pathogen is inserted into a **bacterial plasmid, which is injected directly into the animal** without the need for a carrier organism. The plasmids may be injected by needle (as current veterinary products), administered mucosally (with appropriate protectants) or fired through the epidermis associated with tiny gold particles. The principle of this method involves the **plasmids transfecting host cells at the site of injection,** particularly **APCs**. The pathogen gene is expressed within the APC and the protein enters the processing pathways for MHC expression (**Figure 20.5**). Naked

DNA vaccination triggers a **very potent mixed cell-mediated and humoral immune response** that provides exceptionally effective protection. Such vaccines may be used in young animals **in the face of maternally derived antibody**. The best example of such a product is that used to protect horses from infection by West Nile virus. Naked DNA technology has also been examined experimentally for CDV, FIV

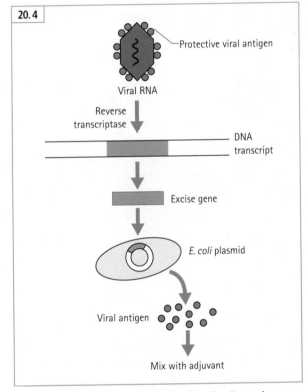

Fig. 20.4 Preparation of a recombinant subunit vaccine. In this example the p45 protein from FeLV is produced in recombinant form for incorporation into a vaccine. The retroviral RNA encoding p45 is first reverse transcribed into DNA and the gene of interest is excised with restriction endonucleases. This gene is then inserted into a bacterial plasmid (typically *E. coli*). The bacteria are cultured in bulk and the secreted protein harvested. Recombinant proteins require an adjuvant to induce a vaccinal immune response.

and rabies virus protection in small animals. A single injection of plasmid incorporating the gene for rabies glycoprotein G, given intradermally into the pinna of beagle dogs, leads to the development of serum neutralizing antibody and affords protection from challenge with virulent virus one year post vaccination. The canine melanoma vaccine described in Chapter 14 is a naked DNA vaccine.

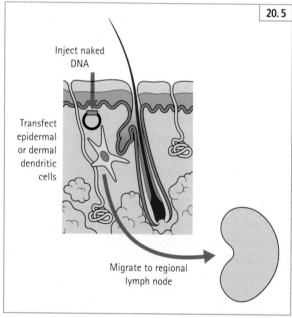

Fig. 20.5 Preparation of a naked DNA vaccine. The gene of interest from a pathogen is incorporated into a bacterial plasmid, which is directly injected into the animal. The plasmid transfects local host cells, including APCs that migrate to the regional lymphoid tissue. Expression of the gene within the APC leads to ready access of the protein to the antigen processing pathways of the cell and effective presentation of peptides for induction of the T-cell response.

VACCINES OTHER THAN FOR INFECTIOUS DISEASE

Traditional vaccines have been designed to protect individuals from the risk of infectious disease and have been highly successful in so doing. The next generation of vaccines will have a range of other applications in the treatment (**therapeutic vaccines**) and prevention of **allergic**, **autoimmune** and **neoplastic diseases**. Vast research effort has been focused on the development of **cancer vaccines**, but of note is the fact that the first commercially available cancer vaccine was for dogs rather than man (see Chapter 14). Another commercially available vaccine is that used to prevent 'boar taint' in pork production. The vaccine induces an immune response to gonadotrophin-releasing hormone (GnRH), which removes the stimulus for production of leuteinizing hormone and follicle-stimulating hormone and, in turn, the effects of these hormones on testosterone production. In effect, the vaccine produces an 'immunological castration', which has welfare benefits when compared with castration practised without anaesthesia or analgesia.

MUCOSAL VACCINES

A number of vaccines used in various species are designed to be delivered across a **mucosal barrier** and, consequently, to stimulate high levels of **local** (as opposed to systemic) **immunity** most relevant to the site of infection by the pathogen (e.g. mucosal IgA production). **Intranasal vaccination** of individual animals is therefore practised in order to protect them from respiratory pathogens such as IBR virus, equine *Streptococcus equi*, canine *Bordetella* and parainfluenza virus, and feline calicivirus and herpesvirus-1. Mucosal delivery has also been used for delivery of vaccines to groups of animals; for example, by **aerosolization** of Newcastle disease vaccine for poultry or **administration in feed or water** for a range of poultry vaccines. Some fish vaccines are administered by **immersion**, allowing uptake by swallowing or absorption via the gills or oral cavity.

NEEDLE-FREE VACCINATION

One FeLV vaccine is currently licensed for delivery using a needle-free system. This apparatus is a modification of one developed for the **transdermal administration** of drugs (e.g. insulin) in man. The vaccine (recombinant canarypox FeLV) is delivered at high pressure transdermally where it can readily transfect APCs for induction of the protective immune response (**Figure 20.6**). The sensitivity of this method is such that a reduced dose of vaccine can be administered and the procedure removes the need for needle administration (at least of this single component). When not properly assembled, the apparatus has been reported to cause femoral fractures in kittens due to detachment of the nozzle when activated. The canine melanoma vaccine (see Chapter 14) is also delivered with this device.

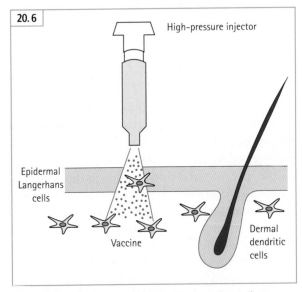

Fig. 20.6 Needle-free vaccination. This procedure utilizes a high-pressure transdermal injection apparatus adapted from human medicine to inject the vaccine (currently the canarypox-vectored FeLV vaccine or canine melanoma vaccine). This specifically targets dendritic cells of the epidermis (Langerhans cells) and dermis for very efficient antigen uptake, processing and presentation.

FUTURE VACCINE DEVELOPMENTS

Numerous developments are likely to occur in the field of vaccinology in the next decades. **More therapeutic vaccines** are likely to be developed and a number of such products are currently in clinical trial for human diseases. **New adjuvants** are likely to be produced that induce more effective Th1 and cytotoxic T-cell responses while attempting to reduce the risks associated with the use of traditional substances such as alum. **Molecular adjuvants** such as recombinant cytokines, cytokine genes incorporated into plasmids or small bacterial nucleotide sequences rich in cytosine and guanidine (CpG motifs) are all potent means of enhancing protective Th1 immune responses.

Novel strategies for vaccination are likely to be introduced; for example the increasing use of **mucosal delivery** with specific '**mucosal adjuvants**' (e.g. bacterially derived toxins) or '**prime-boost**' **protocols** involving priming with a DNA vaccine and then boosting with the equivalent protein product (or vice versa). Another exciting innovation is the delivery of vaccines in foodstuffs. Plants (e.g. bananas or potatoes) can be genetically engineered to express molecules from microorganisms and induce immunity following ingestion of the foodstuff. This has clear benefit for widespread vaccination programmes in developing countries. The approach has already been used in poultry production where it has been possible to genetically engineer a tobacco plant expressing a gene from the Newcastle disease virus. A further innovation in poultry vaccination has been the mechanized delivery of vaccination *in ovo* (i.e. into the egg).

BASIC PRINCIPLES OF VACCINATION

It is beyond the scope of this chapter to give details of all of the currently licensed veterinary vaccines and the recommended schedules by which these are given. Instead, some general principles for vaccination are given below as the '**ten commandments**' **for vaccine use**:

1. **Vaccination is a medical procedure** and the decision on which vaccines to administer to an individual animal or herd should be based on knowledge of local infectious disease risk. **Not every animal necessarily requires every vaccine**. Although vaccines are extremely safe, minimizing vaccine use reduces the risk of any potential adverse consequence of the procedure.

2. In keeping with the concept in (1), vaccines should be considered as 'core' or 'non-core'. A **core vaccine** is one that **every animal of a species should receive**, as the infectious disease that it protects from is widespread and leads to significant morbidity or mortality. **Not every animal requires a 'non-core' vaccine** that protects from a disease that the animal may not be exposed to because of lifestyle or geographical location. Vaccines considered core and non-core for small companion animals are listed in *Table 20.1*.

Some vaccines for which there is little scientific evidence of proven value are regarded as 'not recommended' by expert groups.

3. Vaccines should be administered to **as many animals as possible within a herd or population**. This relates to the concept of **'herd immunity'** whereby a certain level (generally quoted as 75% of a human population) of vaccine protection reduces the likelihood of disease endemics. When vaccine coverage of a population falls below this level, infectious diseases may re-emerge.

4. Maternally derived antibody (MDA) will interfere with the ability of young animals to respond to the majority of currently available vaccines. **Young animals** therefore require a **series of priming immunizations** followed by a **booster vaccine**, generally given 12 months after the priming series or at 12 months of age. The reasons for this approach are discussed in Chapter 18.

TABLE 20.1. CLASSIFICATION OF CANINE AND FELINE VACCINES

	Core	Non-core	Not recommended
Canine vaccines	Distemper	Parainfluenza	Coronavirus
	Adenovirus	*Bordetella*	*Giardia*
	Parvovirus	*Leptospira*	
	Rabies in endemic areas	*Borrelia*	
Feline vaccines	Parvovirus	Feline leukaemia virus	Feline immunodeficiency virus
	Herpesvirus	*Chlamydophila*	Feline infectious peritonitis virus
	Calicivirus	*Bordetella*	
	Rabies in endemic areas		*Giardia*

5. In general, adult animals should be vaccinated as infrequently as legal requirements, current best practice guidelines and quality of the vaccine permits. The revaccination of adult animals currently depends on the licensed 'duration of immunity' (DOI) of a vaccine. DOI is a legal term that describes the length of time after vaccination that an animal is deemed to have protective immunity. This is demonstrated by challenging a group of vaccinated animals with a virulent infectious agent (at a defined time point post vaccination) and determining if they are protected (typically a minimum of 80% of this group must be protected) relative to unvaccinated controls (typically a minimum of 80% of this group must develop disease or die). An indirect measure of DOI for some vaccines is the persistence of a serum antibody titre deemed as 'protective' (for some vaccines there is excellent correlation between protection and serum antibody titre). Most licensed vaccines are supported by studies that demonstrate only the **minimum** rather than the **maximum DOI**. For example, most small companion animal infectious viral vaccines currently carry a legal minimum DOI of 3 or 4 years, when in reality the products provide much longer protection (which may be up to the lifetime of the animal). Regulatory authorities also require 'field studies' of how a vaccine might protect herd animals in a natural farm situation where an infectious disease is endemic.

6. Vaccines should **only** be administered to **pregnant animals** if this procedure is **supported by data sheet recommendations**. If inappropriately used, some vaccines may induce abortion or teratogenic effects. In contrast, the use of some vaccines is indicated during pregnancy in order to ensure good colostral titres of protective antibody.

7. Vaccines should **not be administered to animals that are ill or medically immunosuppressed**. The optimum vaccinal response requires a competent immune system.

8. The decision on which vaccines should be administered should arise from **consultation between veterinarian and client**. Current vaccination **guidelines** from expert groups may conflict with **data sheet recommendations**, as guidelines present up-to-date scientific thinking and data sheets may be historical documents. In most countries, legal advice is that it is possible to use vaccines other than stipulated by data sheets provided that informed client consent is obtained and documented.

9. Always **read and understand the vaccine data sheet** and follow the instructions therein (unless these are modified by current guidelines as in (8)).

10. **Detailed records** should be kept of the vaccines administered to animals (including batch numbers and site of administration). Animals should be monitored for **adverse effects** following vaccination and these should be notified to the appropriate **reporting authority**. By gathering such **pharmacovigilance data** we will learn more about vaccine adverse reactions (see p. 244).

Other vaccine facts that should be considered relate to vaccine formulation and individual variability in response. Veterinarians are often concerned about the **number of components included in some multivalent vaccines** and whether each of these can induce a protective immune response. Experimentally, this is always the case, as multi-component vaccines are not licensed unless protective efficacy can be demonstrated for all components. The immune system is perfectly capable of responding to multiple antigens simultaneously. However, in small companion animals, recent epidemiological data have suggested that the greater the number of components included at one time of vaccination, the greater the likelihood of adverse effects. In canine vaccination it is often questioned why the chihuahua and Great Dane receive the same dose of vaccine when pharmacological products would be given by dose rate. The immunological answer to this question is that the immune repertoire of both breeds is the same and the number of antigen-specific lymphocytes is not greater in larger animals. Breeders of small breed dogs often ask that vaccine doses be split for their animals, but this practice is contrary to data sheet recommendations and should not be encouraged. However, it is of note that small breed dogs do have a higher incidence of adverse effects following vaccination (particularly allergic reactions following the use of adjuvanted bacterins) and appear to make higher serological responses (to rabies vaccine) than larger breed dogs. This latter observation has recently been explored in a study that demonstrated wide differences in breed response to rabies vaccination (**Figure 20.7**). **Breed differences in vaccine responsiveness** may well be related to the MHC background of the dogs as MHC alleles are often strongly restricted in particular purebreeds. It is worth highlighting the rottweiler as a breed known to make poor responses to vaccination (in particular for canine parvovirus).

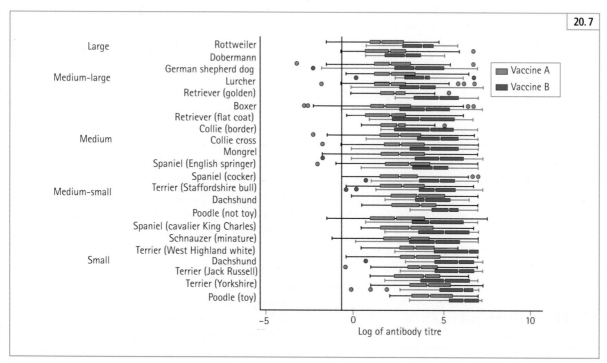

Fig. 20.7 Breed differences in response to rabies virus vaccine. This graph presents the differences in serological titres to rabies vaccination achieved by dogs of different breeds. These were all naïve animals receiving a primary course of vaccine for pet travel from the UK. Small breed dogs make the highest responses and rottweilers and Dobermanns achieve the lowest antibody titres. (Reprinted with permission from Kennedy LJ, Lunt M, Barnes A *et al.* (2007) Factors influencing the antibody response of dogs vaccinated against rabies. *Vaccine* **25**:8500–8507.)

VACCINE HUSBANDRY

The single most common cause for failure of a vaccine to protect an animal from infectious disease (**lack of efficacy**) is not adhering to the manufacturer's recommendations for use and storage of vaccines. Although these are very simple concepts, they are often forgotten in clinical practice. Aspects of 'vaccine husbandry' include:

- Vaccines (and particularly adjuvanted vaccines) have an optimum storage temperature (described on the data sheet), which is usually between 2 and 8°C (domestic refrigerators should be at 4°C). These products should not be frozen or positioned adjacent to the freezer compartment of the refrigerator, and the refrigerator temperature should be monitored regularly. Vaccines transported into the field should also be subject to continuation of the '**cold chain**'.
- Freeze-dried vaccines should be reconstituted immediately before use with appropriate diluent or liquid vaccine given concurrently (as per manufacturer's recommendations). It is not good practice to make up the vaccines anticipated to be used during the day first thing in the morning. Some vaccine components (e.g. CDV, FHV-1) are particularly labile in this regard.
- Vaccines should only be mixed together in the same syringe if this is specified in the manufacturer's data sheets.
- Vaccine injection sites should not be sterilized with alcohol as this may inactivate infectious vaccines.
- Vaccines should be 'in date' and precise details of batch numbers, components and site of injection should be noted in the animal's medical record.

ADVERSE CONSEQUENCES OF VACCINATION

Over the past two decades there has been mounting concern in both human and small companion animal populations about the potential risks of vaccination. In man, these debates have been widely aired by the media and include the erroneous proposed association between multicomponent products (e.g. measles, mumps and rubella) and autism and Crohn's disease. Similar public knowledge concerning specific animal adverse effects, such as FISS and canine IMHA, has been an issue for the veterinary profession.

At the outset it should be emphasized that **adverse effects following vaccination are rare** and that the **benefits of vaccination far outweigh any risks**. In Western countries, millions of animals are vaccinated every year, but very few adverse consequences are reported. It is recognized that the passive nature of reporting schemes is a barrier to gathering high-quality data on adverse effects, but where quantification of risk has been attempted, figures in the region of less than one to 50 adverse effects (no matter how minor) per 10,000 doses of vaccine sold or administered have been calculated.

A wide spectrum of adverse effects is recognized. Those that are generally reported relate to a medical consequence of vaccination. The single most common event is the onset of **transient pyrexia and lethargy** in the immediate few days post vaccination. This effect relates to initiation of the immune response and cytokine production and is not unexpected after a vaccine (particularly an adjuvanted product) has been administered. Surprisingly, there is also some evidence that vaccination may induce a **transient period of immunosuppression** in animals and on rare occasion this might lead to problems such as the emergence of subclinical infection in the vaccinate. Another relatively common occurrence involves a **type I hypersensitivity response within minutes of administration** of a vaccine (**Figure 20.8**). These usually manifest (in cats and dogs) as an acute episode of pruritus or cutaneous oedema (often facial oedema) and are rarely life threatening. Such reactions may occur again with subsequent vaccination. Studies in the dog have revealed that this type of response is related to the **inclusion of excipient proteins** (e.g. bovine serum albumin, BSA) within vaccines. Vaccinated dogs develop both IgE and IgG responses to BSA. Where such responses occur during the primary puppy or kitten vaccination series, it is thought to relate to maternal transfer of these reagenic antibodies.

Vaccines have been associated with a range of other secondary immune-mediated sequelae including examples of type II (e.g. **IMHA or immune-mediated thrombocytopenia**) or type III (e.g. **rabies vaccine-associated cutaneous vasculitis**) hypersensitivity reactions. With few exceptions, the immunopathogenesis of such reactions is poorly defined.

The most serious veterinary vaccine reaction is that of **FISS**. This lesion was first reported in the USA in 1989, but has since been recognized worldwide and continues to be a major problem. FISS is a highly **malignant and deeply invasive sarcoma** that develops in the **skin of cats**, most often at **sites related to previous injection**. Although a range of injectables has been linked to FISS, the **adjuvanted FeLV and rabies vaccines** are most often incriminated. The pathogenesis of these tumours is now thought to involve an initial **chronic inflammatory response, stimulated by adjuvant (Figure 20.9)**, that leads to local **transformation of mesenchymal cells** and development of clinical malignancy. Histologically, these tumours are most often fibrosarcomas, but differentiation of mesenchyme towards other matrix

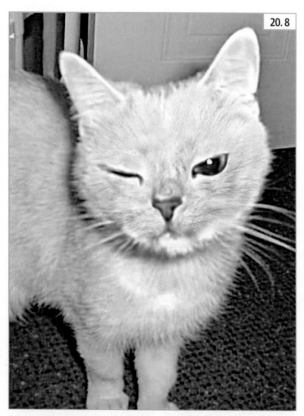

Fig. 20.8 Hypersensitivity response following vaccination. This cat has been very recently vaccinated and developed sudden onset facial oedema. Such reactions are thought to represent IgE-mediated type I hypersensitivity reactions to excipients, such as bovine serum, contained within vaccines, albumin.

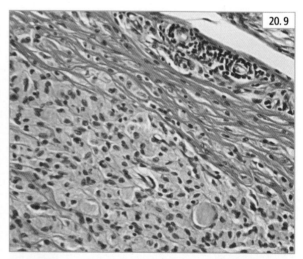

Fig. 20.9 Adjuvant-induced inflammation. This histological section reveals the chronic granulomatous inflammatory response that persists for long periods following administration of adjuvanted vaccine. The grey–blue material within the cytoplasm of macrophages and multinucleate giant cells is alum, the most commonly used adjuvant in human and veterinary vaccines.

elements may occur (**Figures 20.10, 20.11**). The surgical excision of FISS is challenging and the tumours carry a poor prognosis. A novel adjunct immunotherapy for FISS has been described in Chapter 14. The 1996 recommendation of a USA guidelines group that the adjuvanted FeLV and rabies vaccines should be administered distally in a hindlimb appears to have reduced the prevalence of FISS in the interscapular region, which was the traditional predilection site and site of vaccine administration. However, injections to this site are not easy to perform and current guidelines advise that feline vaccines might best be delivered into the skin overlying the abdomen and rotated to different locations on each occasion of vaccination. A recent study has suggested that cats may be vaccinated safely into the skin of the tail and that they show seroconversion to rabies virus and feline parvovirus after that procedure.

A range of other types of adverse reaction to vaccination is recognized in animals and should also be reported to the appropriate authorities. These include '**lack of efficacy**' (i.e. failure of the vaccine to protect from infectious disease), **reversion to virulence** or **batch contamination** (see above).

For further details of current issues and procedures relating to the vaccination of small companion animals the reader is referred to the various **guidelines documents** produced by organizations such as the American Association of Feline Practitioners, the American Animal Hospital Association, the World Small Animal Veterinary Association and the European Advisory Board on Cat Diseases. These guidelines are all readily accessible through the websites of these organizations. A set of equine vaccination guidelines is currently being developed.

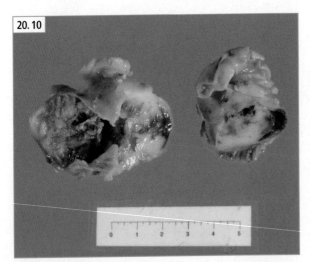

Fig. 20.10 Feline injection site sarcoma. A surgically excised mass from the interscapular region of a cat. The mass consists of firm white tissue with a necrotic cavitated centre. The tumour tissue infiltrates muscle at the margins of the excision.

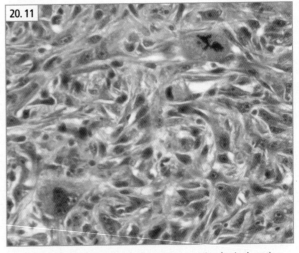

Fig. 20.11 Feline injection site sarcoma. Histological section from the mass shown in **Figure 20.10**. The tumour comprises a highly pleomorphic population of spindle cells including multinucleate cells (bottom left of image). A bizarre mitotic figure is present in one cell (top right of image).

KEY POINTS

- Passive immunization involves administration of pre-formed antibodies to provide immediate protection, typically from the effects of a toxin or venom.
- Active immunization involves administration of an antigen (typically an infectious agent or subcomponent of that agent) in order to induce an immune response and immunological memory.
- The ideal vaccine is cheap to produce, consistent in formulation, stable with a long shelf-life, and able to induce an appropriate and long-lived immune response with good immunological memory, in the absence of side-effects.
- Live virulent infectious vaccines are rare.
- Live attenuated infectious vaccines are common. Attenuation is achieved by growing an organism under unusual conditions or by genetically modifying it to eliminate virulence gene/s.
- A heterologous infectious vaccine is antigenically related to the organism of interest, but adapted to another host species.
- Killed non-infectious vaccines remain antigenically intact, but cannot replicate. Killed vaccines require adjuvant.
- Infectious vaccines are more effective than non-infectious vaccines.
- Subunit non-infectious vaccines contain a relevant structure or secreted molecule from a pathogen and require an adjuvant.
- Recombinant organism vaccines use a benign carrier virus or bacterium to transport a gene encoding an antigen from a pathogen able to induce a protective immune response.
- Naked DNA vaccines use a bacterial plasmid to directly carry the gene encoding a protein of interest from the pathogen. The gene transfects host APCs and is expressed within them.
- Marker vaccines discriminate serological responses due to vaccine from those due to field exposure to the organism.
- Therapeutic vaccines for allergy, autoimmunity and cancer are being developed.
- Not every animal requires every vaccine.
- A core vaccine is one that every animal should receive as the disease that it protects from is widespread and causes significant morbidity or mortality.
- A non-core vaccine protects from a disease that not every animal may be exposed to.
- Herd immunity ensures that an entire population has the greatest chance of resisting infection from endemic pathogens.
- Neonatal vaccination requires multiple immunizations in order to avoid the effects of MDA.
- Vaccines with the longest DOI should be used. DOI is the time after vaccination that the animal remains protected from disease.
- Vaccines should only be used in pregnant animals if licensed for such use.
- Ill or immunosuppressed animals should not be vaccinated.
- Vaccine guidelines are the bridge between current scientific thought and historical data sheet recommendations.
- Detailed records of vaccination should be kept and adverse reactions should be reported.
- Genetic background may determine how individual animals respond to vaccines.
- Vaccines should be stored and reconstituted according to manufacturer's instructions.
- Adverse effects following vaccination are rare.
- Adverse reactions may be mild and transient or severe and life threatening (e.g. FISS).

CHAPTER 21

Immunotherapy

OBJECTIVES

At the end of this chapter you should be able to:
- Discuss the mode of action of glucocorticoids, cytotoxic adjunct immunosuppressive drugs and ciclosporin in the management of immune-mediated disease.
- Appreciate the limited range of veterinary products with immunostimulatory effects.
- Discuss the mode of action of allergen-specific immunotherapy in the management of allergic disease.
- Discuss the mode of action of intravenous immunoglobulin (IVIG) therapy in immune-mediated disease.

- Discuss the basis of recombinant cytokine therapy in human and veterinary medicine.
- Describe the future possibilities for cytokine gene therapy.
- Discuss the use of monoclonal antibody therapy in human medicine.
- Describe new approaches to tolerance induction in autoimmune and allergic diseases of man.
- Discuss the use of gene therapy for treatment of monogenic disorders.
- Give examples of 'alternative' therapies that may modulate immune function.

INTRODUCTION

Preceding chapters have described the wide range of immune-mediated diseases that may affect domestic animals. These are of greatest consequence in companion animal species, which are generally longer lived and have much closer contact with their human owners. There is great demand for medical management of these diseases and a requirement for products that might either suppress (e.g. in autoimmunity or allergy) or amplify (e.g. in immunodeficiency, infectious or neoplastic disease) immune function. Unfortunately, this requirement is poorly met by the availability of safe and effective medicines. The range of immunosuppressive drugs currently used in animals has been adopted from human medicine. These drugs are often used empirically without solid pharmacokinetic studies and most are not specifically licensed veterinary products. There are even fewer options available as a means of stimulating immune function and again most such agents are unlicensed. This chapter reviews these products and also describes recent advances in human immunotherapy that may potentially flow through to veterinary medicine in the future.

IMMUNOSUPPRESSIVE AGENTS

Glucocorticoids

The most widely used immunosuppressive drugs in veterinary medicine are the glucocorticoids. A range of these agents is available (for systemic or local administration); they differ in terms of their **formulation, potency** of their effect and their **duration of action** (*Table 21.1*). Glucocorticoids have both an **anti-inflammatory** and an **immunosuppressive** capacity dependent on the dose rate employed. Glucocorticoids are absorbed through the membrane of the target cell, where they bind to **intracytoplasmic receptor** molecules. The combination of drug and receptor then moves to the nucleus, where **binding to DNA** leads to **activation of genes** with eventual production of proteins involved in cellular function (**Figure 21.1**). Glucocorticoids have effects on a range of leucocytes. They cause **stabilization of the cell membrane** of granulocytes, mast cells and macrophages, thereby inhibiting the production of inflammatory mediators and pro-inflammatory cytokines (i.e. IL-1, IL-6 and TNF-α) by these cells. Glucocorticoids are **inhibitory of T-cell function**, although evidence from rodent models suggests that these effects may sometimes be more subtle and involve altering the balance between the functional T-cell subsets. In contrast, **B cells** are thought to have **greater resistance** to the effects of these drugs, although the inhibition of T-cell help will have indirect consequences for B-cell activation. Glucocorticoids may inhibit the action of complement molecules and interfere with immunoglobulin function by **downregulation of Fc receptor expression** by phagocytic cells.

Much of this information regarding glucocorticoid function is derived from human medicine and studies in experimental rodent systems. There have been surprisingly few investigations specifically addressing the immunological effects of this class of drug in

TABLE 21.1. RELATIVE ANTI-INFLAMMATORY POTENCY OF GLUCOCORTICOIDS

Glucocorticoid	Relative potency	Duration of action
Cortisone	0.8	Short acting
Hydrocortisone	1.0	Short acting
Prednisolone/prednisone	4.0	Intermediate
Methylprednisolone	5.0	Intermediate
Triamcinolone	5.0	Intermediate*
Flumethasone	15.0	Long acting
Dexamethasone	30.0	Long acting
Betamethasone	35.0	Long acting

Short acting, <12 hours; intermediate acting, 12–36 hours; long acting, >48 hours.

* Triamcinolone may act for up to 48 hours.

Prednisone and cortisone must first be activated in the liver to prednisolone and cortisol, respectively.

other animal species. There may be specific species differences with respect to glucocorticoid action; for example, the **cat** is regarded as a relatively '**steroid-resistant**' animal and requires higher doses of these drugs to cause immunosuppression relative to the dose rate for the dog. This difference is thought to relate to a **lower expression of glucocorticoid receptors** in target tissues of the cat.

Two studies have examined the immunological effects of glucocorticoid administration in clinically normal dogs. The first such investigation compared the effects of administering prednisolone (at the immunosuppressive dose rate of 2 mg/kg q12h) with azathioprine (see p. 253), or both drugs in combination, for a 14-day period. The phenotype of blood lymphocytes and concentrations of serum IgG, IgM and IgA were determined after the treatment period. Prednisolone-treated beagles had reduced concentrations of all classes of immunoglobulin and reduction in CD4+ and CD8+ T cells and B lymphocytes within the circulation. No significant changes were seen with azathioprine monotherapy, but this probably relates to the fact that this drug has a 'lead-in' time of around 10 days before any effect becomes manifest. Combination therapy had more subtle effects, with selective reduction in IgG concentration and lowering of CD8+ T cells, with a consequent increase in the CD4:CD8 ratio. The second study examined the effect on lymph node populations of lymphocytes of giving an immunosuppressive dose of prednisone to normal dogs for a 3-day period. Surprisingly, even with this short duration of therapy there was a reduction in T cells (specifically CD4+ cells) within the aspirated population. One study has examined the effect of oral prednisolone (10 mg total dose q24h) on the immune function of healthy cats. The percentage of both CD4+ and CD8+ T cells in blood was reduced as was the ability of blood lymphocytes to respond to mitogen stimulation. Serum IgG and IgA concentrations were unaffected. There was no change in transcription of genes encoding IL-2, IL-4 or IFN-γ, but IL-10 gene expression was increased.

Glucocorticoids have a **wide clinical application** in companion animal medicine. They are used in chemotherapeutic protocols or by intravenous administration in the management of shock. Glucocorticoids at **anti-inflammatory** doses are used to manage the clinical signs of **allergic diseases** of the skin (e.g. AD) or respiratory tract (e.g. feline asthma or canine eosinophilic bronchopneumopathy). In these examples, **topical** (i.e. skin cream or inhaled drug) administration may be used as an alternative to **systemic** dosing. **Immunosuppressive doses** of glucocorticoid are widely used in the management of **autoimmune or idiopathic inflammatory** disorders.

Despite their effectiveness, glucocorticoids have well-recognized **side-effects**. They suppress the function of all T lymphocytes and not just those cells participating in the pathological immune response. This 'blanket immunosuppression' means that the recipient will be susceptible to **secondary infection** (see Chapter 19). Glucocorticoids mimic the metabolic effects of endogenous corticosteroid produced by the adrenal cortex (e.g. gluconeogenesis, protein catabolism and lipolysis) and so with

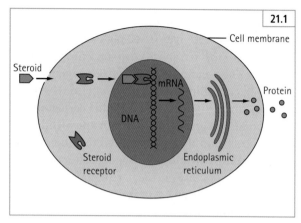

Fig. 21.1 Mechanism of action of glucocorticoids. Glucocorticoids pass through the cell membrane and bind to a cytoplasmic receptor molecule. The combination of drug and receptor passes to the nucleus where binding to DNA initiates gene expression within the cell.

long-term use there may be onset of **iatrogenic hyperadrenocorticism** (Cushing's-like syndrome) involving polyuria/polydipsia, polyphagia/weight gain, accumulation of fat/glycogen within hepatocytes leading to liver dysfunction ('steroid hepatopathy') (**Figure 21.2**), atrophic dermatopathy and secondary diabetes mellitus. **Abrupt withdrawal** of glucocorticoid therapy may lead to clinical signs of **adrenal insufficiency** (hypoadrenocorticism; Addison's-like disease) so the dose of glucocorticoids must always be **slowly tapered** so that the drug is gradually withdrawn (*Table 21.2*).

Some animals may be resistant to the effects of glucocorticoids. In dogs with IBD, the mechanism of such resistance has been proposed to relate to expression of the drug efflux pump p-glycoprotein (encoded by the multidrug resistance 1 gene, *MDR1*) by target mucosal lymphocytes and enterocytes.

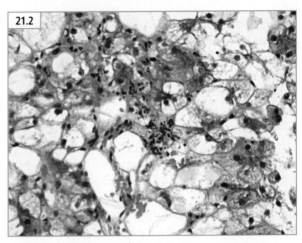

Fig. 21.2 Steroid hepatopathy. One of the side-effects of glucocorticoid therapy involves mobilization of fat reserves and deposition of fat and glycogen within hepatocytes, seen as characteristic multifocal macrovesicular vacuolation of the cytoplasm of these cells.

TABLE 21.2. TAPERING PROTOCOL FOR USE OF IMMUNOSUPPRESSIVE ORAL PREDNISOLONE IN A DOG WITH PRIMARY IMMUNE-MEDIATED DISEASE

Week	Clinical status	Dose of oral prednisolone
0	First diagnosis of immune-mediated disease	1 mg/kg q12h (induction dose)
2–4	Disease controlled with resolution of clinical signs	0.75 mg/kg q12h
6	Clinical resolution maintained	0.5 mg/kg q12h
8	Clinical resolution maintained	0.25 mg/kg q12h
10	Clinical resolution maintained	0.25 mg/kg q24h
12	Clinical resolution maintained	0.25 mg/kg q48h
14	Clinical resolution maintained	Discontinue prednisolone. Continue to monitor clinical progress for the next 12 months

Typical protocol for management of primary immune-mediated (autoimmune) disease in which there is good clinical response to treatment within the first few weeks of treatment. If disease relapses during the tapering protocol, the same or a higher induction dose would be implemented with more prolonged tapering.

Cytotoxic drugs

Three cytotoxic drugs are used in combination with glucocorticoids for an **additive immunosuppressive effect** in animals. These agents have a mode of action that involves **interference with the cell cycle** and therefore the division and replication of lymphocytes. Cytotoxic drugs are also used in chemotherapeutic protocols for management of neoplastic disease. In dogs the cytotoxic agents mostly widely used in immunosuppressive protocols are **azathioprine** and **cyclophosphamide**. **Leflunomide** (an inhibitor of pyrimidine synthesis) and **mycophenolate mofetil** (mode of action similar to azathioprine) are also sometimes employed (but are more expensive drugs), with the latter currently being evaluated for its effect in the management of a range of immune-mediated diseases. The adjunct immunosuppressive agent of choice in cats is **chlorambucil**.

The combination of **glucocorticoid and azathioprine** is used to treat various **immune-mediated (autoimmune) diseases in the dog**. The drugs have an additive immunosuppressive effect so combination therapy is generally used for disease of greater clinical severity. This combination also has a **'steroid-sparing'** effect in that it allows a lower dose of glucocorticoid to be used in the maintenance phase of therapy, thus lowering the risk of glucocorticoid side-effects. As mentioned above, there is a **'lag phase'** between administration of azathioprine and its effect, so the decision to use this combination therapy should be made at the outset.

Azathioprine is a pro-drug of 6-mercaptopurine, which in turn is an analogue of the natural purine hypoxanthine. Hepatic metabolism of azathioprine leads to the formation of nucleotides containing mercaptopurine, which interfere with purine synthesis. Generation of thioinosine monophosphate (thio-IMP) leads to further metabolism to thioguanosine monophosphate (thio-GMP) and thioguanosine triphosphate (thio-GTP). Incorporation of these metabolites into cellular DNA leads to **DNA damage** and **blockade of mitosis and cellular metabolism**. Azathioprine therefore acts on the **S phase of the cell cycle (Figure 21.3)**. The most important immunosuppressive effects of azathioprine are on **T-cell proliferation** and consequently on the provision of T-cell help for B-lymphocyte responses.

The pharmacokinetics of azathioprine involves degradation of the drug to inactive metabolites by enzymes including xanthine oxidase and thiopurine methyltransferase (TPMT). The activity of TPMT is genetically regulated and cats have lower activity of this enzyme than dogs. This means that cats are more sensitive to the side-effects of the drug than are dogs. For this reason, azathioprine is **rarely used in the cat** and in this species chlorambucil is more commonly incorporated into combination immunosuppressive regimes. The most significant **side-effect** of long-term administration of azathioprine is **bone marrow suppression**, and in dogs hepatotoxicity and pancreatitis are also recognized.

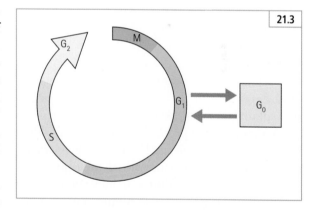

Fig. 21.3 The cell cycle. The cell cycle begins with mitosis (M) and is followed by the gap 1 (G_1) phase during which there is RNA and protein synthesis. The G_1 phase may last for days or weeks depending on the tissue. Cells may then enter a prolonged resting state (G_0) from which they may return to G_1 to continue with the cell cycle. The S phase is relatively short (2 hours) and involves DNA synthesis and there is further RNA and protein synthesis within the subsequent G_2 phase (6–8 hours in duration). The cytotoxic drug azathioprine acts during the S phase of the cell cycle, whereas cyclophosphamide and chlorambucil are not cell cycle specific and act during the mitotic and intermitotic stages.

Mycophenolate mofetil also interferes with purine synthesis in T and B lymphocytes. The drug is metabolized in the liver to mycophenolic acid, which inhibits IMP dehydrogenase, which in turn regulates the synthesis of guanine monophosphate in purine synthesis.

Chlorambucil and **cyclophosphamide** are **alkylating agents** that **alkylate DNA**, leading to breaks or formation of cross-linkages between DNA strands. These changes **inhibit DNA replication and transcription to RNA**. Alkylating agents therefore affect **dividing cells**; however, they also affect cells in the **intermitotic phase** and these drugs are thus **cell cycle non-specific** in action (**Figure 21.3**). In the context of immune-mediated disease, alkylating agents are used for their effects on lymphocytes. The **side-effects** of **chlorambucil** are **bone marrow suppression** and **gastrointestinal disturbance**, and those of **cyclophosphamide** include **leucopenia**, **haemorrhagic cystitis** and **gastrointestinal upset**. All cytotoxic drugs must be handled with care by those administering them, as they are potentially mutagenic, teratogenic and carcinogenic in action.

Ciclosporin

Ciclosporin is a potent immunosuppressive drug developed in the context of human **organ transplantation** and also used as one part of an immunosuppressive protocol for canine and feline kidney transplant recipients. This is the only veterinary immunosuppressive drug for which there are **products licensed for use in the dog**, with indications for the management of AD (systemic administration) and a range of ocular immune-mediated diseases (topical therapy). However, ciclosporin is finding increasing application in the management of a wider range of immune-mediated (autoimmune and idiopathic inflammatory) diseases in the dog and is often used in **combination with a glucocorticoid** in this regard.

Ciclosporin has a more targeted mode of action than the drugs described above and chiefly affects the function of **T lymphocytes**. When absorbed by these cells, ciclosporin binds to a cytoplasmic receptor called **cyclophilin**. The **ciclosporin–cyclophilin complex** then binds to and blocks the action of

another cytoplasmic molecule known as **calcineurin**. In a normal T cell, calcineurin is activated during the influx of Ca^{+2} into the cell that follows ligation of the TCR and stimulation of the CD3 complex. Activated calcineurin binds to the **'nuclear factor of activated T cells'** (NF-AT), which in turn migrates into the nucleus and binds to the **transcription factor AP-1**. The complex of NF-AT and AP-1 induces the **transcription of cytokine genes** by the T cell (**Figure 21.4**). The most important blocking effect is that on **IL-2 production**, which inhibits proliferation of the activated T cell. Although ciclosporin has a selective effect on T cells, the removal of T-cell help leads to indirect suppression of the B-cell response. The related drug **tacrolimus** has a similar effect on T-cell function (through a subtly different cytoplasmic pathway). Tacrolimus is often formulated into a **topical medication** and is now being investigated for efficacy in canine cutaneous immune-mediated

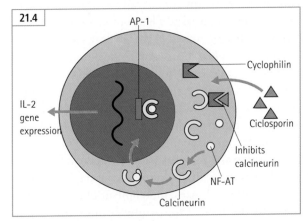

Fig. 21.4 Mode of action of ciclosporin. Ciclosporin enters the cytoplasm of T cells and binds to a receptor called cyclophilin. The drug–receptor complex then binds to and blocks the action of cytoplasmic calcineurin. In a normal T cell, calcineurin binds to the 'nuclear factor of activated T cells' (NF-AT), which in turn migrates into the nucleus and binds to the transcription factor AP-1. The complex of NF-AT and AP-1 induces the transcription of cytokine genes by the T cell. Failure to produce IL-2 impairs the ability of the T cell to become activated and undergo clonal proliferation.

disease. Most of the mechanistic data related to ciclosporin have been extrapolated from human and rodent studies. Few investigations have directly addressed effects on the immune system of normal animals. Incorporation of ciclosporin into cultures of mitogen-stimulated canine lymphocytes led to reduced transcription of genes encoding IL-2, IL-4 and IFN-γ, but not TNF-α. Blood lymphocytes from dogs treated with ciclosporin had reduced cytoplasmic expression of IL-2 and IFN-γ proteins, but there was no effect on IL-4 expression.

A range of **side-effects** is reported with the use of ciclosporin including secondary infection or recrudescence of subclinical infection, anorexia, vomiting, diarrhoea or soft faeces, development of papillomata or gingival hyperplasia, hirsutism or hair shedding, and hepatic and renal toxicity when used at high dosage.

JANUS KINASE INHIBITORS

The JAK–STAT pathway of cellular activation following binding of a cytokine to a cytokine receptor was described in Chapter 8. Novel JAK inhibitors have been developed to block this pathway related to the use of JAK1, 2 and 3 molecules and thereby inhibit the production of a range of cytokines. In human medicine these agents are being developed for the treatment of autoimmune and inflammatory disorders, particularly rheumatoid arthritis. A JAK inhibitor (Apoquel®, Zoetis) has recently been released for the management of pruritus associated with canine allergic dermatitis (e.g. AD). The drug inhibits cytokine production, including that of IL-31, a key mediator of the itch–scratch cycle.

IMMUNOSTIMULATORY AGENTS

Although a selection of immunosuppressive drugs is available (see examples above) and widely used in practice, there are virtually no efficacious and licensed equivalents for stimulating a suboptimal immune response. A number of relatively crude preparations, mostly **extracts from microorganisms or plants**, are sold for their **immune enhancing**

effect, but good data from domestic animal species to support their use are lacking.

During the 1970s and 80s the antiparasitic drug **levamisole** was often used in dogs (particularly animals with severe deep pyoderma) for its immunomodulatory effect. Levamisole was purported to **enhance the function of macrophages** and in fact is still sometimes used as a **vaccine adjuvant** in some products administered to sheep. Levamisole has also been used as an adjunct immunotherapeutic in the management of canine SLE. There are no mechanistic studies that support such applications, and in fact the use of levamisole in dogs is associated with not infrequent **cutaneous drug eruption**, so its use can no longer be recommended. In a similar vein, the antiparasitic drug **ivermectin** was also once examined in order to determine whether it had immunomodulatory properties, but there was no effect on the numbers of canine blood CD4+ or CD8+ T cells or the ability of these cells to respond to mitogens.

A range of **bacterial extracts** has been used in the adjunct management of canine deep pyoderma or for animals with other infectious or even neoplastic diseases. Some of these products are **crude suspensions of bacteria** (e.g. Immunoregulin containing *Propionibacterium acnes*) or **extracts** from a range of bacterial (e.g. Regressin V containing a cell wall extract from *Mycobacterium*; Staphoid AB containing *Staphylococcus aureus* cell wall antigen mixed with staphylococcal α and β toxins; Staphage lysate containing lysed *S. aureus*; muramyl tripeptide or muramyl tripeptide in liposomes containing a mycobacterial cell wall extract) or yeast (e.g. *Serratia marcescens*) species.

A similar basis is found in the practice of **autogenous vaccination** for the management of **canine deep pyoderma**. In this practice the causative *Staphylococcus* organism is isolated from lesions on the patient and cultured organisms in suspension are given by repeated subcutaneous injection over a number of weeks in order to stimulate the antigen-specific immune response. One published clinical trial reported clinical efficacy of this approach in 50% of cases.

There is a logical basis to the use of **mycobacterial derivatives** as immunoenhancing agents, as these bacteria are known to be potent **stimulators of a Th1 immune response**. There is clear evidence from rodent studies that administration of mycobacteria or mycobacterial extracts can skew a pathological Th2 allergic response towards a Th1 response with clinical improvement. A recent study has suggested a similar effect may occur in dogs with **AD**. A single intradermal injection of heat-killed *Mycobacterium vaccae* led to clinical improvement in dogs with moderately severe AD.

Acemannan is an extract from the aloe vera plant with purported immunoenhancing properties. It has been injected directly into tumours (e.g. fibrosarcoma) or given systemically in animals with a range of other neoplasms or used to enhance immune function in cats with retroviral infection.

The single licensed product in this category of immunomodulatory drugs is one containing **inactivated *Parapoxvirus ovis***; it has a spectrum of actions that collectively enhance innate immune function. Originally produced in Europe as Baypamune®, the drug is now named Zylexis® and is licensed as an aid to the management of stress-related respiratory disease in horses.

ALLERGEN-SPECIFIC IMMUNOTHERAPY

ASIT (hyposensitization) is widely practised for the management of canine (and, less frequently, feline) **AD**. In a referral setting this process may be efficacious in up to 80% of patients. ASIT has been practiced in human medicine since the early 1900s. The procedure involves identification of causative allergens (see Chapter 17) and then repeated injection of these allergens in increasing dose increments over a number of weeks until a maintenance phase is reached. Allergens are formulated in **aqueous suspension** or may be **adjuvanted with alum (Figure 21.5)** and there are several different protocols by which each may be administered. The precise mode of action

of ASIT is not completely understood, but it likely involves the generation of **'blocking' IgG antibody** that competes with mast cell-bound IgE for allergen in addition to the **activation of Treg cells** that inhibit the function of allergen-reactive Th2 and Th1 effector cells (**Figure 21.6**). There is evidence for both mechanisms in canine AD patients treated by ASIT in which elevation in allergen-specific IgG and IL-10 gene transcription is reported. Refinements of the ASIT procedure are currently being evaluated. These include **'rush immunotherapy'**, where the process is compacted into hours rather than weeks, and the **mucosal administration** of allergens, particularly by the **sublingual** route. The first commercially produced sublingual immunotherapy (SLIT) is now available for the management of canine atopic dermatitis.

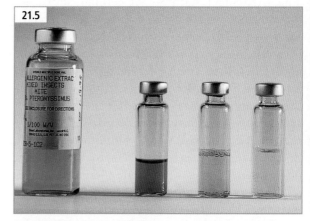

21.5

Fig. 21.5 Allergen-specific immunotherapy. The allergens to which an individual patient is reactive are formulated into aqueous solutions of differing concentration (the darker vials are more concentrated). ASIT involves repeated administration of these allergens in increasing dose increments over an induction period of many weeks. Maintenance therapy requires less frequent administration. Allergens may also be alum adjuvanted and given by alternative protocols.

INTRAVENOUS IMMUNOGLOBULIN THERAPY

IVIG therapy has been adopted from human medicine for the management of an increasing array of immune-mediated diseases. The process involves the **intravenous injection** of a high concentration of **purified human immunoglobulin**. This product is prepared from donated blood and in human medicine is used for the management of primary immunodeficiency disease. Although it would be optimum to have access to purified canine or feline immunoglobulin (in order to avoid the potential for hypersensitivity to these foreign proteins), such preparations are not commercially available. IVIG therapy has been remarkably successful in the management of **canine IMHA and immune-mediated thrombocytopenia (IMTP)**. In these disorders the clinical effect likely relates to the **binding** of the human Ig to the **macrophage FcR**, thereby blocking the receptors and preventing interaction with antibody-coated erythrocytes or platelets. IVIG therapy has also proven of benefit in the management of challenging cases of **autoimmune skin diseases** (particularly erythema multiforme), where the effect most likely relates to **inhibition of apoptosis** of target keratinocytes by blocking the **CD95–CD95 ligand** (Fas–Fas ligand) interaction. The human immunoglobulin is also thought to contain a range of antibodies that can bind to various other lymphocyte surface molecules, leading to inhibition of lymphocyte function (**Figure 21.7**), although recent studies have suggested that the product might also induce activation of Treg cells in human patients with autoimmune diseases. IVIG therapy has also been used successfully in the management of dogs with the peripheral neuropathy known as polyradiculoneuritis.

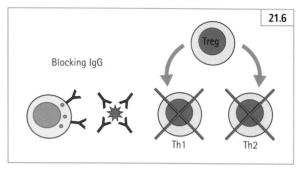

Fig. 21.6 Mode of action of ASIT. Animals undergoing ASIT develop increased titres of allergen-specific IgG antibodies. These compete with mast cell-bound IgE for allergen and are termed 'blocking antibodies'. Additionally, ASIT is likely to act by inducing IL-10-producing Treg cells that inhibit the function of allergenic Th2 or Th1 cells.

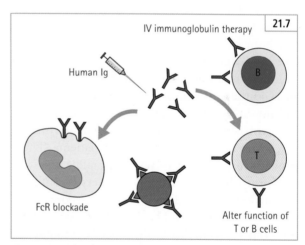

Fig. 21.7 Mode of action of intravenous human immunoglobulin therapy. A single large dose of human immunoglobulin allows these molecules to bind to and block Fc receptors expressed by phagocytic cells. In patients with IMHA or IMTP this prevents antibody-coated red cells or platelets from being removed from the circulation. Some antibodies within the immunoglobulin preparation are able to bind to surface molecules expressed by lymphocytes and thus inhibit the function of these cells.

RECOMBINANT CYTOKINE THERAPY

A major recent advance in human medicine has been the commercial production of recombinant versions of a range of immunoregulatory cytokines. These can be directly injected into patients to manipulate the immune response for clinical benefit. For example, **recombinant human IFN-γ** (rHuIFN-γ) would mimic the effect of Th1-derived cytokine and thus be beneficial in a wide range of **infectious or neoplastic disorders**. In fact, rHuIFN-γ is now used as an adjunct to antiparasitic medical therapy in the treatment of **human leishmaniosis** and intralesional injection of rHuIFN-γ is efficacious in reducing the size of the lesions of **lepromatous leprosy**. **Recombinant human IL-10** (Tenovil®) is of benefit in the management of **psoriasis** and can prolong remission in patients with **Crohn's disease** after surgical removal of lesional intestine.

The benefits of recombinant cytokine therapy have also been applied in veterinary medicine. One of the first applications was the use of **recombinant human granulocyte colony-stimulating factor** (rHuGCSF) or **recombinant human granulocyte–monocyte colony-stimulating factor** (rHuGMCSF) as a means of increasing bone marrow production of these leucocytes in canine chemotherapy patients. These products (e.g. Neupogen®) are able rapidly to restore subnormal blood neutrophil numbers, but if used repeatedly they will induce an immune response to the foreign human protein. The **dog anti-human GCSF antibody** will neutralize further injected recombinant cytokine.

Moreover, as there is antigenic cross-reactivity between the canine and human molecules, this antibody can also potentially neutralize any endogenous canine GCSF present (**Figure 21.8**). **Recombinant human IFN-α** (rHuIFN-α; type I or antiviral interferon) has also been widely used in cats with retroviral or FIP virus infections, but similar risks of developing an anti-human cytokine immune response exist.

The successful application of recombinant cytokine therapy to animals would therefore necessitate production of species-specific molecules. In fact, **recombinant canine GCSF and GMCSF** have both been produced, but not commercially. **Recombinant**

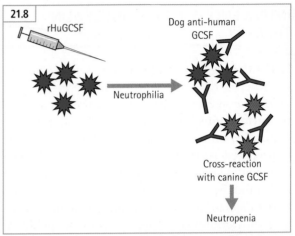

Fig. 21.8 Risk of using recombinant human cytokines in animals. rHuGCSF may enhance bone marrow production of neutrophils in a neutropenic animal. Repeated injections of rHuGCSF will lead to production of antibodies that can neutralize further recombinant protein, but may also cross-react with endogenous protein and further compound the initial problem.

canine IFN-γ (**Interdog®**) has also been prepared and is licensed in Japan for the treatment of canine AD. Another licensed animal recombinant cytokine is **feline interferon omega** (Virbagen Omega®), which is indicated for the adjunct therapy of **dogs with parvovirus** infection (there is cross-reactivity between the canine and feline molecules) and **cats with retroviral infection**.

CYTOKINE GENE THERAPY

Although not yet routinely undertaken in human medicine, the next advance in this area would be the use of **cytokine genes** incorporated into **bacterial plasmids** and directly injected into the patient. This procedure is not dissimilar to the use of naked DNA vaccines (see Chapter 20). The cytokine gene would be expressed within host cells and the local production of cytokine may direct the nature of the immune response. These effects might occur within lymphoid tissue or at the site of an infectious or neoplastic lesion. The use of virus-vectored IL-2 gene therapy in cats has been described in Chapter 14.

MONOCLONAL ANTIBODY THERAPY

The production of monoclonal antibodies has been described in Chapter 9. These highly specific antibodies have found wide application in human medicine because, when injected systemically, they are able to **target and block** many stages of the immune response from antigen presentation to T-cell activation, cytokine production, lymphocyte homing and effector function (**Figure 21.9**). Numerous such products are now licensed for routine use in human medicine. One of the first such products was Campath 1 (Alemtuzumab®), a monoclonal antibody that binds to the leucocyte surface molecule CD52 and depletes these cells. This antibody has found wide application in the management of chronic lymphocytic leukaemia, rheumatoid arthritis, multiple sclerosis (MS) and in immunosuppressive protocols for transplantation. Another very successful product is Infliximab®(also Remicade®), which is a monoclonal antibody with specificity for the cytokine TNF-α. Injection of this monoclonal antibody leads to neutralization of the pro-inflammatory cytokine and the procedure is of clinical benefit in the management of psoriasis, rheumatoid arthritis and Crohn's disease. The monoclonal antibody Natalizumab® binds the α_4 component of the leucocyte homing receptor $\alpha_4\beta_7$ and prevents interaction of circulating cells with the endothelial mucosal addressin cell adhesion molecule (MAdCAM). This binding prevents the migration of leucocytes from the circulation into the intestinal lamina propria and has proven successful in the management of inflammatory enteropathy. Not all such products have had the expected efficacy; for example, an IL-5 neutralizing reagent used in patients with allergic disease to inhibit eosinophil recruitment has had limited success.

Monoclonal antibody therapy is not, however, without risks. Most such antibodies are of murine origin (see Chapter 9) and so repeated use in a human patient is likely to lead to immunological **sensitization and the risk of anaphylaxis**. In order to prevent this possibility, molecular biologists have engineered **'humanized' monoclonal antibodies** in which the murine Fc portion of the immunoglobulin is replaced by human Fc. The relatively small murine

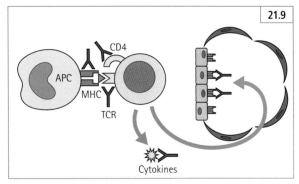

Fig. 21.9 Targets for monoclonal antibody therapy.
Monoclonal antibodies may be designed to inhibit many stages of an immune response including antigen presentation, T-cell activation, cytokine binding to receptors and the process of lymphocyte homing and recruitment into tissue.

antigen-binding regions escape detection by the patient immune system. Such therapy may also have unforeseen complications. During a recent human safety trial for such a reagent (an anti-CD28 antibody), the test subjects responded with a severe and unexpected 'cytokine storm' related to the target of the antibody, that led to severe multisystem organ failure and death. Monoclonal antibody therapy was employed in one comparative therapeutic study of exfoliative CLE in German shorthaired pointers in an experimental setting. The human TNF-α inhibitor Adalimumab® failed to have a clinical effect on the disease. The production of therapeutic monoclonal antibodies specific for animal molecules has not yet been attempted, but it should be entirely feasible and it is already possible to synthesize hybrid (e.g. canine–murine) monoclonal antibodies.

ANTIGEN-SPECIFIC IMMUNOTHERAPY

The ultimate advance in immunotherapy would be the ability to selectively neutralize or destroy those specific lymphocytes responsible for an allergic or autoimmune reaction, perhaps by inducing regulatory populations that might control pathogenic cells. This process requires detailed knowledge of the specificity of the target lymphocytes in terms of their recognition of antigenic peptide and presenting MHC molecule.

Experimental rodent studies have clearly shown that such 'tolerance induction' is feasible and that the most effective means of inducing it is to deliver **target peptides** across **mucosal barriers** (peptide specific therapy), in particular the nasal mucosa. For example, small peptides derived from mice with experimental autoimmune encephalomyelitis (EAE; a model for human MS) may be instilled into the nasal cavity to induce IL-10-producing Treg cells that may either inhibit the experimental induction of EAE or ameliorate ongoing CNS inflammation (**Figure 21.10**). The transition of such therapy from experimental models to clinical medicine has now begun. Clinical trials in MS patients have shown benefit from peptide immunotherapy, although such peptides must be selected for individual patients with an understanding of that individual's MHC background. Similar trials in humans with allergic disease have shown the benefit of instilling allergenic peptides across the mucosa with induction of Treg cells able to control the pathogenic lymphoid cells. Of note is the fact that oral tolerance (see Chapter 15) has already been applied to the development of a novel (unlicensed) product for the management of chronic arthritis. It is suggested that feeding a source of bovine collagen induces Treg cells, which may inhibit collagen-specific autoreactive cells mediating joint damage.

In addition to administration of antigenic peptides, another approach to allergen-specific selective immunotherapy lies at the molecular level and involves **administration of the gene encoding the causative allergen**. This approach has again already been investigated experimentally in dogs. Laboratory beagles sensitized to the Japanese cedar allergen Cry j1 develop IgE antibodies to this allergen and clinical signs of allergic disease on subsequent antigenic challenge. If sensitized beagles are given a bacterial plasmid containing the Cry j1 gene, and are subsequently challenged with allergen, they have reduced serum allergen-specific IgE concentrations, lower reactivity to allergen on intradermal administration, reduced bronchial hyperreactivity and a lower number of pulmonary mast cells (**Figure 21.11**). The same therapy appears beneficial in dogs with spontaneously arising AD caused by Cry j1 exposure.

PARASITE THERAPY

It has long been recognized that in man there is an inverse relationship between susceptibility to allergic disease and the presence of an intestinal nematode burden. For example, people in developing nations where such endogenous parasitism may be present have a low prevalence of allergic disease. There is now excellent experimental evidence that the presence of **intestinal nematodes** is a potent means of **inducing IL-10-producing Treg cells**, and many rodent models of allergic or autoimmune disease can be manipulated by establishing such an infection. Clinical trials in humans with allergic disease or inflammatory enteropathies have now also shown the therapeutic benefit of this approach (see Chapter 17). Parasites such as *Trichuris suis* or hookworms are used as they have an incomplete life cycle in the human intestine, but provide the appropriate stimulus for induction of regulatory cells. A study of parasite therapy in dogs with AD is summarized in Chapter 17. **Probiotic bacteria** within the intestinal microbiota are thought to have similar effects and again may be used to modulate experimental disease in rodents.

GENE THERAPY

Gene therapy holds great promise for the **treatment of monogenic disorders** in man. This procedure involves inserting a functional copy of a **normal gene** into a **viral vector** and giving this to the affected patient or incubating the vector with stem cells derived from the patient. The gene should insert into host cells and permit repopulation by this competent population. The dog is often used as a model for studies of gene therapy. For example, dogs with haemophilia B (factor IX deficiency) have been treated by administration of adenoviral or retroviral vectors incorporating a functional copy of the factor IX gene. Treated animals begin to produce factor IX and show clinical improvement, although the effects are transient because the dog eventually recognizes the protein as a foreign antigen. Such therapies must be coupled with a mechanism for inducing tolerance to the protein. Gene therapy has also been used to treat dogs with X-linked SCID (X-SCID) or cyclic haematopoiesis (see Chapter 19) (**Figure 21.12**).

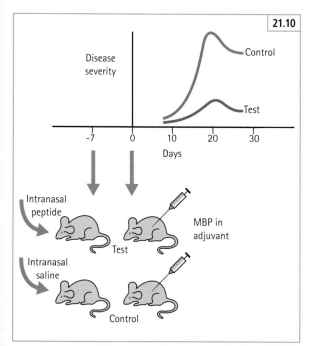

Fig. 21.10 Peptide immunotherapy. Administration of small peptides derived from allergenic or autoantigenic proteins via the nasal mucosa can lead to the induction of Treg cells and amelioration of disease. In this experimental example, mice were given a peptide (residues 1–11) derived from myelin basic protein (MBP) by intranasal deposition (100 mg) and 7 days later were immunized with entire MBP in adjuvant subcutaneously. The severity and incidence of disease (EAE) was markedly reduced relative to control animals that did not receive intranasal peptide.

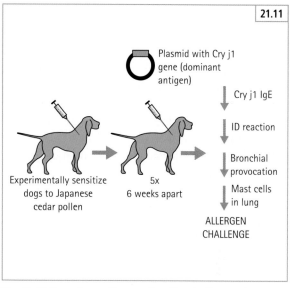

Fig. 21.11 Gene imunotherapy for allergic disease. An alternative approach to administration of allergen by ASIT (**Figure 21.6**) may be administration of the gene encoding that allergen. In this model, dogs are sensitized to the Japanese cedar pollen (Cry j1) by repeated injection of allergen in adjuvant. Some dogs then receive multiple injections of bacterial plasmid containing the Cry j1 gene. When challenged with allergen, the dogs receiving the plasmid have reduced severity of immunopathology.

Fig. 21.12 Gene therapy. Canine monogenic diseases, including primary immunodeficiencies, have been studied as models for gene therapy. A retroviral vector incorporating the gene encoding the γ chain of the IL-2 receptor gene was injected intravenously into a group of pups with X-SCID. Treated dogs had normalization of T- and B-cell number and function and serum IgG concentration and were able to respond serologically to vaccination.

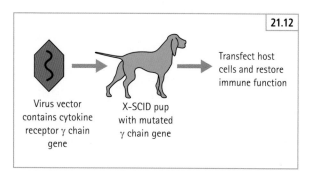

STEM CELL THERAPY

Bone marrow or mesenchymal stem cells are able to differentiate into mature cells of various phenotypes when appropriately cultured *in vitro* or injected into tissue *in vivo*. Stem cell therapy is therefore an active area of research and has already been incorporated into veterinary medicine. Allogeneic stem cells may be cultured and then injected into sites of tendon injury in horses, and such therapy is commercially available. Stem cell therapy has also been investigated for the treatment of primary immunodeficiency disease (**Figure 21.13**).

ADJUNCT IMMUNOTHERAPY

Numerous unconventional methods of modulating immune function have been tested in experimental and human systems. Some may have a scientific basis and some may prove to have clinical benefit. Procedures such as acupuncture or the use of Chinese herbal medicines are being actively investigated for potential immunomodulatory effects. The use of various plant extracts or dietary supplements of antioxidants or diets with altered omega 3:omega 6 fatty acid ratios have already received wide attention in companion animal medicine.

Fig. 21.13 Stem cell therapy. Stem cell therapy has many clinical applications and is already used in equine medicine for tissue repair in musculoskeletal disease. Stem cell therapy is another approach to the treatment of primary immunodeficiency disease in man and CLAD has been used as a model to study this technique. A pup with CLAD received whole body irradiation and then bone marrow (including stem cells) was transplanted from an unaffected littermate. The recipient dog was maintained on immunosuppressive medication, but it developed functionally normal neutrophils able to migrate from the circulation into tissues.

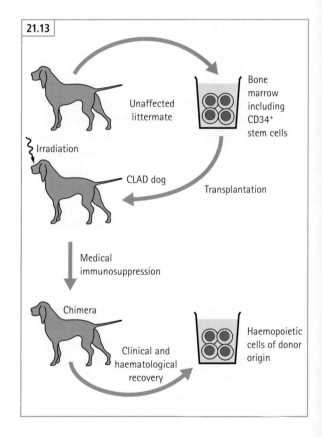

KEY POINTS

- Glucocorticoids differ in formulation, potency and duration of action.
- Glucocorticoids may be anti-inflammatory or immunosuppressive.
- Glucocorticoids bind an intracytoplasmic receptor. The drug–receptor complex moves to the nucleus to associate with DNA, leading to gene activation.
- Cats are relatively 'steroid resistant' compared with dogs, as they may have a lower expression of glucocorticoid receptors within tissue cells.
- Prednisolone can decrease blood lymphocyte numbers and the concentration of serum IgG, IgM and IgA in normal dogs.
- Prednisolone can decrease blood lymphocyte numbers, but not IgG or IgA concentration, in normal cats. Transcription of the IL-10 gene increases in treated animals.
- Prolonged use of glucocorticoids may lead to iatrogenic hyperadrenocorticism.
- Glucocorticoids must be slowly tapered as abrupt withdrawal may lead to signs of hypoadrenocorticism.
- Azathioprine is used in conjunction with glucocorticoid for additive immunosuppressive and steroid-sparing effects.
- Azathioprine interferes with the S phase of the cell cycle.
- Cats are sensitive to azathioprine as they have lower activity of TPMT.
- Prolonged use of azathioprine may cause bone marrow suppression.
- Chlorambucil and cyclophosphamide alkylate DNA and act in a non-cell cycle-specific manner.
- Ciclosporin inhibits T-cell activation via blocking cytokine (particularly IL-2) gene transcription.
- There are almost no effective immunostimulatory drugs licensed in veterinary medicine. Numerous crude extracts of plants or animals are used for their immunoenhancing effects.
- Allergen-specific immunotherapy may have an effect in AD by inducing blocking IgG antibodies and IL-10-producing Treg cells.
- IVIG therapy may be effective in IMHA/IMTP by blocking macrophage Fc receptors and in other immune-mediated diseases by binding to lymphocyte surface molecules and inhibiting the function of these cells.
- Recombinant human cytokines may induce a neutralizing antibody response in animals.
- Recombinant feline interferon omega is commercially available for use in dogs and cats in some countries.
- Monoclonal antibodies are used to block numerous stages of the immune response in human medicine. Such products are not yet produced for animals.
- The goal of immunotherapy is to selectively inhibit those lymphocytes responsible for allergic or autoimmune diseases. This may be achieved by methods such as peptide-specific therapy.
- Gene therapy and stem cell therapy has been used successfully to correct monogenic disorders in experimental dogs.

Case Studies in Clinical Immunology

INTRODUCTION

The purpose of this final chapter is to place the fundamental knowledge presented previously into a clinical context. To that end this chapter introduces some key aspects of clinical immunology and presents 17 simple clinical case studies, each of which provides an example of an aspect of immunology as it relates to veterinary practice. The information given on each case cannot be exhaustive, instead the major clinical and laboratory diagnostic features are presented together with a discussion of the fundamental immunological mechanism and, where appropriate, the therapy employed.

THE BASIS OF IMMUNE-MEDIATED DISEASE

The four major categories of immune-mediated disease (**hypersensitivity** [allergic] diseases, **autoimmune** diseases, **primary immunodeficiency** diseases and **immune system tumours**) have been discussed in earlier chapters. The common basis for all of these disorders is that they are **multifactorial** in aetiology and have a pathogenesis that reflects a **disturbance in normal immune system homeostasis**.

A helpful way of thinking about immune-mediated disease is using the **analogy of the iceberg** (**Figure 22.1**). An iceberg has the main part of its structure hidden beneath the waterline with the peaks of the structure visible from the surface. In this model, the 'body' of the iceberg (beneath the waterline) represents the immune system. The immune system is surrounded by a 'sea' of triggering and predisposing factors; these, when present in appropriate combination, can act on the immune system to dysregulate it. The clinical expression of immune system dysregulation, or the visible peak of the iceberg, is immune-mediated disease. The iceberg model also helps to explain the interrelationship between immune-mediated diseases. There are many examples of concurrent or temporally distant immune-mediated diseases occurring in a single individual. These instances (e.g. the concurrence of IMHA with underlying lymphoma) are situations where the surrounding factors have led to immune system dysregulation, which is expressed in two

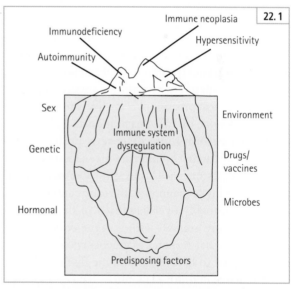

Fig. 22.1 The iceberg model of immune-mediated disease. In this model the 'body' of the iceberg (beneath the waterline) represents the immune system. Predisposing and trigger factors (in the sea surrounding the iceberg) impinge on the immune system, leading to its dysregulation. Immune system dysregulation is expressed clinically as one or more of the four types of immune-mediated disease (seen as peaks of the iceberg above the waterline) occurring contemporaneously or sequentially in the patient.

distinct fashions (as two peaks of the iceberg protruding above the waterline). The nature of these predisposing factors and the way in which they impact upon the immune system to cause dysregulation have been discussed in earlier chapters.

HOW COMMON IS IMMUNE-MEDIATED DISEASE?

It is important to leave a course in veterinary immunology with an appreciation of the clinical relevance of different types of immune-mediated disease. For example, although **primary immunodeficiency** diseases are fascinating and help to explain aspects of the immune response, they are **relatively rare** conditions and many practitioners may not encounter one of these diseases throughout their practice career. In contrast, **allergic diseases** are of **major clinical importance** and the majority of small companion animal practitioners will spend consultation time every day in dealing with patients affected by flea allergy or AD.

Autoimmunity and immune system neoplasia fall between these two ends of the spectrum. **Immune system neoplasia** (lymphoma, leukaemia or mast cell neoplasia) is **relatively common** in small companion animals and most practitioners are likely to make such a diagnosis once or twice each month. Laboratory confirmed **autoimmune disease** is probably **less common**, but in first opinion practice a few cases each year of diseases such as IMHA, IMTP or pemphigus foliaceus might be diagnosed. In reality, autoimmune disease is probably overdiagnosed in first opinion practice. Many animals with a vague collection of clinical signs that respond to glucocorticoid therapy are suggested to have 'autoimmune disease', but in the absence of definitive laboratory data or a specific diagnosis such definition is at best nebulous.

However, having made these generalizations it is important to realize that they are backed up by little epidemiological evidence. There are few studies that present the true prevalence of these immune-mediated diseases, but such data might be derived from analysis of large multipractice computerized databases and this type of investigation is now being undertaken. Hopefully, in the future more accurate figures might be presented.

IMMUNODIAGNOSIS

Earlier chapters in this book have described the range of **immunodiagnostic procedures** that may be used to support a diagnosis of immune-mediated disease. The veterinary student should also be aware that many such tests are **difficult to access** from veterinary practice. Most commercial clinical pathology laboratories will offer serological detection of allergen-specific IgE or some form of Coombs test. Specialist laboratories may offer molecular diagnostic tests for primary immunodeficiency, measurement of serum immunoglobulin concentration and flow cytometric phenotyping of leukaemic cells, but such tests are often difficult to source, relatively expensive and sometimes require samples that are not readily shipped over long distances. Veterinarians are cautioned against sending animal samples to local human medical diagnostic laboratories. Those immunological tests that are based on the use of antisera generally require the use of species-specific reagents and the interpretation of immunodiagnostic tests for animals is a specialized skill that should not (and legally cannot) be undertaken by unqualified individuals.

CASE 1: CANINE IMMUNE-MEDIATED HAEMOLYTIC ANAEMIA

Signalment
Six-year-old, male English springer spaniel (**Figure 1a**; photo courtesy S Warman).

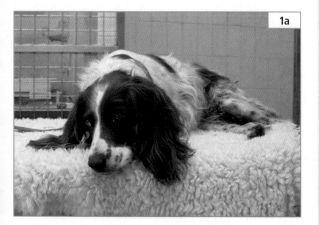

1a

Parameter	Value	Normal range
PCV	0.13	0.35–0.55 l/l
Haemoglobin	50	120–180 g/l
Red blood cells	1.68	5.4–8.0 × 10^{12}/l
MCV	80.1	65–75 fl
MCHC	373	340–370 g/l
MCH	29.8	22–25 pg
Absolute reticulocytes	280	≤60 × 10^9/l
Platelets	251	170–500 × 10^9/l
White blood cells	19.8	5.5–17 × 10^9/l
Neutrophils	15.5	3–11.5 × 10^9/l
Band neutrophils	1.67	0–0.3 × 10^9/l
Lymphocytes	0.84	0.7–3.6 × 10^9/l
Monocytes	1.68	0.1–1.5 × 10^9/l
Eosinophils	0.3	0.2–1.4 × 10^9/l
Basophils	0.0	0–0.1 × 10^9/l
Nucleated red blood cells	2.9 × 10^9/l	

History and physical examination
The dog is presented with a 2-week history of increasing lethargy, weakness and reduced appetite. There have been no recent changes to the lifestyle of the animal and no recent administration of drugs or vaccines. The dog has lived all of its life in northern Europe in an area non-endemic for arthropod-borne infectious diseases such as babesiosis, ehrlichiosis and leishmaniosis. Clinical examination reveals pallor of the oral and conjunctival mucous membranes, mild pyrexia and mild elevation in heart and respiratory rate. Abdominal palpation reveals enlargement of the spleen.

Diagnostic procedures
Routine haematology, serum biochemistry and urinalysis are performed initially. Haematological examination (see below) reveals a strongly regenerative anaemia and leucocytosis due to a left shift neutrophilia and mild monocytosis. Examination of the blood smear reveals polychromasia, anisocytosis and spherocytosis with prominent nucleated erythrocytes (**Figure 1b**).

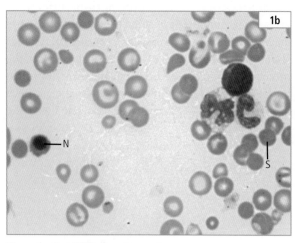

1b

N, nucleated RBC; S, spherocyte.

Serum biochemistry and protein electrophoresis reveal the presence of a mild polyclonal hypergammaglobulinaemia, but there is no significant elevation in serum bilirubin or liver enzymes. Urinalysis is unremarkable. Survey radiographs of the thorax and abdomen are obtained, but they reveal no abnormalities apart from the diffuse enlargement of the spleen identified on clinical examination. On the basis of the haematological data, a Coombs test and a serum ANA are performed. The Coombs test is positive (see below) and the ANA test is negative.

Antiserum	Titre at 37°C	Titre at 4°C
Polyvalent Coombs reagent	640	1,280
Anti-dog IgG	2,560	2,560
Anti-dog IgM	0	0
Anti-dog complement C3	0	0

Diagnosis and immunopathology

Springer spaniels have a recognized genetic predisposition to IMHA. Common underlying trigger factors (drugs, vaccination, infectious disease or neoplasia) are ruled out by historical and diagnostic investigation. The haematological findings are strongly suggestive of IMHA, in particular the presence of spherocytosis. This suspicion is confirmed by the Coombs test, which demonstrates the presence of a warm-reactive IgG antibody associated with the red cells in this dog.

This dog has primary idiopathic (autoimmune) IMHA in which IgG antibody attached to the surface of erythrocytes mediates removal and partial phagocytosis (leading to the formation of spherocytes) by macrophages within the spleen/liver (extravascular haemolysis). This is an example of a type II hypersensitivity reaction (see Chapter 12). The diffuse splenomegaly in this dog is likely attributed to the combination of erythrocyte removal and extramedullary haematopoiesis. The anaemia is strongly regenerative and the dog has a relatively chronic-onset disease for which it compensates physiologically (elevated heart and respiratory rate). Serum hypergammaglobulinaemia likely reflects immune activation.

Treatment and prognosis

This dog was treated with an immunosuppressive dose of oral prednisolone. A good response to therapy was observed and the drug was slowly tapered and eventually withdrawn (see Chapter 21). The owner was warned that the pattern for IMHA is of a relapsing disease, so the dog should be closely monitored by regular PCV checks.

CASE 2: CANINE IMMUNE-MEDIATED THROMBOCYTOPENIA

Signalment

Five-year-old, neutered female English cocker spaniel (**Figure 2a**; photo courtesy S Warman).

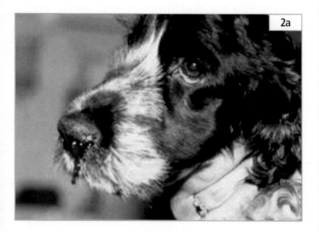

2a

Parameter	Value	Normal range
PCV	0.22	0.35–0.55 l/l
Haemoglobin	75.7	120–180 g/l
Red blood cells	2.82	5.4–8.0 × 10^{12}/l
MCV	76.5	65–75 fl
MCHC	350	340–370 g/l
MCH	26.8	22–25 pg
Absolute reticulocytes	Not counted	≤60 × 10^9/l
Platelets	2.0	170–500 × 10^9/l
White blood cells	8.11	5.5–17 × 10^9/l
Neutrophils	4.71	3–11.5 × 10^9/l
Band neutrophils	0.0	0–0.3 × 10^9/l
Lymphocytes	1.30	0.7–3.6 × 10^9/l
Monocytes	1.46	0.1–1.5 × 10^9/l
Eosinophils	0.0	0.2–1.4 × 10^9/l
Basophils	0.0	0–0.1 × 10^9/l
Nucleated red blood cells	0.5 × 10^9/l	

History and physical examination

The dog is presented with acute onset epistaxis, haematuria, melaena and haematemesis. There have been no recent changes to the lifestyle of the animal and no recent administration of drugs or vaccines. There is no known contact with anticoagulant rodenticides. The dog has lived all of its life in Northern Europe in an area non-endemic for arthropod-borne infectious diseases such as babesiosis, ehrlichiosis and leishmaniosis. Clinical examination reveals pallor of the oral and conjunctival mucous membranes, mild pyrexia and petechial haemorrhages of the oral mucous membranes and ventral abdominal skin.

Diagnostic procedures

Routine haematology, serum biochemistry, urinalysis and coagulation profile are performed initially. Haematological examination (see below) reveals a moderate regenerative anaemia and severe thrombocytopenia.

Examination of the blood smear reveals polychromasia, anisocytosis and the presence of nucleated erythrocytes. Serum biochemistry reveals mild elevation in ALP and AST. Urinalysis is unremarkable. There is no abnormality in prothrombin time (PT) or activated partial thromboplastin time (APTT). Survey radiographs of the thorax and abdomen reveal no abnormalities. On the basis of the haematological data, a Coombs test and a serum ANA are performed, but both are negative. The laboratory does not provide an antiplatelet antibody test.

Diagnosis and immunopathology

Cocker spaniels have a recognized genetic predisposition to developing immune-mediated cytopenias. Common underlying trigger factors (drugs, vaccination, infectious or inflammatory disease or neoplasia) are ruled-out by historical and diagnostic investigation. The haematological findings are strongly suggestive of IMTP with secondary blood loss anaemia. There is no widely available test for antiplatelet antibodies, so IMTP generally remains a diagnosis of exclusion.

This dog has primary idiopathic (autoimmune) IMTP in which IgG antibody attached to the surface of platelets mediates removal by macrophages within the spleen/liver or intravascular complement-mediated platelet lysis. This is an example of a type II hypersensitivity reaction (see Chapter 12). The virtual absence of platelets means that the dog is unable to form a primary platelet plug at the site of vascular damage, resulting in the observed haemorrhages.

Treatment and prognosis

The dog was treated with an immunosuppressive dose of oral prednisolone and an injection of vincristine. Vincristine enhances bone marrow thrombopoiesis and inhibits macrophage removal of antibody-coated platelets. The dog made no response to therapy and continued to deteriorate. Three days after presentation the owners elected for euthanasia. A necropsy examination was performed, which revealed severe gastric haemorrhage with blood clot overlying the gastric mucosa (**Figure 2b**). There was active erythropoiesis and plentiful megakaryocytes within the bone marrow, spleen and liver.

IMTP is a severe disease and a number of animals (as in this case) will fail to respond to therapy. Those animals that recover may have relapses of IMTP or develop other autoimmune diseases later in life.

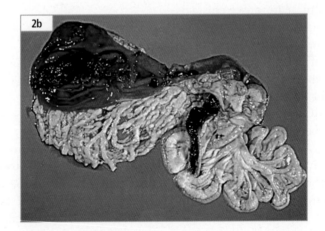

CASE 3: CANINE SYSTEMIC LUPUS ERYTHEMATOSUS

Signalment
Seven and a half-year-old, male English cocker spaniel (**Figure 3a**).

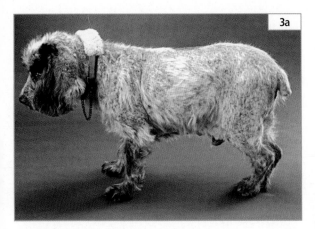

History and physical examination
This dog was presented with a history of chronic skin disease that had developed progressively over the past 11 months. Nine months previously the dog had been diagnosed with keratoconjunctivitis sicca (KCS) and was being treated for that condition with topical ciclosporin. Physical examination revealed the presence of severe generalized crusting skin lesions with areas of alopecia. Additionally, there was conjunctival discharge, otitis externa and generalized lymphadenomegaly. The dog had pale ocular and oral mucous membranes. The owner reported removing several ticks from the dog one month before the onset of the skin disease. The dog lives in Northern Europe in an area non-endemic for arthropod-borne infectious diseases such as babesiosis, ehrlichiosis and leishmaniosis.

Diagnostic procedures
A swab taken from the external ear canal revealed the presence of mixed bacterial species. Schirmer tear test readings confirmed the presence of KCS. Skin punch biopsies demonstrated the formation of subcorneal pustules filled by eosinophils and acanthocytes (**Figure 3b**; from Foster AP, Sturgess CP, Gould DJ *et al.* [2000] Pemphigus foliaceus in association with systemic lupus erythematosus with subsequent lymphoma in a Cocker Spaniel dog. *Journal of Small Animal Practice* **41**:266–270, with permission). These features are consistent with pemphigus foliaceus and the presence of IgG antibody associated with the desmosomes of the keratinocytes was confirmed by immunohistochemistry.

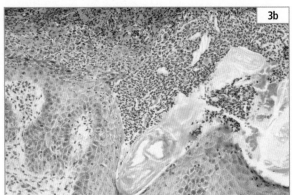

Haematological examination revealed a mildly regenerative anaemia, a marked thrombocytopenia and leucocytosis due to a left shift neutrophilia, monocytosis, lymphocytosis and eosinophilia (see overleaf). Serum biochemical abnormalities included hypoalbuminaemia and hypergammaglobulinaemia. Urinalysis was unremarkable.

Parameter	Value	Normal range
PCV	0.25	0.35–0.55 l/l
Haemoglobin	109	120–180 g/l
Red blood cells	2.93	5.4–8.0 × 10^{12}/l
MCV	86.6	65–75 fl
MCHC	431	340–370 g/l
MCH	37.2	22–25 pg
Absolute reticulocytes	83.0	≤60 × 10^9/l
Platelets	9.0	170–500 × 10^9/l
White blood cells	43.7	5.5–17 × 10^9/l
Neutrophils	22.3	3–11.5 × 10^9/l
Band neutrophils	2.19	0–0.3 × 10^9/l
Lymphocytes	6.12	0.7–3.6 × 10^9/l
Monocytes	3.93	0.1–1.5 × 10^9/l
Eosinophils	9.18	0.2–1.4 × 10^9/l
Nucleated red blood cells	Sparse on blood film	

Antiserum	Titre at 37°C	Titre at 4°C
Polyvalent Coombs reagent	40	640
Anti-dog IgG	640	1,280
Anti-dog IgM	0	0
Anti-dog complement C3	0	0

On the basis of these findings a Coombs test and serum ANA and RF were performed. The Coombs test was positive (see below) and the ANA titre was 10,240 with homogeneous nuclear staining. RF was negative. Antiplatelet antibody testing was not available. The concentrations of serum IgG, IgM and IgA were measured and the hypergammaglobulinaemia attributed to a selective elevation in IgG.

A bone marrow aspirate was taken. This revealed a normal myeloid:erythroid ratio but with a prominent population of eosinophil precursors. Biopsy of an enlarged lymph node demonstrated reactive and inflammatory change. A screen for arthropod-borne infectious diseases (serology and PCR) revealed no evidence of exposure to *Bartonella*, *Rickettsia*, several *Ehrlichia* spp. or *Borrelia*. Survey radiographs of the thorax and abdomen showed no abnormality.

Diagnosis and immunopathology

This dog has at least four concurrent manifestations of autoimmunity affecting three body systems: KCS, pemphigus foliaceus, IMHA and IMTP. Two of these are proven to be associated with the presence of autoantibody (interepithelial IgG within the skin and positive Coombs test). It is likely that antiplatelet antibodies would have been demonstrated had testing been possible. KCS is likely to involve infiltration of cytotoxic lymphocytes into lacrimal glandular tissue. These immune responses involve a combination of type II and type IV hypersensitivity mechanisms (see Chapter 12). Additionally, the dog has a very high-titre serum ANA. These findings readily satisfy the criteria for SLE. Cases of true SLE are very rare in veterinary medicine; many animals may only partially satisfy the diagnostic criteria and are considered to have an 'SLE overlap syndrome'. At the time of diagnosis this dog was considered to have primary idiopathic multisystemic autoimmune disease. There was no historical or diagnostic evidence of underlying trigger factors (drug or vaccine administration, neoplasia, infection) and the cocker spaniel breed has a recognized susceptibility to autoimmune disease.

Treatment and prognosis

The dog was treated with glucocorticoid therapy, medicated baths, covering antimicrobials and ocular ciclosporin and tear replacement. There was response to therapy within 3 weeks. Seven months after initial presentation the dog was re-presented with marked enlargement of peripheral lymph nodes together with enlargement of thoracic and abdominal nodes and diffuse splenomegaly. At this time lymph node biopsy and immunohistochemistry confirmed a diagnosis of B-cell lymphoma. A histological section from the biopsy sample is shown in **Figure 3c** and immunohistochemical labelling of the tumour cells with antibody to the B-cell marker CD79a is shown in **Figure 3d**. The owner elected for no further treatment and the dog died 2 months later. This fascinating case demonstrates two distinct 'peaks of the iceberg' (autoimmunity and immune system neoplasia) appearing successively in this dog (see Chapter 21).

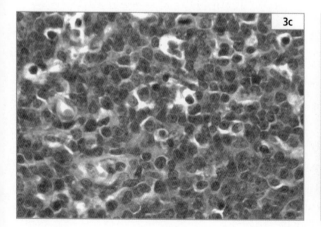

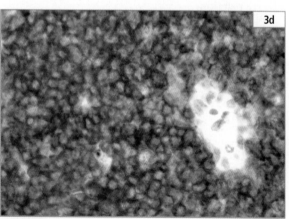

CASE 4: FELINE BLOOD TRANSFUSION

Signalment
Four-year-old, male British shorthair cat.

History and physical examination
This cat is currently being investigated because of a primary problem of chronic non-regenerative anaemia. While hospitalized the PCV has decreased from 0.15 l/l to 0.1 l/l (15% to 10%). The clinician decides that a supportive whole blood transfusion is required.

Diagnostic procedures
Feline blood transfusion carries a relatively high risk of transfusion reaction. For that reason, all blood transfusions in cats should be based on both blood typing and cross-matching. The cat has a relatively simple blood group antigen system (summarized below).

The prevalence of blood type varies by breed and geographical location (and therefore gene pool). The British shorthair is one breed in which there is a recognized higher prevalence of the B blood group. It is therefore very important to ensure that this patient receives compatible blood, as the cat may have high-titre anti-A alloantibody and a mismatched transfusion of type A or AB blood would lead to an adverse reaction.

The blood type of the recipient may be determined by submitting a sample to a specialist immunohaematology laboratory or by the use of a rapid in-house test kit. Feline blood typing cards (see Chapter 4) are widely used in practice. This patient was typed using a new tube-based test. The plastic card comprises a set of small columns containing a gel matrix impregnated with typing reagent. A small volume of washed patient erythrocytes is loaded to the top of the column and the card is centrifuged. If the erythrocytes carry a surface antigen reactive with the reagent in the gel, they are unable to pass through the matrix and form a band at the upper surface of the gel. In a negative reaction the cells pass through the gel and button at the base of the column. In this instance it can be seen that the cat (number 322 on the card) is of blood type A (**Figure 4a**).

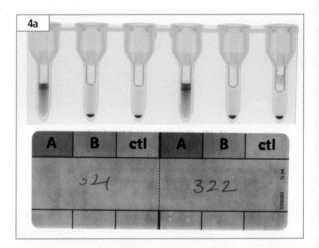

Phenotype (blood group)	Genotype	Inheritance	Alloantibody
A	AA, Aa^{ab} or Ab	A is dominant over B	Some may have low-titre anti-B
B	bb	B is recessive to A	All have high-titre anti-A
AB	a^{ab}b or a^{ab}a^{ab}	Determined by a third allele a^{ab} that is recessive to A and dominant over b	Have no alloantibody
Mik		Some type A cats are Mik⁻, but most are Mik⁺	Mik⁻ cats may have alloantibody to Mik

As this cat is of blood group A, it should be able to safely receive whole blood from a type A donor. However, it remains possible that there may be minor incompatibilities (for example related to the Mik antigen) and so a cross-match should still be performed. The aim of the cross-match is to determine whether serum from the recipient cat contains antibody that might react with antigens expressed on the erythrocytes of the donor (major cross-match). The reverse possibility, that donor serum transfused into the recipient might contain antibodies able to react with recipient erythrocytes (minor cross-match), is also tested. Blood from several possible donors is normally evaluated. There are a number of methods of performing a cross-match ranging from a simple emergency slide agglutination test to a more complex procedure performed in microtitration plates with the addition of complement. An in-practice card-based cross-match test is also available commercially. The basic procedure for the plate test involves the incubation of serum with a suspension of washed erythrocytes (summarized below).

In this instance a cross-match was performed with blood from a panel of known type A donor cats and a suitable donor animal identified.

Treatment and prognosis

Blood was collected from the type A donor cat (**Figure 4b**; photo courtesy S Warman) and successfully transfused into the recipient animal, leading to elevation of PCV in the recipient. Subsequent diagnosis revealed that the non-regenerative anaemia in this patient was likely to be related to FeLV infection and so the long-term prognosis was guarded.

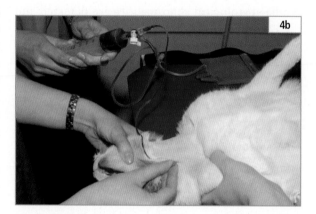
4b

Reaction number	Components	Nature of test
1	Recipient serum + donor RBC	Major cross-match
2	Recipient serum + recipient RBC	Control
3	Donor serum + recipient RBC	Minor cross-match
4	Donor serum + donor RBC	Control

CASE 5: FELINE MULTIPLE MYELOMA

Signalment
12-year-old, neutered female domestic shorthair cat.

History and physical examination
This cat is presented with a 3-week history of intermittent vomiting and diarrhoea. An endoscopic examination is scheduled for further investigation of the problem and initial screening samples taken for haematological and biochemical examination.

Diagnostic procedures
No haematological abnormalities are detected and the cat is negative for FeLV and FIV by standard serological testing (see Chapter 4). The main elements of the serum biochemistry data are presented below.

Parameter	Value	Normal range
Urea	9.8	6.5–10.5 mmol/l
Creatinine	129	133–175 µmol/l
Total protein	104.1	77–91 g/l
Globulin	77.5	21–51 g/l
Albumin	26.6	24–35 g/l
A:G ratio	0.34	0.4–1.3
Alanine aminotransferase	24	15–45 IU/l
Alkaline phosphatase	33	15–60 IU/l
Total bilirubin	9.9	0–10 µmol/l
Fasting bile acids	15.1	0–15 µmol/l
Calcium	2.69	2.3–2.5 mmol/l

The finding of elevated globulins necessitates further evaluation by serum protein electrophoresis and a densitometric scan of this analysis is presented (**Figure 5a**). This reveals the presence of a striking monoclonal gammopathy. Differential diagnoses for this change in cats include multiple myeloma (see Chapter 14) and occasional cases of FIP virus infection, ehrlichiosis or leishmaniosis. This cat does not clearly have FIP (although there is currently no reliable antemortem diagnostic test for this infection) and it has not travelled beyond Northern Europe into an area endemic for the relevant arthropod-borne infectious diseases.

Given that multiple myeloma often arises within bone marrow, survey radiography is performed but does not reveal the presence of classical 'punched out' osteolytic foci. A bone marrow aspirate does not reveal any abnormality in haemopoietic precursors and only a low number of plasma cells are noted. The imaging examination does, however, reveal marked enlargement of the spleen and mesenteric lymphadenomegaly. Urinalysis is performed (some cases of multiple myeloma have urine Bence-Jones protein) and although there is a mild proteinuria, the urine protein:creatinine (UPC) ratio is normal. A simple agar gel diffusion test with serum from the patient confirms that the monoclonal gamma globulin is an IgG antibody.

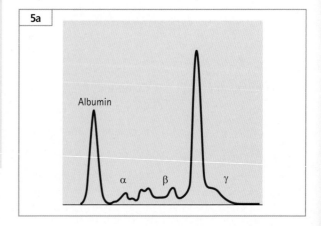

5a

Exploratory laparotomy confirms the splenomegaly (**Figure 5b**) and lymphadenomegaly and the liver is noted to have a mottled red–tan parenchyma. A splenectomy is performed and biopsy samples are taken from the mesenteric lymph nodes and liver. Endoscopic biopsy samples of the gastrointestinal mucosa are also collected.

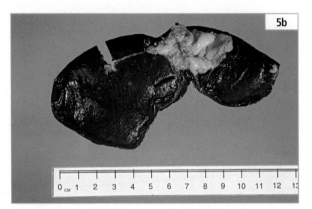

5b

Histopathological examination reveals mild pyogranulomatous enteritis, reactive hyperplasia of the mesenteric lymph nodes, peliosis hepatis (blood-filled spaces in the liver parenchyma) and diffuse infiltration of the spleen by pleomorphic, occasionally multinucleate and mitotic plasma cells (**Figure 5c**).

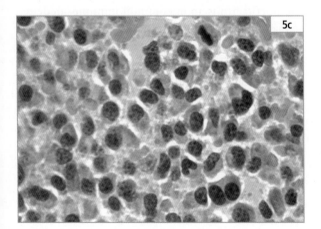

5c

Diagnosis and immunopathology

The final diagnosis in this case is multiple myeloma with IgG paraproteinaemia. The tumour appears primarily to involve the spleen rather than bone marrow and there is no significant hypercalcaemia of malignancy in this case. It is increasingly recognized that feline myeloma more commonly affects abdominal soft tissue than bone.

Treatment and prognosis

In this cat the monoclonal gammopathy began to resolve soon after splenectomy, suggesting that the primary neoplasm and source of the paraprotein had been removed. A follow-up serum protein electrophoresis is shown (**Figure 5d**).

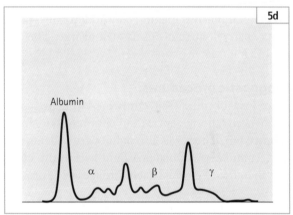

5d

Albumin

α   β   γ

CASE 6: EQUINE PURPURA HAEMORRHAGICA

Signalment
Eight-month-old Thoroughbred colt.

History and physical examination
The animal was presented with a 4-day history of progressive facial swelling. Clinical examination confirmed that this was subcutaneous oedema. The colt was also pyrexic and had an elevated pulse rate. Parenteral penicillin was administered and there was an initial reduction in pyrexia and facial oedema. However, 2 days later there was return of facial oedema that now also involved the ventral cervical and thoracic area. The colt was pyrexic, had an elevated pulse rate and petechial haemorrhages were present on the oral mucous membranes. Additionally, there was a bilateral sanguineous nasal discharge. The colt died 12 hours later.

Diagnostic procedures
Necropsy examination confirmed the presence of marked anteroventral subcutaneous oedema (**Figure 6a**). There was also pulmonary oedema and an accumulation of oedema fluid within the chest and abdomen. Petechial haemorrhages were present

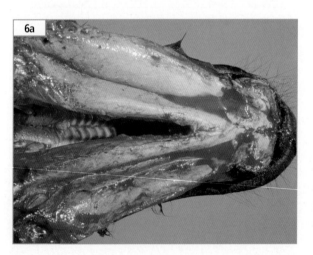

over the mucous membranes and the epicardial and endocardial surfaces of the heart. Blood clots were present within the nasal cavity (**Figure 6b**).

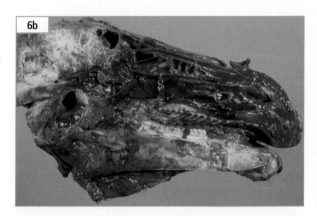

There was enlargement of the submandibular and retropharyngeal lymph nodes with cream-coloured pus noted on sectioning these structures. *Streptococcus equi* was cultured from this material. Histological examination confirmed the presence of lymphadenitis and vasculitis affecting the nasal mucosa.

Diagnosis and immunopathology
The diagnosis is this case was equine 'strangles' caused by infection with *Streptococcus equi* ssp. *equi*, with secondary purpura haemorrhagica. Purpura haemorrhagica is an uncommon immune-mediated sequela to strangles infection; it arises in 1–2% of cases within weeks of the primary infection. The streptococcal M protein forms immune complexes with IgG or IgA antibody and these complexes circulate and deposit within the walls of blood vessels throughout the body (antigen excess type III hypersensitivity; see Chapter 12). This establishes a leucocytoclastic vasculitis leading to fluid loss or haemorrhage. The clinical presentation of this colt followed the classical distribution reported for these lesions. Some animals also develop an immune complex glomerulonephritis, but there was no evidence of this in the present case.

CASE 7: BOVINE THYMIC LYMPHOMA

Signalment
12-month-old Friesian heifer.

History and physical examination
The heifer was presented with loss of body condition and marked subcutaneous oedema affecting the ventral cervical and anterior thoracic region. No other animals in the herd were affected. On clinical examination there was an elevated heart rate and dyspnoea.

Diagnostic procedures
Given the severity of the clinical signs the farmer elected for euthanasia of the animal. A necropsy examination was permitted. The main finding was the presence of a very large, solid, cream-coloured mass of 30 cm diameter within the anterior mediastinum. The mass had caused displacement and compression of the heart and lungs within the thoracic cavity. The mass, bisected with the two cut halves lying anterior to the heart and lungs, is shown (**Figure 7a**). An enlarged cervical lymph node may be seen just above the mass.

Microscopic examination confirmed that the mass comprised a closely packed sheet of neoplastic lymphocytes. Immunohistochemical examination revealed that these were of T-cell lineage (**Figure 7b**).

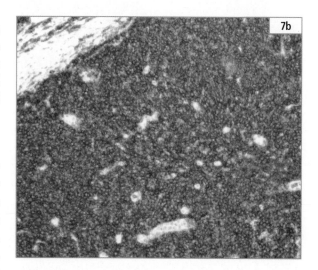

Diagnosis and immunopathology
The final diagnosis in this case was of thymic T-cell lymphoma (see Chapter 14). The presence of the large mediastinal mass was responsible for the observed clinical signs. The direct compression of heart and lungs led to dyspnoea and elevated heart rate, while occlusion of draining lymphatic vessels was responsible for the observed anteroventral subcutaneous oedema. There may also have been compromise of the ability of the animal to swallow, thus contributing to the loss of body condition. This case was notified to the government authority, but it tested negative for bovine leukaemia virus, which may cause multicentric lymphoma in older cattle.

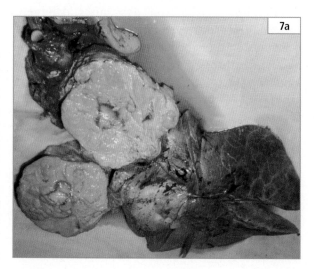

CASE 8: CANINE ATOPIC DERMATITIS

Signalment
Three-year-old, male English setter (**Figure 8a**).

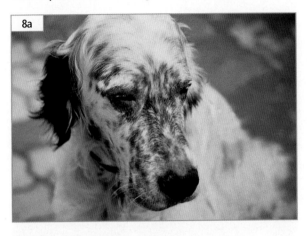

8a

History and physical examination
The dog is presented with severe pruritic skin disease that began 6 months previously and has progressively worsened. The dog continually rubs its face and chews its front paws. Clinical examination reveals erythema and alopecia affecting the face, the inner surface of the pinnae and the axillary and inguinal skin. There is conjunctivitis and cheilitis (inflammation of the lips) and particularly severe lesions with lichenification (thick and fissured skin) of the dorsal surface of the front paws (**Figure 8b**). Some of the lesions appear to have secondary infection and 'tape strip' cytology reveals the presence of coccoid bacteria and yeasts with the appearance of *Malassezia*. *Staphylococcus* is subsequently cultured from the lesions.

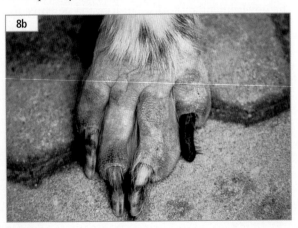

8b

Diagnostic procedures
A thorough clinical history is obtained. The owner uses appropriate and effective flea control and there is no evidence of fleas or flea dirt on the hair coat. The dog lives indoors and is exercised in a suburban environment. The patient's diet is commercial dry kibbles supplemented with occasional canned food and treats. Three months ago the owner switched to a commercially available hydrolysed protein hypoallergenic diet. After feeding this for 3 weeks with no change in the skin disease the owner returned the dog to the standard diet.

After discussion with the owner an IDST is performed (see Chapter 17). This reveals strong positive reactions at 20 minutes to house dust, mattress dust and the two house dust mites *Dermatophagoides pteronyssinus* and *Dermatophagoides farinae*.

Diagnosis and immunopathology
The final diagnosis is of AD with secondary bacterial and yeast infection. The causative allergens are primarily the house dust mites. This is a classical type I hypersensitivity reaction (see Chapter 12) involving a genetically predisposed dog of young age, with lack of sufficient Treg cell function, becoming sensitized to allergens derived from dust mites. Allergen-specific IgE coats dermal mast cells, leading to their degranulation on subsequent percutaneous absorption of allergen through a defective epidermal barrier. With chronicity and secondary infection the disease extends to involve a Th1-mediated inflammatory response.

Treatment and prognosis
The approach to management of this case is complex and long term, requiring excellent owner compliance. The initial clinical signs are managed with topical antimicrobial baths, systemic antibiotics and a combination of an anti-inflammatory dose of glucocorticoid and essential fatty acid supplementation. Ongoing flea control is maintained. Once these signs are controlled, long-term management with ASIT can be considered (see Chapter 22). In this patient, ASIT proved successful (but this is not always the case).

CASE 9: EQUINE SEVERE COMBINED IMMUNODEFICIENCY

Signalment
Three-month-old Arabian foal.

History and physical examination
The foal was born normally and took in adequate colostrum within the first 24 hours of life. For the first 8 weeks of life the foal was clinically normal and appeared to develop appropriately. Over the past 2 weeks the foal had been lethargic and developed diarrhoea. Physical examination also revealed pyrexia, conjunctivitis, laboured breathing and an elevated heart rate.

Diagnostic procedures
The onset of this collection of clinical signs in an Arabian foal of this age creates a high index of suspicion for SCID. In a stud environment the breeder may be asked whether similar problems have been recognized in the past, particularly with the mating of the current dam and sire. Routine haematological examination reveals leucopenia and marked lymphopenia, with virtually no lymphocytes detected on a blood smear. Serum biochemistry and protein electrophoresis reveals hypogammaglobulinaemia. Traces of maternal IgG may still be present and detected by techniques such as SRID (see Chapter 18), but serum IgM will be undetectable.

Diagnosis and immunopathology
These clinical and laboratory findings are consistent with equine SCID and the diagnosis can now be unequivocally confirmed by use of a PCR-based test. This test detects the 5 base pair deletion in the gene encoding DNA-dependent protein kinase involved in the VDJ recombination event that forms TCRs and BCRs. The test allows detection of both homozygous affected foals and heterozygous carrier animals of this autosomal recessive mutation. Affected foals are unable to form functional T and B lymphocytes and therefore have hypoplastic lymphoid tissue and inadequate immune defences. The animals readily succumb to multisystemic infection, which is commonly most severe in the respiratory tract with development of a complex mixed viral and bacterial pneumonia.

Treatment and prognosis
There is no practical treatment for this disease. Affected foals may be treated symptomatically, but most die by five months of age. Experimentally, one animal was kept alive for 12 months with a bone marrow transplant. This foal died and was subject to necropsy examination. There was severe pneumonia with anteroventral consolidation and abscessation of the lung (**Figure 9a**). Lymphoid tissue was profoundly hypoplastic, as evidenced by the width of the cross-section of spleen (**Figure 9b**).

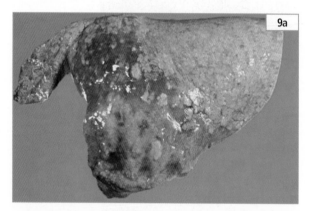

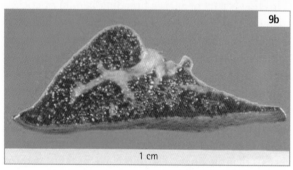

The molecular diagnostic test should be used to screen Arabian breeding stock for this mutation and controlled breeding programmes instigated. Surveys conducted in 1997 revealed that the mutation was carried by 8% of Arabian horses in the USA and up to 5% in the UK. It is likely that the current prevalence is now considerably lower.

CASE 10: CANINE LYMPHOCYTIC THYROIDITIS

Signalment

Nine-year-old, female English cocker spaniel (**Figure 10a**).

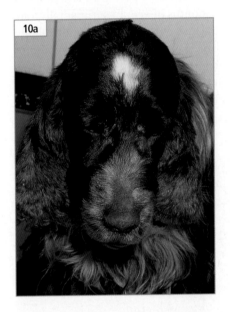

Parameter	Value	Normal range
PCV	0.31	0.35–0.55 l/l
Haemoglobin	50	120–180 g/l
Red blood cells	5.0	5.4–8.0 × 10^{12}/l
MCV	67.0	65–75 fl
MCHC	350	340–370 g/l
MCH	23.0	22–25 pg
Platelets	260	170–500 × 10^9/l
White blood cells	12.0	5.5–17 × 10^9/l
Neutrophils	8.0	3–11.5 × 10^9/l
Lymphocytes	2.0	0.7–3.6 × 10^9/l
Monocytes	1.0	0.1–1.5 × 10^9/l
Eosinophils	0.5	0.2–1.4 × 10^9/l

History and physical examination

This dog is part of a large breeding kennel of cocker spaniels. Within the colony there is a high prevalence of immune-mediated disease of various types. Two years ago this bitch was diagnosed with Coombs-positive IMHA and was successfully treated with a course of immunosuppressive glucocorticoid therapy. The dog has now been presented because of clinical signs of increasing lethargy and the breeder is concerned that this may be a relapse of IMHA. Physical examination reveals that the dog is also obese, has areas of truncal alopecia and scaling and a 'puffy' face with partial closure of the eyelids.

Diagnostic procedures

Routine haematological and serum biochemical examinations are performed initially and these data are presented below. There are no significant changes to erythrocyte morphology on evaluation of a blood smear.

Parameter	Value	Normal range
Urea	6.1	2.0–7.0 mmol/l
Creatinine	115	100–133 µmol/l
Total protein	85	63–71 g/l
Globulin	47.5	20–35 g/l
Albumin	33.8	32–38 g/l
A:G ratio	0.70	0.6–1.5
Alanine aminotransferase	24	20–60 IU/l
Alkaline phosphatase	33	0–110 IU/l
Total bilirubin	2.0	0–10 µmol/l
Glucose	5.2	3.5–5 mmol/l
Cholesterol	14.0	3.5–7 mmol/l
Creatine kinase	114	77–280 IU/l
Calcium	2.3	2.3–2.5 mmol/l

The main findings of these tests are a mild anaemia, hyperglobulinaemia (determined by protein electrophoresis to be a polyclonal hypergammaglobulinaemia) and hypercholesterolaemia. The clinical history and presenting signs, together with these laboratory findings, are suggestive of hypothyroidism.

Further specific tests of thyroid function are performed. There is a low serum T4 concentration and injection of exogenous TSH fails to elevate this concentration on repeated sampling 6 hours after injection. At the time of examination, testing for serum TSH concentration (which would be expected to be elevated) was not available.

At this time the dog had a negative Coombs test, but serum autoantibody to thyroglobulin was demonstrated and there was a positive serum ANA (titre 640 with speckled nuclear staining).

Diagnosis and immunopathology

This dog is of a breed and familial group highly predisposed to autoimmune disease and it has a previous history of IMHA. The current clinical presentation is consistent with hypothyroidism. This is almost certainly caused by lymphocytic thyroiditis, an infiltration into the thyroid gland of cytotoxic autoreactive T cells with destruction of follicular epithelium (**Figure 10b**).

Thyroglobulin autoantibodies may also have a pathogenic role as they are often detected in advance of clinical disease in susceptible dogs. The clinical signs and laboratory findings in this bitch all relate to depressed metabolism caused by insufficiency of thyroid hormone. The observed lethargy, obesity and hypercholesterolaemia are a direct consequence of this altered metabolism. The cutaneous signs (alopecia and scaling) reflect an atrophic dermatopathy with telogen arrest of follicles and hyperkeratosis. The facial puffiness is due to 'myxoedema', an accumulation of mucopolysaccharide matrix within the dermis. The observed mild anaemia is due to bone marrow suppression rather than haemolysis. The autoimmune nature of the disease is confirmed by the presence of serum thyroglobulin and nuclear autoantibodies, but this case does not satisfy the criteria for SLE.

Treatment and prognosis

Management of lymphocytic thyroiditis involves simple supplementation with L-thyroxine sodium (a synthetic mimic of T4). Despite the fact that this is an autoimmune process, patients are not treated with immunosuppressive drugs.

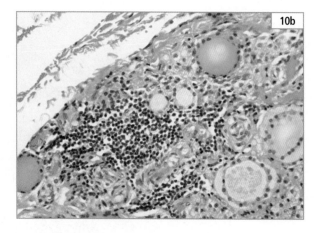

CASE 11: CANINE IMMUNE-MEDIATED POLYARTHRITIS

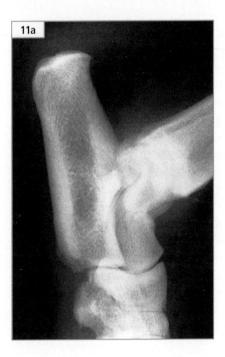

Signalment
Four-year-old crossbred dog.

History and physical examination
The dog is presented because the owner has noticed an increasing reluctance to exercise and a slow and stiff gait when the dog first rises from rest. The problem is described as not continuous, with 'some days being better than others'. Physical examination reveals mild pyrexia and swelling and heat related to the carpal and tarsal joints. Pain is elicited when these joints are manipulated. There has been no recent history of drug administration or vaccination and the dog has not travelled from Northern Europe. The owner lives in the countryside and the dog is exercised in nearby woodland.

Diagnostic procedures
Initial diagnostic procedures include radiography and routine haematological and serum biochemical examination. There are similar radiographic changes in both carpal and tarsal joints characterized by increased soft tissue density around the joints with synovial effusion (**Figure 11a**). There are no bony changes or damage to articular surfaces. No visceral abnormalities are present on thoracic or abdominal radiographs.

Haematological examination reveals leucocytosis with neutrophilia (19.8×10^9/l; normal range 3–11.5) and monocytosis (3.2×10^9/l; normal range 0.1–1.5) and there is mild polyclonal hypergammaglobulinaemia recognized on biochemical investigation.

A sample of synovial fluid is collected from one carpal and one tarsal joint. The 'mucin clot' is friable, consistent with damage to hyaluronic acid, and there is a high nucleated cell count (82×10^9/l). Cytological examination reveals a dominance of neutrophils with some vacuolated macrophages and a background of blood contamination (**Figure 11b**). There are no bacteria associated with these cells or within the fluid.

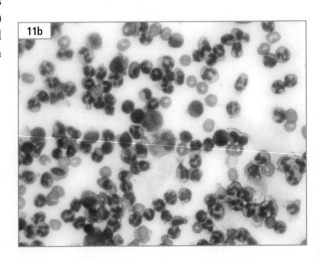

The dog has negative serum ANA and RF tests and there is no serological or molecular (PCR) evidence of infection by *Borrelia* (Lyme disease) or *Anaplasma phagocytophilum* (*Ixodes*-transmitted organisms endemic in the local area).

Diagnosis and immunopathology

The final diagnosis in this case is type I idiopathic polyarthritis. There are four subtypes of canine idiopathic polyarthritis (summarized below). This dog has no history of exposure to known trigger factors, no evidence of underlying systemic disease or neoplasia, and no evidence of infection by arthropod-borne agents known to lead to joint disease. The pathogenesis of this disease is poorly understood, but is thought to relate to a mixed type III and IV hypersensitivity reaction within the synovium (see Chapter 12).

Treatment and prognosis

The dog was treated with a course of immuno-suppressive glucocorticoid therapy and it made an uneventful recovery. Although the prognosis is relatively good, the owner was warned about the relapsing/remitting nature of immune-mediated diseases and the potential for recurrence.

Type of disease	Clinical association
Type I	Joint disease alone
Type II	Joint disease with infectious disease of other body systems ('reactive arthritis')
Type III	Joint disease with gastrointestinal disease ('enteropathic arthritis')
Type IV	Joint disease with underlying neoplasia ('arthritis of malignancy')

CASE 12: BOVINE ALLERGIC RHINITIS

Signalment
A herd of 50 milking Jersey cows established 6 years ago with calves bought in from three different farms.

History and physical examination
Fifteen of the cows have recently shown signs of snorting, coughing, nasal discharge and being seen to push their noses onto sticks. The herd is up-to-date with its vaccination against IBR.

Diagnostic procedures
One of the affected animals (a 5-year-old female) is culled and a postmortem examination conducted. The nasal passages are oedematous, with mucosal nodular swellings and a mucopurulent exudate (**Figure 12a**). Large fragments of stick are removed from the nasal cavity and the mucosa underlying these is ulcerated and haemorrhagic (**Figure 12b**).

Samples of the nasal mucosa are examined histologically. There is hyperplasia, ulceration and inflammation of the mucosal epithelium with oedema and inflammation of the underlying lamina propria. There is marked infiltration of eosinophils into the affected mucosa.

Diagnosis and immunopathology
The clinical presentation and pathological findings are consistent with the condition known as 'allergic nasal granuloma' or 'allergic rhinitis'. The aetiopathogenesis is unconfirmed, but the disease is believed to have an allergic basis (most likely type I hypersensitivity), as it occurs when animals are at grass and generally resolves over winter. Bovine allergic rhinitis has been documented most often in Australia and New Zealand as sporadic or herd outbreaks.

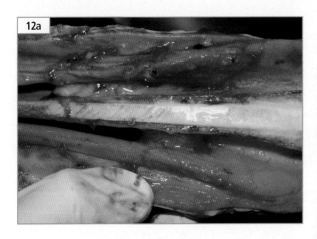

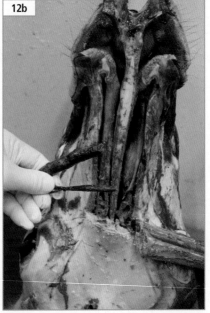

CASE 13: CANINE DRUG REACTION

Signalment

Ten-month-old, female Neapolitan mastiff (**Figure 13a**; photo courtesy P. Mellor).

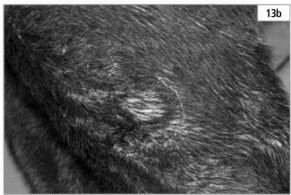

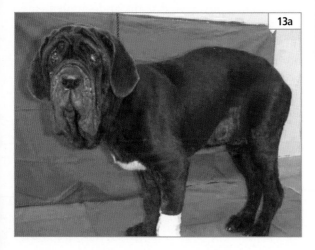

History and physical examination

This dog had surgical correction of bilateral entropion (inversion of the eyelid margin) 15 days ago. Immediately before surgery the dog had been on a course of cephalexin and immediately after surgery had been placed on a course of co-amoxiclav and the anti-inflammatory drug carprofen. The dog had received both antimicrobials at different times earlier in its life. Seven days ago there was a sudden onset of extensive generalized skin eruptions and since that time the dog had become increasingly weak and lethargic with periods of collapse.

Physical examination at presentation revealed that the lesions were alopecic, erythematous and ulcerated and many had a distinctive 'target ring' appearance (**Figure 13b**; from Mellor PJ *et al*. [2005] Neutrophilic dermatitis and immune-mediated haematological disorders in a dog: suspected adverse reaction to carprofen. *Journal of Small Animal Practice* **46**:237–242, with permission). The dog also had generalized peripheral lymphadenomegaly, pale mucous membranes and an elevated heart rate with a systolic heart murmur.

Diagnostic procedures

Initial diagnostic procedures included cardiac imaging, routine haematology and serum biochemistry, urinalysis and skin biopsy. Haematological data are presented below.

Parameter	Value	Normal range
PCV	0.08	0.37–0.55 l/l
Haemoglobin	36.5	120–180 g/l
Red blood cells	1.19	5.5–8.5 × 10^{12}/l
MCV	73.6	60–77 fl
MCHC	305	340–370 g/l
MCH	41.5	32–37 pg
Absolute reticulocytes	0	≤60 × 10^9/l
Platelets	63	150–500 × 10^9/l
White blood cells	8.97	6–17.5 × 10^9/l
Neutrophils	5.1	3–11.5 × 10^9/l
Lymphocytes	1.5	1–4.8 × 10^9/l
Monocytes	2.3	0.2–1.5 × 10^9/l
Eosinophils	0.04	0.05–1.3 × 10^9/l
Basophils	0.0	0–0.5 × 10^9/l

There is a marked non-regenerative anaemia, thrombocytopenia (confirmed on evaluation of the blood smear) and monocytosis. There were no abnormalities on serum biochemistry and urinalysis revealed the presence of haemoglobinuria. No cardiac abnormalities were detected on imaging examination and the heart murmur was attributed to being of haemic origin. Skin biopsy revealed the presence of a neutrophilic vasculitis.

These observations were suggestive of a multisystemic immune-mediated process indicating further specific diagnostic procedures. An EDTA blood sample showed autoagglutination of red cells, which was not dispersed by the addition of saline (positive in-saline agglutination test). This was considered presumptive evidence for IMHA, but a Coombs test was not performed. A direct immunofluoresence test demonstrated antibody associated with the patient's platelets. Serum ANA was negative and immunohistochemistry did not demonstrate immunoglobulin or complement associated with the cutaneous vascular lesions.

Diagnosis and immunopathology

The history, clinical presentation and laboratory findings in this dog were consistent with an immune-mediated drug reaction. There was evidence for IMHA, IMTP (type II hypersensitivity) and cutaneous vasculitis (type III hypersensitivity). The pathogenesis of this disease may involve the causative drug acting as a hapten and binding to host carrier protein. The dog had received three drugs in the period immediately before the onset of disease and both antimicrobials had been given in the past, thus providing an opportunity for sensitization. In fact, once this dog had clinically recovered blood was taken and extracted lymphocytes were cultured *in vitro* in the presence of both antimicrobials. Although the lymphocytes were able to respond to mitogen (see Chapter 10), there was no proliferative response to either drug. This was interpreted as presumptive evidence that the causative agent may have been carprofen.

Treatment and prognosis

The dog was given an infusion of polymerized bovine haemoglobin (as oxygen-carrying support) and started on a course of immunosuppressive prednisolone and azathioprine. A new covering antimicrobial (enrofloxacin) was administered and the dog was given topical medicated baths and supplemented with essential fatty acids. There was rapid clinical improvement with erythroid regeneration, normalization of platelet count, resolution of the heart murmur and reduced severity of skin lesions at discharge 9 days after presentation. The dog was well at a recheck examination 7 months later.

CASE 14: CANINE TRAPPED NEUTROPHIL SYNDROME

Signalment

Eight-month-old, female border collie (**Figure 14a**). The dog lives on a farm and has been bred to be a working animal.

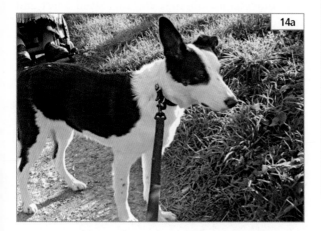

14a

Parameter	Value	Normal range
PCV	0.32	0.35–0.55 l/l
Haemoglobin	109	120–180 g/l
Red blood cells	4.64	5.4–8.0 × 10^{12}/l
MCV	69.4	65–75 fl
MCHC	337	340–370 g/l
MCH	23.4	22–25 pg
Platelets	295	170–500 × 10^9/l
White blood cells	2.57	5.5–17 × 10^9/l
Neutrophils	0.05	3–11.5 × 10^9/l
Lymphocytes	0.77	0.7–3.6 × 10^9/l
Monocytes	0.72	0.1–1.5 × 10^9/l
Eosinophils	0.0	0.2–1.4 × 10^9/l
Basophils	0.0	0–0.1 × 10^9/l

History and physical examination

The owner reports that this young dog has always been 'small for its breed' and since a young age has had episodes of inappetence, vomiting, diarrhoea, lethargy and apparent pain on walking. These episodes appeared to begin at around the time of the second in the puppy series of vaccinations. Although not currently diarrhoeic, the dog does have pyrexia, conjunctivitis and cheilitis and apparent joint pain on manipulation of the limbs.

Diagnostic procedures

Initial investigations include routine haematology, serum biochemistry, urinalysis and radiographs of major joints. Haematological data are presented below.

The most significant haematological findings are leucopenia with profound neutropenia and a mild anaemia. There are no abnormalities on serum biochemistry or urinalysis. Radiographs do not reveal active joint pathology and survey radiographs of the thorax and abdomen are considered normal. Samples of joint fluid from the carpal and tarsal joints have low cellularity and normal mucin clot formation. Bacteriological culture of these fluids leads to no significant growth. PCR fails to identify infection with either *Borrelia* or *Anaplasma* and serum ANA and RF are negative.

Further blood samples confirm that the neutropenia is persistent and so a bone marrow core biopsy is collected. This is markedly cellular with profound elevation in the myeloid:erythroid ratio. The majority of cells are of the granulocytic lineage (**Figure 14b**).

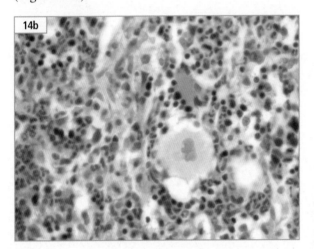

14b

Diagnosis and immunopathology

The main features of the disease in this young dog are a severe neutropenia (predisposing to multisystemic infectious/inflammatory disease), but plentiful granulocytic precursors within the bone marrow. Given the breed of dog and clinical history, the most likely diagnosis is 'trapped neutrophil syndrome of border collies'. This inherited primary immunodeficiency disorder is also known as myelokathexis and is essentially a failure of the bone marrow to release neutrophils into the circulation.

Treatment and prognosis

There is no effective cure for this disease. A PCR molecular diagnostic test for the causative gene mutation is marketed by the University of Sydney. Data from that laboratory suggest that this autosomal recessive mutation is widespread in this breed throughout the world. The present case was not tested.

CASE 15: FELINE LYMPHOID LEUKAEMIA

Signalment

Six-year-old, neutered female domestic shorthair cat.

History and physical examination

The cat is presented with a 5-day history of anorexia and lethargy. On physical examination the cat is seen to be in thin bodily condition and lethargic and with pale mucous membranes and increased heart and respiratory rates (**Figure 15a**; photo courtesy Feline Centre, University of Bristol).

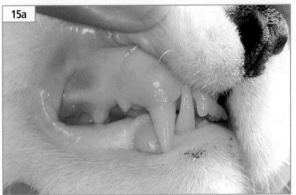

15a

Diagnostic procedures

Initial diagnostic procedures include routine haematology, serum biochemistry and urinalysis and evaluation of retroviral status. Haematological data are presented below.

Examination of the blood smear also reveals the presence of a population of atypical lymphoblastic cells. The only abnormality on serum biochemistry is elevation of alkaline phosphatase (71 IU/l; normal range 0–20) and urinalysis is normal. The cat is negative for FeLV and FIV.

Parameter	Value	Normal range
PCV	0.4	0.27–0.50 l/l
Haemoglobin	14	80–150 g/l
Red blood cells	0.85	5.5–10.0 × 10^{12}/l
MCV	47.1	40–55 fl
MCHC	350	310–340 g/l
MCH	16.5	13–17 pg
Platelets	<5 per × 100 field	
Neutrophils	1.5	2.5–12.5 × 10^9/l
Lymphocytes	3.9	1.5–7.0 × 10^9/l
Monocytes	0.1	0.0–0.8 × 10^9/l
Eosinophils	0.0	0.0–1.5 × 10^9/l

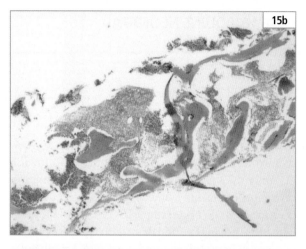

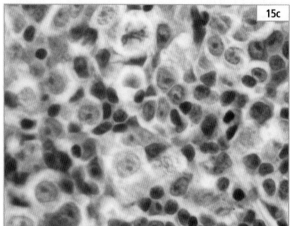

The major findings are, therefore, a severe anaemia, thrombocytopenia and neutropenia (pancytopenia) associated with the presence of atypical lymphoid cells within the circulation. These observations are consistent with bone marrow disease and presumptive leukaemia. Survey radiographs of the thorax and abdomen do not reveal visceral disease. A bone marrow core biopsy is taken. The marrow is hypercellular with haemopoietic tissue almost entirely replaced by a monomorphic population of pleomorphic and mitotic lymphoblastic cells (**Figures 15b** and **15c**).

Diagnosis and immunopathology

The diagnosis is chronic lymphocytic leukaemia of bone marrow origin with neoplastic cells seeding to the blood. It is also possible that these cells had started to colonize the liver and spleen. The tumour does not appear to be FeLV associated in this case. The severity of disease in this cat might seem at odds with the relatively late clinical presentation, but it is a good example of the propensity of this species to compensate and present with relatively subtle clinical signs.

Treatment and prognosis

The cat was placed onto a combination chemotherapeutic protocol, but the long-term prognosis must be guarded in this case.

CASE 16: EQUINE NEONATAL ISOERYTHROLYSIS

Signalment
One-day-old Thoroughbred foal.

History and physical examination
The foal was born normally in the afternoon and was seen to take in adequate colostrum. The following morning the foal is collapsed. Physical examination reveals pallor (but not jaundice) of mucous membranes (**Figure 16**) and a urine sample has red discolouration. The foal is not pyrexic and there is no clinical evidence of sepsis. There is an elevated heart rate, a weak pulse and occasional 'yawning' is observed. This is the second foal born to this mare by the same stallion. The first foaling was uneventful.

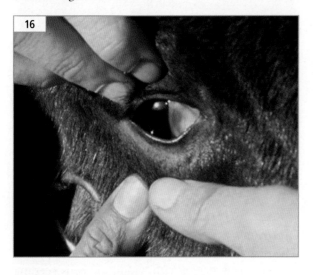

Diagnostic procedures
A blood sample reveals severe anaemia with a PCV of 0.8 l/l (18%) (normal range for adult horse 0.32–0.53 [32-53%]). Platelet and leucocyte counts are normal. Analysis of the urine sample confirms that the discolouration is due to the presence of haemoglobin. A Coombs test performed with equine polyvalent Coombs reagent is positive (titre 320 at 37°C) and when serum from the mare is mixed with a suspension of washed foal erythrocytes, there is also a strong agglutination reaction, which titrates *in vitro* to a titre of 1,280.

Diagnosis and immunopathology
The foal has neonatal isoerythrolysis (see Chapter 18). The mare became sensitized to foreign blood group antigens from the first foal and developed antibodies to these molecules. These antibodies concentrated in the colostrum that was taken in by the foal. The absorbed antibody has rapidly attached to the foal's red cells, resulting in peracute onset, severe IMHA. The most likely blood group antigen incompatibility in this case is with respect to the Aa antigen (which the stallion likely expresses but not the mare). The disease may also have an acute (2–4 days old) or subacute (4–5 days old) onset, with progressively less severe clinical signs and greater likelihood of icterus at presentation.

Treatment and prognosis
This foal must immediately be prevented from further access to milk from the mare for the remainder of that day. A foster mother or milk replacement should be used, but after 48 hours it should be safe to permit the foal to suck the mare. The severity of anaemia in this foal means that the prognosis should be guarded. The foal requires a blood transfusion. A whole blood transfusion must be cross-matched and this can be done by testing serum from the mare against potential donor erythrocytes. A second transfusion may be required depending on the degree of elevation of the foal's PCV. The stud should be warned not to mate these parent animals in the future. For future pregnancies, it would be wise to test the mare's serum with the stallion's erythrocytes during the final 2 weeks of pregnancy. Any reaction would indicate that the foal should be fostered or hand-reared using alternative colostrum.

CASE 17: IMMUNOLOGICAL ASPECTS OF A HERD OUTBREAK OF BOVINE VIRAL DIARRHOEA VIRUS INFECTION

Signalment

Full-term calf born dead with diffuse cataracts and cerebellar hypoplasia.

History and physical examination

This 30-cow dairy herd has a history of multiple abortions (especially in first calf heifers), weak calves at birth and calves developing pneumonia and ringworm infection during the first few months of life.

Diagnostic procedures

Blood and tissue samples were collected and tested from an aborted fetus and a 2-week-old calf by IFA testing and virus isolation. Tissue samples were positive for BVDV by IFA testing. At necropsy examination, the fetus and calf both had multiple gross abnormalities. The fetus had cerebellar hypoplasia (**Figures 17a** and **17b**) and thymic aplasia. The calf also had thymic aplasia and hypoplasia of all lymphoid tissues. All cattle were ear notched and tested by ELISA for the presence of BVDV. This test is specifically designed to detect animals persistently infected with BVDV. Persistently infected animals develop when fetuses from conception to 120 days are infected *in utero* with a non-cytopathic strain of BVDV. The animals often fail to develop an immune response (cellular and/or humoral) because the immune system considers the BVDV to be self rather than non-self.

Diagnosis and immunopathology

This herd did not have a history of vaccination with the cattle viral core vaccines specific for BVDV, IBR, parainfluenza-3 and bovine respiratory syncytial virus. It was also not a closed herd and three 4–9-month-old heifers had been purchased during the past year. It is very likely that one or more of those heifers were persistently infected with BVDV. The persistently infected animal is infected for life and although many will die by 1 to 3 years of age, some cattle have been known to survive for more than 10 years.

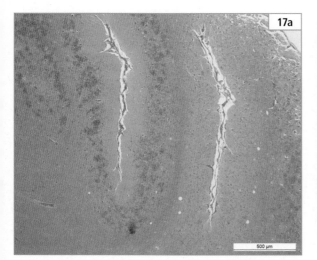

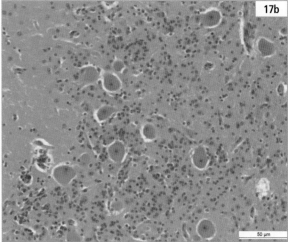

Treatment and prognosis

Acutely infected animals often require antibiotic treatment for secondary bacterial infections due to the immunosuppressive effects of the virus causing the animal to be at greater risk for bacterial diseases, especially gastrointestinal and respiratory diseases. Additional supportive therapy (e.g. fluids) is often necessary since diarrhoea is common. An animal found to be persistently infected must be removed from the herd and sent to slaughter as it cannot be permitted to remain in the herd of origin or go into another herd. All new animals entering the herd need to be tested for BVDV before they are brought in and all herd animals need to be vaccinated as calves and then revaccinated with the cattle core vaccines every 3 or more years to maintain herd immunity. If these recommendations are followed, the herd should not develop similar problems in the future.

Active immunization   Injection of antigen to stimulate an immune response and induce immunological memory.

Acute phase proteins   Group of proteins found in the blood during the early stages of an infectious/inflammatory response.

Adaptive   A form of immunity that is specifically stimulated by antigen, resulting in clonal selection of antigen-relevant lymphocytes. This provides a more potent immune response to support non-specific innate immunity. The adaptive immune response generates immunological memory. Also 'acquired immunity'.

ADCC   Cytotoxic destruction of a target cell coated by antibody that is recognized by an Fc receptor on the surface of the cytotoxic cell.

Adhesion molecule   Mediates the binding of cells to each other, or cells to matrix proteins.

Adjuvant   Substance that enhances the immune response. Traditional adjuvants are non-specific in their effect or they may have a 'depot effect' causing sustained release of antigen. Modern adjuvants may have a more targeted effect on the immune response (e.g. cytokine adjuvants, CpG motifs).

Adult tolerance   Induction of tolerance to an antigen in an adult animal.

Aeroallergen   Airborne allergen that can be inhaled or absorbed percutaneously.

Afferent lymphatic   Lymphatic vessel draining lymph from tissue to the regional lymph node.

Affinity   Strength of binding of one molecule to another; specifically the binding of a single antigenic epitope to a single Fab binding site within an immunoglobulin.

Affinity maturation   Process of acquiring somatic mutations in the BCR to increase the affinity of the receptor.

Agammaglobulinaemia   Absence of B cells and immunoglobulin.

Agglutination   Aggregation of particulate antigens by antibodies; in particular multivalent antibodies such as IgA and IgM.

Alarmin   Molecule released by damaged tissue cells that triggers innate immunity and inflammation.

Allele   Two or more alternative forms of a gene.

Allergen   Antigen that induces an allergic or hypersensitivity reaction.

Allergy   See 'hypersensitivity'.

Alloantigen   Tissue antigen derived from a genetically dissimilar individual of the same species. Typically stimulates an immune response following incompatible grafting of tissue or cells.

Allograft   Transplant of tissue or organ between genetically dissimilar individuals of the same species.

Alopecia   Loss of the hair coat by failure to grow or interference with the hair cycle after growth.

Alum   Adjuvant based on the use of aluminium phosphate or hydroxide.

Amastigote   Stage of protozoal life cycle. That form of *Leishmania* found within tissue macrophages.

Amino acid   Building block of protein.

Anaphylaxis   Systemic type I hypersensitivity reaction.

Anergy   Failure of an immune response to a presented antigen due to lack of co-stimulation by the APC. Patients are 'anergic' when they fail to respond to an antigen by mounting a DTH response.

Anaphylotoxin   Substance capable of directly degranulating a mast cell; typically C3a and C5a of the complement pathway.

Anchor residues   Specific points of contact between an antigenic peptide and an MHC or TCR molecule.

Anorexia   Reduced appetite for food.

Antibody   Protein that binds specifically to an antigen. Antibodies are secreted by plasma cells and can bind to pathogens to target them for removal. Each antibody has unique antigen binding capacity, but shares structure with other antibodies or immunoglobulins.

Antigen Substance that initiates a specific immune response; technically a molecule that can bind to specific antibody, although some antigens do not elicit antibodies as part of the immune response.

Antigen presentation Expression of small peptide fragments derived from an antigen (by antigen processing) on the surface of an APC within the binding groove of an MHC class I or II molecule.

Antigen processing Breakdown of antigen to small peptide components within the cytoplasm of an APC via either the endogenous or exogenous pathway.

Antinuclear antibody Autoantibody with specificity for one of the components of the nucleus of a cell.

Antiserum Serum collected from an individual following exposure to an antigen. Contains antibody that can be utilized in serological assays. A polyclonal antiserum contains multiple antibodies specific for different epitopes of the antigen. In contrast, a monoclonal antibody is an antibody of a single type that recognizes a single epitope.

Aplasia Failure of an organ or tissue to develop.

Apoptosis Cell death resulting from activation of an 'internal death programme' within the cell leading to DNA degradation, nuclear degeneration and condensation and phagocytosis of the cell remains. Also 'programmed cell death'.

Arthus reaction Local tissue type III hypersensitivity reaction involving immune complex formation in a sensitized individual following local exposure to antigen.

ASIT See 'hyposensitization'.

Asthma Respiratory disease that may have several causes, one of which is type I hypersensitivity to aeroallergens.

Atopic dermatitis Skin disease that may have several causes, one of which is type I hypersensitivity to aeroallergens that are percutaneously absorbed. Likely to have a genetic basis.

Attenuation Reduction in virulence of an infectious agent so that it retains antigenic structure and limited replicative capacity, but cannot produce disease (live attenuated vaccine; infectious vaccine).

Autoantigen Antigen derived from self-tissue that stimulates an autoimmune response.

Autogenous vaccination Culture of a pathogen from a patient and injection of a crude preparation of that pathogen subcutaneously to promote the immune response to the organism.

Autoimmunity Generation of an immune response to self-antigen resulting in tissue pathology and autoimmune disease.

Autophagy Degradation of dysfunctional or unnecessary cellular components via the lysosomal pathway. Such components are contained within autophagosomes, which then fuse with lysosomes for degradation of their content.

Avidity Strength of overall binding of two molecules that contact at multiple sites; specifically the binding of multiple antigenic epitopes by multiple Fab binding sites within an immunoglobulin.

BALT Unencapsulated mucosal lymphoid aggregate associated with the bronchial mucosa.

BCR Immunoglobulin receptor for antigen on the surface of a B lymphocyte.

Bence-Jones protein Free immunoglobulin light chains that may be produced in multiple myeloma and pass through the glomerular filter into the urine (Bence-Jones proteinuria).

Bronchoconstriction Narrowing of the diameter of a bronchus following contraction of the bronchial smooth muscle. May be mediated by mast cell or basophil contents in a type I hypersensitivity reaction.

Bursa of Fabricius Specialized organ associated with the cloaca that is the primary site of B-cell development in birds.

Bystander suppression Non-specific suppression of a local immune response not directly related to that being controlled by a suppressor lymphocyte.

Carrier protein Protein that when linked to a hapten can initiate an immune response to the hapten in addition to responses to its own 'native' epitopes.

CD Nomenclature used to define immune cell surface molecules.

CH$_{50}$ An *in-vitro* test of the function of the classical and terminal pathways of complement.

Chediak–Higashi Syndrome Abnormal granulation in the cytoplasm of neutrophils of blue smoke

Persian cats. May be associated with functional impairment of these cells.

Chemokine Soluble protein released from a cell to form a chemotactic gradient responsible for the chemoattraction of specific leucocytes (e.g. into tissue from the circulation).

Chemotaxis Migration of a leucocyte along a chemotactic gradient of increasing concentration of a chemoattractant.

Chromatin The substance of the chromosomes within the cell nucleus; includes DNA and histone proteins.

CLAD Genetic mutation resulting in failure to express leucocyte adhesion molecules involved in the migration of leucocytes (in particular neutrophils) from blood to tissue. Occurs in Irish setters.

Clonal deletion Removal by apoptosis of autoreactive lymphocytes bearing receptors specific for self-antigens. May occur within the thymus or bone marrow for T and B cells, respectively (central deletion), or may occur within secondary lymphoid tissue (peripheral deletion).

Clonal differentiation Following activation of a lymphocyte by antigen, there are repeated rounds of cell division (clonal proliferation) during which the cells may acquire specific functional or effector characteristics.

Clonal proliferation Exponential expansion of a clone of lymphocytes following activation by antigen.

Clonal selection Selection (for activation) of antigen-relevant lymphocytes from the entire repertoire on exposure to antigen.

CMI That type of immune response mediated by lymphocytes and typically involving cytotoxic destruction of target cells (e.g. infected cells, neoplastic cells or incompatible graft cells).

Complement Series of plasma proteins which, when activated, interact sequentially, forming a self-assembling enzymatic cascade and generating biologically active molecules that mediate a range of end processes.

Complementarity determining region Hypervariable regions within the variable regions of TCRs and BCRs that bind to antigenic peptides or epitopes, respectively.

Conformation Three-dimensional tertiary structure of a molecule.

Constant region Portion of an immunological molecule in which there is conserved amino acid sequence in the polypeptide chain that is shared by different molecules.

Contact allergy Type IV hypersensitivity reaction to percutaneously absorbed allergen.

Coombs test Agglutination test used to detect the presence of immunoglobulin and/or complement on the surface of erythrocytes in IMHA.

Core (vaccine) Vaccine that all animals should receive, as it protects from a serious infectious disease that is prevalent in that geographical location.

Cortex Outer zone of an organ; in immunology, specifically of the lymph node and thymus.

Co-stimulation Co-stimulatory signals are required to fully activate a lymphocyte following recognition of antigen. Co-stimulatory signals may be delivered by molecular interaction between lymphocyte and APC, or cytokine released from the APC and binding cytokine receptor on the lymphocyte.

CpG motif Sequence of bacterial DNA rich in cytosine and guanidine nucleotides that is a potent stimulus for Th1 immune responses.

CR1–4 Cell surface receptors that bind complement components.

Cross-link Joining together (i.e. cross-linkage) of two mast cell surface Fcε receptors by allergen binding two individual receptor-bound IgE molecules.

Cross-reactive Two antigens may share common or similar epitopes, enabling recognition by more than one antigen receptor (immunoglobulin or TCR).

Cross-regulation Regulation of the function of one cell by another; typically the mutually antagonistic effects of Th1 and Th2 lymphocytes.

Cyclic haematopoiesis Genetic mutation in grey collie dogs resulting in cyclic cytopenia and susceptibility to infectious/inflammatory disease.

Cytokine Soluble protein secreted by one cell that binds to a specific cytokine receptor expressed by another cell, leading to a change in function of the target cell. Cytokines are considered intercellular messengers of the immune system. A generic term for molecules including interleukins, monokines and lymphokines.

Cytolysis Lysis of a cell (e.g. by the effects of the complement pathway).

Cytotoxicity   Destruction of a target cell by a cytotoxic effector cell.

D region   Gene segment that links the joining and constant regions of immunoglobulin heavy chain and TCR chain loci.

DAMP   Damage-associated molecular pattern. Molecules derived from damaged cells that activate inflammation and immunity by binding to PPRs on APCs.

Data sheet   Package insert that accompanies a drug or vaccine giving details of its formulation, use and potential side-effects. In Europe, the 'summary of product characteristics', SPC.

Deep pyoderma   Staphylococcal infection of the hair follicles of the dog.

Defensin   Antimicrobial peptide secreted from epithelial surfaces.

Degranulation   Release of cytoplasmic granules containing biological mediators following activation of a mast cell or basophil.

Delayed-type hypersensitivity   Type IV hypersensitivity reaction involving activation of mononuclear cells and production of cytokines inasensitized individual re-exposed to antigen. Takes 24–72 hours to become manifest clinically.

Dendritic cell   Major APC for a primary immune response. Undertakes antigen capture, processing and presentation to T cells. Characteristic morphology with cytoplasmic dendrites.

Determinant   See 'epitope'.

Diapedesis   Process by which leucocytes squeeze between endothelial cells to enter tissue from a blood vessel.

Dietary hypersensitivity   Hypersensitivity to food-derived allergen (see also 'food allergy'). Presents as cutaneous or alimentary disease. Most likely a type I hypersensitivity reaction.

Dimer   Complex of two individual units (e.g. an IgA dimer).

Domain   Conformational region of a polypeptide that may have specific function (e.g. the domain structure of the immunoglobulin molecule).

Downregulation   Suppression.

Duration of immunity   Period after vaccination in which an immune response to vaccine can be detected (by experimental challenge or serologically).

Ectoparasite   Parasite of the external surface of the body.

Effector cell   Cell that actively participates in an immune response (e.g. by producing antibody or destroying a target cell via cytotoxicity).

Efferent lymphatic   Lymphatic vessel draining lymph from a lymph node to the common thoracic duct.

Efficacy (vaccine)   Measure of how well a vaccine works, by preventing infection and/or the tissue pathology and clinical signs of disease. Determined experimentally by challenge of vaccinated versus unvaccinated animals with virulent organism. May also be studied in the field where there is natural exposure to the organism.

Eicosanoids   Family of inflammatory mediators derived from arachidonic acid.

ELISA   An *in-vitro* serological test used to determine the concentration of either antigen or antibody. Based on detection by an enzyme-conjugated secondary antiserum and demonstrated by providing an appropriate substrate that leads to a colour change, which may be measured spectrophotometrically.

Endogenous antigen   Antigen produced within the cytoplasm of an APC (i.e. a self-antigen or viral antigen).

Endoparasite   Parasite that lives within the body of the host.

Endoplasmic reticulum   Folded membrane sheets within the cytoplasm that are sites of protein synthesis. Site of interaction between endogenous peptide and MHC class I in antigen processing.

Endosome   A cytoplasmic compartment formed by invagination of the cell membrane around an antigenic substance during the process of antigen uptake by an APC. See also 'phagosome'.

Endotoxin   Toxin derived from the cell wall of gram-negative bacteria (e.g. *E. coli*), which is absorbed to mediate systemic endotoxaemia.

Enterocyte   Epithelial cell lining the intestinal tract.

Enterotoxin   Toxin produced by enteric pathogenic bacteria that binds to receptors on enterocytes and mediates osmotic diarrhoea.

Eotaxin Chemokine that attracts eosinophils into tissue. Includes eotaxin-1, eotaxin-2 and eotaxin-3.

Epitheliotropic lymphoma Lymphoma of skin or mucosae where the neoplastic lymphocytes infiltrate the epithelium. Also known as 'mycosis fungoides'.

Epitope Site on an antigen that may be recognized by an antibody or TCR. The nature of epitopes bound by these two types of receptor is different. Also called an antigenic 'determinant'.

Epitope spreading Spreading of the immune response to other epitopes within an antigen (generally an autoantigen) after the response is initiated by presentation of one epitope.

Erythema Redness of the skin due to increased blood flow. One of the cardinal signs of inflammation.

Exogenous antigen External antigen taken up by an APC.

Exon The nucleotide sequence of a gene that is represented in the mRNA.

Fab Fragment antigen binding. Antigen binding site at the N terminal end of the immunoglobulin molecule.

Fc Fragment crystallizable. Heavy chains at the C terminal end of the immunoglobulin molecule.

Fc receptor Cell surface receptor that binds immunoglobulin.

Flea allergy dermatitis Type I hypersensitivity to antigens within flea saliva.

Fluorescence Colour emitted by a fluorochrome when activated by light of a specific wavelength (usually ultraviolet). Fluorochromes such as fluorescein isothiocyanate (FITC) may be coupled to antibodies to detect molecules within tissue (immunofluorescence) or on the surface of cells (by flow cytometry).

Follicle Area of lymphoid tissue within which B lymphocytes reside. Follicles are found within lymph nodes, spleen and mucosal lymphoid tissue. Primary follicles are inactive, whereas secondary follicles with a germinal centre and mantle zone reflect activation of the immune system by antigen.

Food allergy An immunological reaction to dietary antigens. Most often considered a type I hypersensitivity reaction. (See also 'dietary hypersensitivity').

Frustrated phagocytosis Situation where a phagocytic cell cannot ingest a large antigen, but is able to release cytoplasmic granule contents adjacent to the particle to produce surface damage to that target.

GALT Unencapsulated lymphoid tissue associated with the alimentary mucosa. Includes tonsils, gastric lymphoid follicles, Peyer's patches and colonic lymphoid aggregates.

Gene conversion Generation of BCR diversity in animals and birds by incorporation of V region pseudogenes into the expressed V region segment.

Gene therapy Delivery of normal functional gene copies into an individual with an inherited mutation of that gene.

Genome The entire complement of genetic material contained within a haploid set of chromosomes.

Germinal centre Central region of a secondary lymphoid follicle where antigen-activated B lymphocytes divide.

Germline repertoire Theoretical number of different immunoglobulin or TCR molecules that can be generated from the multiple gene segments encoding variable domains inherited by an individual. The repertoire can be further expanded by variable recombination or somatic mutation.

Giant cell Aggregate of macrophages formed during a chronic inflammatory (granulomatous) response.

Golgi apparatus Cytoplasmic organelle consisting of flattened sacs (cisternae) and vesicles involved in protein synthesis. Thought to have a role in the processing and presentation of endogenous antigen. Plasma cells have a distinct cytoplasmic 'Golgi zone'.

Granuloma Distinct arrangement of inflammatory cells formed in response to a persistent stimulus. Typically a necrotic centre surrounded by concentric layers of macrophages, then lymphocytes and plasma cells.

Granulomatous inflammation Chronic inflammation characterized by diffuse infiltration of macrophages without formation of distinct granulomas.

Grave's disease Human autoimmune disease involving binding of autoantibody to TSH receptor leading to uncontrolled thyroid activation and hyperthyroidism.

Haematopoiesis Generation of haemopoietic cells, normally in the bone marrow. Also 'haemopoiesis'.

Haplotype   Linked set of genes associated with one haploid genome. Used to describe a set of linked MHC genes inherited as a haplotype from one parent.

Hapten   Small chemical group which by itself cannot elicit an immune response, but when bound to a 'carrier protein' is capable of generating an antibody or T-cell response.

Hassall's corpuscle   Epithelial structure in the medulla of a thymic lobule.

Heavy chain   One of two large polypeptides making up the immunoglobulin molecule.

Herd immunity   Protection of a population from an infection by ensuring the maximum number of individuals in that population are vaccinated.

Heterologous (vaccine)   Use of an antigenically similar, related infectious agent that lacks virulence to cross-protect against another more virulent pathogen.

HEV   Structural modification of venular endothelial cells such that they take on a cuboidal morphology, thus creating local turbulent flow to maximize the chance of interaction with leucocytes.

Hinge region   Portion of an immunoglobulin molecule between Fab and Fc that permits movement of the 'arms' of the Y-shaped structure.

Histocompatibility   Immunological similarity between individuals. Determined by the cellular expression of histocompatibility molecules and forms the basis of tissue matching before transplantation.

Histiocyte   Tissue macrophage.

Histiocytic sarcoma   Malignant proliferation of histiocytic cells (dendritic cells in this context) that may be either localized or disseminated.

Histiocytoma   Benign cutaneous neoplasm of epidermal Langerhans cells in the dog.

Homing receptor   Molecule expressed by leucocytes that enables interaction with specific endothelial vascular addressins to allow that leucocyte to enter tissue at particular anatomical locations.

Humanized monoclonal antibody   Genetically engineered monoclonal antibody with human Fc region and murine antigen binding region. Avoids initiation of anti-murine responses when used therapeutically in people.

Humoral immunity   Immunity mediated by antibodies.

Hybridoma   A cell arising from the fusion of an antigen-specific plasma cell with an immortal myeloma cell. Hybridoma cells secrete monoclonal antibodies.

Hygiene hypothesis   States that the western lifestyle with high sanitation and reduced exposure to microbes underlies susceptibility to allergic and autoimmune disease in humans.

Hypercalcaemia of malignancy   Elevated blood calcium concentration due to the ability of some tumours (e.g. lymphoma, myeloma) to produce PTH-like peptides that mediate osteoclast resorption of calcium from bone.

Hypergammaglobulinaemia   Elevation in serum gamma globulin concentration.

Hyperplasia   Increase in size of a tissue or organ due to an increase in the number of constituent cells (e.g. reactive hyperplasia of a lymph node due to antigenic stimulation of the lymphoid cells in that node).

Hypersensitivity   State of immunological sensitization to an innocuous antigen that leads to an excessive (symptomatic) immune response on re-exposure to the antigen. See also 'allergy'.

Hypervariable   Portion of an antigen-binding molecule with the greatest variability in amino acid sequence. Typically forms the contact residues with antigen. Found in antibodies, TCRs and histocompatibility molecules. See also 'complementarity determining region'.

Hypogammaglobulinaemia   Decrease in the concentration of serum gammaglobulin.

Hypoplasia (e.g. thymic)   Reduced size of an organ or tissue from birth (i.e. a congenital defect due to incomplete development).

Hyposensitization   Repeated injection of gradually increasing quantities of antigen to which an individual is sensitized diminishes the immune response on subsequent natural exposure to antigen. Used in the management of atopic dermatitis (see also 'ASIT').

Iatrogenic hyperadrenocorticism   Induction of hyperadrenocorticism by prolonged medical administration of glucocorticoids.

IBD   Chronic diarrhoea of unknown aetiology that responds clinically to immunosuppressive therapy.

Idiopathic   Of undetermined cause.

IgA deficiency   Lack of IgA in serum and at mucosal surfaces with resulting predisposition to infectious and immune-mediated disease. In man and dogs is a relative, rather than absolute, deficiency and does not involve genetic mutation of genes encoding the IgA molecule.

Immediate hypersensitivity   Occurs in a sensitized individual within minutes of re-exposure to antigen. Involves type I hypersensitivity.

Immune adherence   Adherence of complement C3b-coated particles to macrophages bearing CR1 receptors. A mechanism for clearance of circulating antigen within the bloodstream. C3b-coated particles are bound by CR1 on erythrocytes and subsequently removed from the red cell by macrophages within the spleen.

Immune complex   Complex of antigen and antibody with or without complement. Aggregated immunoglobulin can also form an immune complex in the absence of antigen.

Immune deviation   Polarization of the immune response to a specific antigen such that the response is predominantly regulated by Th1 (CMI) or Th2 (humoral) cells.

Immune surveillance   Surveillance of the entire body by the immune system for encounter with potential pathogens, damage to tissue or emergence of neoplastic clones.

Immunity gap   Period of time when there is insufficient maternally derived immunoglobulin to protect a young animal from infection, but sufficient maternal immunoglobulin to prevent onset of the endogenous immune response in that animal. Also termed the 'window of susceptibility'.

Immunodeficiency   Failure of part/s of the immune system due to inherited gene mutations (primary immunodeficiency) or acquired suppression of immune function (secondary immunodeficiency).

Immunodominant   Those epitopes within an antigen that are most likely to engender an immune response.

Immunofluorescence   See 'fluorescence'.

Immunogen   A substance that induces an adaptive immune response following injection into an individual.

Immunoglobulin   A general term for all antibody molecules. There are five classes of immunoglobulin: IgD, IgM, IgG, IgA and IgE.

Immunoglobulin class switch   Commitment of an antigen-activated B lymphocyte to express a single immunoglobulin class (IgA, IgG or IgE) instead of the combination of IgM and IgD that characterizes the naïve B cell.

Immunoglobulin superfamily   Relatedness of a series of immunological molecules that likely arose through gene duplication during evolution. There are conserved regions of structure between immunoglobulins, TCRs, MHC antigens and other CD molecules.

Immunohistochemistry   Use of antibodies to probe a tissue section for the presence of a specific molecule. The binding of antigen and antibody is visualized by conjugating the antibody to either a fluorochrome (immunofluorescence) or enzyme (immunoperoxidase). Multiple layers of reagents can be used to amplify the signal intensity.

Immunological ignorance   Tolerance of a lymphocyte due to failure to present the cognate antigen.

Immunological synapse   Point of contact between the cell membranes of an APC and T cell formed by multiple intercellular molecular interactions with the TCR–MHC–peptide interaction at the core.

Immunopathology   Tissue pathology caused by an immune response. The hypersensitivity reactions may also be considered immunopathological mechanisms.

Immunoperoxidase   A type of immunohistochemistry involving conjugation of the enzyme peroxidase to an antibody used to probe tissue sections for the presence of a specific molecule. Upon subsequent incubation with hydrogen peroxide and a chromogenic substrate there is colour deposition (usually brown) within the tissue section at the site of the reaction.

Immunoregulation   Control of the immune response; may be a positive effect (upregulation) or suppressive effect (downregulation).

Immunosenescence   Decline in immune function with advancing age.

Immunosuppression   Damping down or switching off an active immune response.

Induced suppressor   A suppressor T cell (Treg) induced as part of an immune response.

Inflammation   A localized protective response to a stimulus (e.g. infection or trauma) that contains and removes the injurious agent. The cardinal signs of inflammation are heat, redness, swelling, pain and loss of function. Inflammation may be acute or chronic.

Innate   That form of more primitive immunity that is evolutionarily older and provides continuous protection of body surfaces.

Interferon   A type of cytokine. The type I interferons (e.g. IFN-α, IFN-β) are antiviral molecules, whereas type II interferon (IFN-γ) is a key immunological molecule.

Interleukin   A type of cytokine secreted by one leucocyte that binds a receptor expressed by another leucocyte.

Intradermal (skin) test   Intradermal injection of a small quantity of antigen to which an individual is sensitized. Formation of a local area of erythema and oedema (wheal) within minutes after injection is consistent with a type I hypersensitivity response. A local area of erythema and induration that arises 48–72 hours post injection suggests a delayed (type IV) hypersensitivity response. The procedure is used diagnostically to determine causative allergens in allergic disease.

Intron   Portion of DNA that does not code for protein. The intervening sequence of nucleotides between coding sequences (exons).

Invariant chain   Molecule that wraps around an MHC class II molecule within a cytoplasmic endosome that is broken down by acid proteases, allowing peptides to associate with the variable region of the MHC molecule.

IVIG   Intravenous injection of immunoglobulin in the management of immune-mediated disease.

J chain   Joining chain that links together monomers of IgA or IgM via their heavy chains.

Joining region   Gene segment that links the variable and constant regions of an immunoglobulin or TCR locus.

Keratoconjunctivitis sicca   Lymphocytic destruction of the lacrimal glands leading to reduced production of tears and 'dry eye'.

Killed vaccine   Vaccine containing an organism that has been killed but retains antigenic structure (a non-infectious vaccine).

Langerhans cell   A type of dendritic APC located within the epidermis.

Late-phase response   Occurs 24 hours after an immediate hypersensitivity reaction and involves the infiltration of eosinophils into affected tissue.

Leptin   An example of a cytokine produced by adipocytes (adipokine) that has immunomodulatory functions in addition to a role in regulation of body mass.

Lethal acrodermatitis   Putative immunodeficiency disease affecting bull terrier dogs.

Ligand   Molecule that binds to another (e.g. the ligand for a specific receptor).

Light chain   One of two small polypeptides making up the immunoglobulin molecule.

Lupus erythematosus   Group of autoimmune diseases involving either the skin (e.g. CLE) or multiple body systems (SLE). Name derives from the facial cutaneous rash that characterizes humanSLE (lupus – 'wolf like').

Lymphadenomegaly   Enlargement of lymph nodes.

Lymphadenopathy   Pathological change in lymph nodes; often used to describe lymph node enlargement in clinical setting.

Lymphoblast   Antigen-activated lymphocyte.

Lymphoid leukaemia   Neoplasia of lymphocytes that begins within the bone marrow with subsequent release of neoplastic cells into the circulating blood.

Lymphoma   Tumour of lymphocytes presenting as diffuse infiltration or mass lesions of the viscera.

Lysosome   Structure within the cytoplasm of a phagocytic cell that contains a collection of potent proteolytic enzymes.

Lysozyme   An enzyme found in secretions that disrupts the cell wall of bacteria.

M cell   Microfold cell. Specialized cell found within the epithelial surface of the 'dome' of an intestinal Peyer's patch. Thought to 'sample' antigen from the overlying intestinal lumen and transfer it to lymphoid cells below.

MAC   Collection of terminal pathway complement components that form a channel through the membrane of a target cell and lead to osmotic lysis.

MALT   Unencapsulated lymphoid tissue associated with the mucosal surfaces of the body.

MAMP A conserved antigen expressed by any microorganism (pathogen or part of the microbiome), which is recognized by the PRR on the dendritic cell. See also PAMP.

Mantle zone Outer region of a secondary lymphoid follicle comprised of small lymphocytes.

Marginal zone Region at the edge of splenic white pulp that incorporates both the PALS and follicles.

Marker (vaccine) Vaccine containing a modified organism that induces an immune response that may be distinguished from the natural immune response made to field strains of the organism.

Memory Ability of the adaptive immune system to recall a previous encounter with an antigen and to make a more potent secondary immune response on re-encounter. Underlies the process of vaccination.

MHC Complex of genes encoding molecules that mediate histocompatibility and antigen presentation. Highly polymorphic and broadly divided into class I, II and III genes.

Microarray Molecular technique used to determine the gene expression profile in a tissue.

Mitogen Substance (often plant derived) that can non-specifically stimulate lymphocytes by binding to other than the antigen-specific lymphocyte receptor.

Molecular adjuvant Gene (e.g. cytokine gene) or nucleotide sequence (e.g. CpG motif) incorporated into a molecular vaccine to enhance the immune response to the protein encoded by the vaccinal gene, or to direct the nature of the ensuing immune response (e.g. Th1 or Th2).

Molecular mimicry Shared structure or sequence of an epitope expressed by a pathogen and a self-molecule. Infection by such pathogens may give rise toautoimmunity.

Monoclonal Immune response specific for a single antigenic epitope mediated by a single lymphocyte clone.

Monoclonal antibody Antibody of a single specificity produced *in vitro* in large quantity for research, diagnostic or therapeutic purposes.

Monoclonal gammopathy Single species of immunoglobulin derived from neoplastic plasma cells in multiple myeloma (or rarely B cells in lymphoma) that presents as a 'spike' in the gamma globulin region

on serum protein electrophoresis. May occasionally occur in some infectious diseases (e.g. monocytic ehrlichiosis or leishmaniosis).

Monomer Single unit (i.e. of antibody).

Mononuclear cells Leucocytes with a large round to oval nucleus (e.g. monocytic and lymphocytic cells). Often used to refer to these populations in the circulation (PBMCs).

Mucocutaneous junction Junction between haired skin and mucous membrane.

Mucosal Pertaining to surfaces of the body lined by a mucosa and in direct contact with the external environment; specifically the conjunctiva, respiratory tract, alimentary tract, urogenital tract and mammary gland.

Mucosal adjuvant Substance that enhances the immune response to antigen delivered via a mucosal surface (e.g. cholera toxin). In some instances (depending on dosage regime) the same adjuvant may enhance the development of mucosal tolerance to the antigen.

Multiple myeloma Malignant tumour of plasma cells. May target bone or soft tissue and is associated with paraproteinaemia.

Myasthenia gravis Autoimmune disease in which autoantibody binds the acetylcholine receptor at the neuromuscular junction. Inhibition of acetylcholine binding leads to muscle weakness.

Myeloid Of the bone marrow or referring to leucocytes of the myeloid series (granulocytes and monocytes).

Myxoedema Accumulation of mucinous matrix within the dermis resulting in thickened skin. Characteristic of canine hypothyroidism.

Naïve Pertaining to a lymphocyte that has not previously encountered the antigen that its receptor is programmed to recognize. Also 'virgin lymphocyte'.

Naïve CD4$^+$ T cell A CD4$^+$ helper T lymphocyte that is a precursor to mature Th1, Th17 and Th2 cells.

Naked DNA (vaccine) Vaccination with plasmid containing a gene of interest leads to direct transfection of host APC with expression of peptides derived from the protein encoded by the gene. Induces a powerful humoral and cell-mediated immune response in the recipient.

Nasal tolerance   Induction of tolerance (systemic non-responsiveness to antigen) by previous exposure of the antigen through the nasal mucosa. Akin to oral tolerance.

Natural killer cell   Lymphoid cell with granular cytoplasm that mediates cytotoxicity of targets via NK-cell receptors or Fc receptor. See also 'ADCC'.

Natural suppressor   Suppressor cell naturally active in the body; important in controlling responses to self-antigens.

Needle-free vaccination   Delivery of a vaccine other than by injection. Includes oral, intranasal and percutaneous administration. The latter may be via a purpose-designed apparatus that delivers vaccine under high pressure; this can pass through the epidermis to target dermal dendritic cells.

Negative selection   Selection of those developing T lymphocytes within the thymus that bear a TCR able to recognize self-antigen with high affinity. These cells are deleted by apoptosis within the thymus.

Neonatal isoerythrolysis   Situation where the colostrum of the dam contains antibodies with specificity for blood group antigens carried by erythrocytes of the newborn offspring. Absorption of these antibodies leads to haemolytic anaemia in the newborn animal.

Neonatal tolerance   Failure of immune response to an antigen in adult life due to exposure to that antigen *in utero* or during the early neonatal period.

Non-core (vaccine)   Vaccine not recommended for every individual, perhaps because it has poor efficacy, or the infection is not prevalent in the geographical area in which the individual lives, or the lifestyle of that individual is unlikely to bring them into contact with the infectious agent.

Nucleotide   The building blocks of DNA: adenine, thymine, guanine and cytosine.

Oedema   Accumulation of fluid within tissue; immunologically this generally follows vasodilation as part of an inflammatory response.

Oncogene   Gene encoding molecules involved in regulation of cell growth and division. Mutation or inappropriate activation of such genes underlies neoplastic transformation.

Opsonization   Coating of a particle with antibody and/or complement to enhance the effectiveness of phagocytosis.

Oral tolerance   Experimental phenomenon. When antigen is first fed to an animal and the same antigen is subsequently delivered systemically in an immunogenic dose, the immune system fails to respond to the antigen. The same effect can be induced by primary antigen exposure at other mucosal surfaces (e.g. nasal tolerance).

PALS   Area of white pulp of the spleen in which T lymphocytes reside. In three dimensions, the T cells form a cylindrical sheath that surrounds an arteriolar blood vessel.

PAMP   A conserved antigen expressed by pathogenic microbes, which is recognized by the PRR on the dendritic cell. See also MAMP.

Paracortex   Intermediate area of a lymph node that envelopes the cortical follicles. Area of the lymph node in which T lymphocytes reside.

Paraprotein   Abnormal immunoglobulin secreted by neoplastic plasma cells (multiple myeloma) or, rarely, B cells. Results in a monoclonal gammopathy within serum.

Passive immunization   Transfer of pre-formed antibody to provide immediate protection.

Pathogen   Organism that causes disease or tissue damage when it infects a host.

PCR   A means of amplifying a particular portion of DNA *in vitro*.

Pelger–Hüet anomaly   Genetically mediated hyposegmentation of neutrophil nuclei of no apparent clinical significance.

Pemphigus   A group of autoimmune blistering skin diseases characterized by the formation of vesicles/pustules within the epidermis.

Peptide   Short stretch of amino acids.

Perforin   A molecule released from a cytotoxic cell that polymerizes to form a pore within the cell membrane of the target cell, allowing the influx of other cytotoxic molecules, ions and water.

Peristalsis   Directional motility of the intestinal tract responsible for the transit of ingesta through the system.

Peyer's patch   Area of organized but unencapsulated lymphoid tissue within the small intestinal mucosa.

Phagocytosis   Internalization of a particle by a phagocytic cell (e.g. neutrophil or macrophage).

Phagolysosome   Digestive vacuole within the cytoplasm of a phagocytic cell formed by the fusion of the phagosome with the enzyme-rich lysosome.

Phagosome   Membrane-bound vesicle within the cytoplasm of a phagocytic cell containing the phagocytosed material. See also 'endosome'.

Pharmacovigalence   Monitoring adverse reactions to drugs and vaccines to identify patterns of such reactions and those products with suboptimal safety.

Phenotype   The outward appearance; immunologically the identity of a cell as determined by the expression of a range of surface molecules or cellular function.

Plasma cell   Late stage of differentiation of a B lymphocyte. The cell that synthesizes and secretes immunoglobulin.

Plasmacytoma   A localized, benign tumour of plasma cells usually involving the skin or mucous membranes.

Polarization   Of an immune response, where the response to a specific antigen may be dominated by antibody production or CMI.

Polyarthritis   Inflammation of several joints.

Polyclonal   An immune response activating multiple clones of lymphocytes specific for numerous epitopes of an antigen.

Polymeric Ig receptor   Receptor expressed at the basolateral surface of mucosal epithelial cells for the capture of IgA or IgM and transfer of these immunoglobulins across the mucosal barrier.

Polymorphic   As related to genetic loci; many different possible alleles at any one locus.

Positive selection   Selection of developing T lymphocytes within the thymus that bear a functional TCR able to recognize antigen in the context of major histocompatibility molecules.

Precipitation   Interaction of soluble antigen and antibody to form a lattice-like precipitate in solution or a line of precipitation in an agar gel.

Predictive value   Positive predictive value of a diagnostic test: the probability that an animal with a positive test actually has the disease under question. Negative predictive value of a diagnostic test: the probability that an animal with a negative test is actually free of the disease under question.

Primary immune response   Immune response made by an individual on first encounter with a foreign antigen.

Pro-inflammatory   Enhancing the inflammatory response (e.g. pro-inflammatory cytokines amplify inflammation).

Proliferative response   Measure of the ability of lymphocytes to respond to antigen or mitogen *in vitro* by dividing. Generally performed using mononuclear cells derived from the blood.

PRR   Receptor on the surface (or in the cytoplasm) of dendritic cells that recognizes specific conserved antigens expressed by pathogenic microbes (PAMPS). Some are known as 'Toll-like receptors'.

Pruritus   Itching. A sign of a cutaneous type I hypersensitivity reaction, manifest in animals by scratching and self-trauma.

Pseudogene   DNA sequence resembling a gene, but containing codons that prevent transcription into full-length RNA.

Pyogranulomatous inflammation   Mixed chronic inflammatory response involving infiltration of both macrophages and neutrophils.

Pyrexia   Fever.

Rearrangement   Of DNA. The process of looping out and deleting introns via the action of recombinase enzymes.

Receptor editing   Rearrangement of genes of an immature B cell to create a new BCR following contact with self-antigen during B-cell development.

Recirculation   Movement of lymphocytes between interstitial tissue, lymphoid tissue, lymphatics and the vasculature. Allows lymphocytes wide access to areas of the body to maximize the change of encounter with the antigen that they have been pre-programmed to recognize.

Recombinant (vaccine)   Pure source of protein produced *in vitro* by inserting a gene into a vector (e.g. bacterial, insect or mammalian cell). The gene is expressed and the protein released from the cells into the culture medium. Such recombinant proteins can form the basis for vaccines.

Recombination   In genetics, recombination of genes by crossing-over between chromosomes during cell division.

Recruitment   Particular cell types may be recruited to tissue to participate in any immune response (e.g. eosinophils may be recruited into the site of a nematode infection for their antiparasitic action).

Regulation   Of an immune response; may be either positive (to amplify the response) or negative (to switch the response off).

Repertoire   Immunologically, the complete range of antigen-specific receptors that may be generated within an individual.

Rheumatoid factor   Typically an IgM autoantibody with specificity for IgG. Found in the serum and synovial fluid of patients with autoimmune polyarthropathies.

RT-PCR   Means of quantifying mRNA in a sample by extracting RNA and reverse transcribing it to cDNA for the PCR reaction.

Rush immunotherapy   Hyposensitization protocol in which incremental doses of allergen are administered over hours rather than weeks.

SCID   Genetic mutation resulting in lack of functional T and B lymphocytes and severe immune impairment.

Secondary immune response   Immune response made by an individual on secondary re-encounter with antigen. The secondary immune response is typically induced more rapidly, is more powerful and persists for a longer period.

Secretory component   Portion of the polymeric Ig receptor that wraps around the Fc portion of an IgA molecule when it is released from a mucosal surface and that protects the molecule from enzymatic degradation.

Self-tolerance   Failure of the normal animal to respond immunologically to self-antigens.

Sensitivity   The probability that a diagnostic test will correctly identify those animals in a population that are affected by a particular disease.

Sensitization   Repeated exposure to an antigen over time. A sensitized individual may make a hypersensitivity response on re-exposure to the antigen.

Serology   The study of antigen–antibody interactions *in vitro*.

Seropositive   Having serum antibodies against a specific antigen as detected by a serological test.

Single radial immunodiffusion   Serological technique based on the principle of precipitation of antigen and antibody. Often used to measure the concentration of immunoglobulin in serum.

SLE   Multisystemic autoimmune disease often involving the skin, joints, blood and renal glomerulus. Characterized by the presence of high-titre serum ANA.

Somatic mutation   Mutations that spontaneously arise in genes in somatic cells (e.g. nucleotide substitutions or deletions) giving rise to diversity in the encoded proteins.

Specificity   The probability that a diagnostic test will correctly identify those animals in a population that do not have the disease under consideration.

Splenomegaly   Enlargement of the spleen.

Subunit (vaccine)   Vaccine containing an antigenic fragment of an organism rather than the entire organism itself.

Superantigen   Molecule that can activate T or B cells non-specifically by binding to their receptors in a non-antigen-specific fashion. Typically derived from microbes.

Suppressor cell   Lymphocyte that functions to suppress the actions of other (effector) lymphocytes to switch off an immune response.

Tc   A cytotoxic T cell, usually CD8+, which mediates destruction of a specific target cell.

TCR   Two-chain molecule (or chains) on the surface of a T lymphocyte that recognizes antigenic peptide combined with major histocompatibility molecule on the surface of the APC.

Th1   A CD4+ helper T lymphocyte that preferentially produces IFN-γ and stimulates cellular immunity.

Th2   A CD4+ helper T lymphocyte that preferentially produces IL-4, IL-5, IL-9 and IL-13 and stimulates humoral immunity.

Th3   An induced CD4+ Treg cell that preferentially produces TGF-β and may be important in mediating oral tolerance.

Th17   A CD4+ T lymphocyte that preferentially produces IL-17A, IL-17F, IL-21 and IL-22 and has pro-inflammatory effects.

Thoracic duct   Major lymphatic vessel of the body into which all lymphatics flow. The thoracic duct in turn empties into the bloodstream to permit the recirculation of leucocytes within the body.

Thymic aplasia   Congenital defect resulting in absence of the thymus. Often associated with hairlessness and results in impairment of T-cell-mediated immunity.

Titre   Measure of the concentration of specific antibody produced in an immune response. In a serological test, the titre is the inverse of the last serum dilution giving an unequivocally positive reaction in the test system.

Tolerance   Failure of the immune system to respond to an antigen.

Toll-like receptor   See PAMP.

Tr1   An induced CD4+ Treg cell that preferentially produces IL-10 and mediates immunosuppression.

Transcription   Synthesis of messenger RNA from a DNA template.

Transduction (of signal)   Following occupation of a cell surface receptor, a positive or negative signal is delivered to the cell via cell membrane transduction molecules that activate cytoplasmic pathways, leading to gene activation.

Translation   Synthesis of polypeptide from the mRNA template.

Transmembrane   Molecule on the surface of a cell that is anchored through the cell membrane into the cytoplasm.

Transporter protein   Molecule that allows entry of a peptide derived from a proteasome into the endoplasmic reticulum for association with an MHC class I molecule.

Treg cell   A CD4+ T lymphocyte that mediates suppression. There are two categories of Treg cells: natural and induced.

Tumour suppressor cell   Regulatory T cell that mediates immunological tolerance to the presence of a tumour.

Tumour suppressor gene   Encodes a protein that inhibits the cell cycle and promotes apoptosis.

Mutations in these genes permit neoplastic transformation of the cell.

Ubiquitin   Molecule that 'tags' a cytoplasmic protein allowing it to enter the proteasome for degradation and entry into the MHC class I antigen presenting pathway.

Urticaria   Cutaneous reaction characterized by the sudden appearance of erythematous and oedematous foci (wheals). Most often secondary to a type I hypersensitivity reaction.

Vaccination   Induction of an adaptive immune response with immunological memory by deliberate exposure to an antigen. Typically, the antigen is an attenuated or killed pathogen and the process of vaccination induces an immune response that can protect the individual from field exposure to virulent pathogen.

Valence   The number of antigen binding sites carried by an Ig (e.g. IgG has a valence of two).

Variable region   Portion of an immunological molecule in which there is variability in amino acid sequence when the polypeptide chains of different molecules are compared.

Vascular addressin   Molecules expressed by HEVs that are unique to the anatomical location of that venule. Only leucocytes bearing corresponding 'homing receptors' can interact with these endothelia and migrate into the local tissue.

Vasculitis   Inflammation of the wall of a blood vessel leading to increased permeability of the vessel. Often induced by deposition of circulating immune complex within the wall.

Vasodilation   Dilation of a blood vessel with increased permeability between endothelial cells allowing egress of fluid, protein and cells into the surrounding tissue.

Vectored (vaccine)   Insertion of a specific gene into a carrier organism (bacteria or virus) such that the organism expresses the protein encoded by the gene and thus acts as a 'vector' for transport of the protein. Such recombinant organisms have been used in vaccination.

Virulent   The form of an infectious agent capable of producing tissue pathology and clinical disease.

Western blotting Serological technique used to determine the components of an antigen to which antibody responses are made. Involves separation of the constituent parts of an antigen by polyacrylamide gel electrophoresis and transfer to a membrane (e.g. nitrocellulose), which is then incubated with serum. Also called 'immunoblotting'.

Wheal A small raised, erythematous and oedematous focus within the skin. Most often associated with type I hypersensitivity reactions.

Xenoantigen A tissue antigen derived from another species. May induce an immune response following transplantation of an incompatible tissue xenograft.